www.harcourt-international.com

Bringing you products from all Harcourt Health Sciences companies including Baillière Tindall, Churchill Livingstone, Mosby and W.B. Saunders

- **Browse** for latest information on new books, journals and electronic products

- **Search** for information on over 20 000 published titles with full product information including tables of contents and sample chapters

- **Keep up to date** with our extensive publishing programme in your field by registering with eAlert or requesting postal updates

- **Secure online ordering** with prompt delivery, as well as full contact details to order by phone, fax or post

- **News** of special features and promotions

If you are based in the following countries, please visit the country-specific site to receive full details of product availability and local ordering information

USA: www.harcourthealth.com

Canada: www.harcourtcanada.com

Australia: www.harcourt.com.au

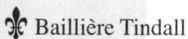 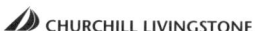 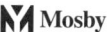 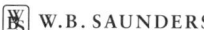

PHARMACEUTICAL MEDICINE DICTIONARY

Commissioning Editor: Timothy Horne
Project Manager: Fiona Conn
Designer: Erik Bigland

PHARMACEUTICAL MEDICINE DICTIONARY

Amer Alghabban MSc (Pharmacol) BSc (Hons) DipBioSci
Pharmacovigilance Coordinator
Medicines Control Agency
London, UK

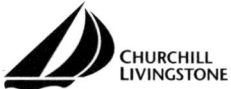

EDINBURGH LONDON NEW YORK PHILADELPHIA ST LOUIS SYDNEY TORONTO 2001

CHURCHILL LIVINGSTONE
An imprint of Harcourt Publishers Limited

© Harcourt Publishers Limited 2001

D is a registered trademark of Harcourt Publishers Limited

The right of Amer Alghabban to be identified as author of this work has been asserted by him in accordance with the Copyright, Designs and Patents Act 1988

All rights reserved. No part of this publication may be reproduced, stored in a retrieval system, or transmitted in any form or by any means, electronic, mechanical, photocopying, recording or otherwise, without either the prior permission of the publishers (Harcourt Publishers Limited, Harcourt Place, 32 Jamestown Road, London NW1 7BY), or a licence permitting restricted copying in the United Kingdom issued by the Copyright Licensing Agency, 90 Tottenham Court Road, London W1P 0LP.

First published 2001

ISBN 044306475X

British Library Cataloguing in Publication Data
A catalogue record for this book is available from the British Library

Library of Congress Cataloging in Publication Data
A catalog record for this book is available from the Library of Congress

Note
Medical knowledge is constantly changing. As new information becomes available, changes in treatment, procedures, equipment and the use of drugs become necessary. The author and the publishers have taken care to ensure that the information given in this text is accurate and up-to-date. However, readers are strongly advised to confirm that the information, especially with regard to drug usage, complies with the latest legislation and standards of practice.

Printed in China

Preface

It usually requires a considerable time to determine with certainty the virtues of a new method of treatment and usually still longer to ascertain the harmful effects

Alfred Blalock 1899–1964

Pharmaceutical medicine is the medical discipline specializing in the discovery, research, and development of new drugs, vaccines, medical devices and diagnostics. It is a truly multidisciplinary profession comprising medicine, pharmaceutical sciences, marketing, medical communications, experimental pathology, pharmacology, medical laboratory sciences, clinical research methodology, medicinal chemistry, managed care, pharmacoepidemiology, pharmacogenetics, health economics, statistics, epidemiology, governmental health and licensing law.

The main goals of professionals working in this discipline are: studying the efficacy and monitoring of safety of medicines, teaching their appropriate and safe use and supporting their ethical promotion.

Due to the rapid and continuous evolution of these medical sciences, and consequently pharmaceutical medicine, hundreds of new terms are born every year. Additionally, terms in these disciplines are not always clear, can vary from one country to another and very often from one organization to another. Some terms are only applicable to certain countries; others involve different concepts in different, but related, disciplines. This situation is bound to leave the professionals involved very distracted if not confused, particularly newcomers to pharmaceutical medicine who soon realize the multiplicity of its facets.

Having worked in the pharmaceutical industry, medical publishing, and currently working for a regulatory authority, I recognized the acute need for an aid for the professionals working in such a challenging environment, and decided to compile this dictionary to aid communication between all those professionals involved in the industry. While compiling the book, I also tried to keep in mind the needs of students pursuing studies in pharmaceutical medicine and related areas; those working within drug companies, research and clinical trials organizations, marketing organizations; government regulatory agencies; departments of health; and NHS and HMO (US) executives.

I have tried to cover the terms and abbreviations commonly used in pharmaceutical medicine and its allied sciences worldwide. The dictionary defines approximately 3,500 terms, but inevitably, it will not include all terms or abbreviations. If you discover any omissions, please let me know.

A.A.
2000

Acknowledgements

I would like to thank the numerous people, organizations, and regulatory authorities who helped and supported me writing this dictionary. Although too many to mention, I would like to record my thanks to:

The European Medicines Evaluation Agency (EMEA), Medicines Control Agency (MCA), Association of British Pharmaceutical Industry, HMSO, The NHS Confederation, The Office of Health Economics, The UK Prescription Pricing Authority, The US Food and Drugs Administration, The University of Sheffield School of Health and Related Research, Professor John Gay of Washington State University, Institute of Public Health, Centre for Evidence-Based Child Health, The Royal Pharmaceutical Society of Great Britain, the Commonwealth Pharmaceutical Association, British Medical Association, The Safety and Efficacy Register of New Interventional Procedures (SERNIP), European Federation of Pharmaceutical Industries Association, European Society of Regulatory Affairs, European Union Drug Regulatory Authorities, US Center for Drugs Evaluation and Review, US Department of Health and Human Services, the US Agency for Health Care Policy and Research (AHCPR).

I would also like to thank the publishers of the numerous sources, books, reports, and journals used to create this book for giving permission to quote certain definitions. I would like to particularly thank Radcliffe Medical Press and International Thomson Publishing Services Ltd.

The creation of this book would have not been possible without the dedication and efforts of its publisher, Churchill Livingstone.

I would also like to thank my daughter, Thanna, for her love and support and my best friend, Andrew Williams.

If I have forgotten to individually thank anyone, I do apologize.

A.A.

Foreword

At last we have a comprehensive book bringing together the many terms and abbreviations used in pharmaceutical medicine.

The Pharmaceutical Medicine Dictionary represents a major undertaking which, due to the diligence of the author, will benefit all of us by providing an easy reference source for our work. All doctors, pharmacists, scientists and administrators working in pharmaceutical medicine will find this a helpful companion on their desks. It will be particularly useful for those entering pharmaceutical medicine for the first time, those starting in a new area of the discipline, as well as, those taking exams.

Although we may be familiar with the terminology used in our own countries or regions, terminology use abroad is frequently different and therefore confusing. The Pharmaceutical Medicine Dictionary includes terminology from around the world and will be a valuable asset in helping to interpret documents originating in other countries. As a result the Pharmaceutical Medicine Dictionary is relevant internationally.

Dr Peter Arlett
Acting Head
National Pharmacovigilance and Epidemiology Team
Medicines Control Agency, UK

Abbreviations used

Cf.	Compare
(Clinical Trials)	Clinical trials term
Gr.	Greek
Pl.	Plural
(Statistics)	Statistical term
(UK)	Applicable in the United Kingdom
(US)	Applicable in the USA

Note: throughout the book, emboldened type has been used in entries to indicate terms that are defined in full elsewhere in the dictionary.

A

α see **maximum agonist effect**.

AAA see **Annual Accountability Agreement**.

AADA (US)
Abbreviated Antibiotic Drug Application (**Food and Drug Administration**).

AAFP see **American Academy of Family Physicians**.

AAPP see **American Academy of Pharmaceutical Physicians**.

AAPS see **American Association of Pharmaceutical Scientists**.

Abbreviated New Drug Application (ANDA) (US)
An abbreviated and simplified version of a New Drug Application (NDA). It is the application for a marketing authorization if a drug has already received approval under a previous conventional NDA. Important drug properties such as **toxicity** and **safety**, have therefore already been documented. It is allowed for duplicates of **drug products** (e.g. generics) which were first approved before 10 October 1962 and for certain other drugs which are described in the **Code of Federal Regulations**. 'Duplicate products' refer to products with the same **active ingredient**(s), route of administration, **labelling**, dosage form, strength, or condition of use that may be made by different **manufacturers**.

For ANDA, reports of non-clinical laboratory studies and clinical investigations (except for those pertaining to *in vivo* **bioavailability** of the drug product and all the information on chemistry and manufacturing controls found in a NDA) are not required. It must, however, contain evidence that the duplicate drug is bioequivalent to the previously approved drug.

See also **bioequivalence, duplicate products**.

abbreviated protocol (Clinical Trials)
A summary **protocol** containing brief information about the study which may be used as a **concept document** to get internal approval to start the planning phase of a study. It may also be used as an initial discussion document for a meeting with a prospective principal **investigator**.

ABEMIP
Association Belge des Médicins de l'Industrie Pharmaceutique, see **Belgian Society of Pharmaceutical Physicians**.

ABHI (UK)
Association of British Healthcare Industries.

abnormality
A **sign, symptom**, or laboratory result not within **normal range** or, as applied to **clinical trials**, not characteristic of those seen in either **normal volunteers** or patients participating in a clinical trial.

abortifacient
A drug or agent that can induce expulsion of a **fetus**.

ABPI see **Association of the British Pharmaceutical Industry**.

ABPI Code of Practice for the Pharmaceutical Industry (UK)
A code administered and operated by the **Prescription Medicines Code of Practice**

Authority (PMCPA), independently from the **Association of the British Pharmaceutical Industry** (ABPI) itself, for the pharmaceutical industry. The Code has been regularly revised since its inception in 1958 and is drawn up in consultation with the **British Medical Association**, the **Royal Pharmaceutical Society of Great Britain** and the **Medicines Control Agency**. Members of the ABPI must abide by the Code. The PMCPA provides advice, guidance and training on the use of the Code, which consists of 20 clauses and applies to the promotion of ethical **prescription only medicines**, but not **over-the-counter drugs** to the health professionals and their administrative staff, and to the information provided to the public in the UK. The Code prohibits the promotion of medicines prior to obtaining a **marketing authorization** (MA), and following which it dictates that promotion must be strictly in accordance to the terms (e.g. **indications** and **dose**) of the MA (as listed in the **Summary of Product Characteristics**). It also provides guidance to ensure good standards of advertising and deals with complaints or claims of breach of the Code by other companies.

In the event a company is found in breach of this Code, the PMCPA communicates with the company to ensure compliance, e.g. withdrawing the promotional material that is in breach of the Code.

See also **Association of the British Pharmaceutical Industry**, **Prescription Medicines Code of Practice Authority**.

ABPI Compendium of Data Sheets and SPCs (UK)

A book comprised of the **Summary of Product Characteristics** (prepared and supplied by pharmaceutical companies) that are compiled by the **Association of the British Pharmaceutical Industry**. Participation is open to all companies supplying **medicinal products** intended for use under medical supervision. The book is intended for members of the health and pharmaceutical profession.

abridged licensing

Licensing for products that contain **active ingredients** already licensed by the **regulatory authority** (RA) in similar or other pharmaceutical forms and where the clinical data are largely established. The data requirements, by the RAs are generally less; full results of tests and trials are not required since the product is essentially similar to the one already licensed in that country (or the constituents of the product have a well established medicinal use).

Compare **Abbreviated New Drug Application.**

absolute risk reduction (ARR)

The absolute arithmetic difference in the event (or outcome) rate between control group (CER) and experimental (or treated) group (EER): ARR = CER − EER.

Where: CER = control event rate; EER = experimental event rate.

Also called risk difference.

absorption

The removal of antibodies from a mixture by the addition of soluble antigens, or the removal of soluble antigens from a mixture by the addition of antibodies.

abstergent

A cleansing application or medicine.

AC

1. *Ante cibos* (before meal), drug or medicine to be taken before a meal.
2. Audit Commission.

accelerated approval (US)
A highly specialized mechanism intended to speed **approval** of drugs promising significant benefit over existing therapy for serious or **life-threatening** illnesses. It incorporates elements aimed at making sure that rapid review and approval is balanced by safeguards to protect both the public health and the integrity of the regulatory process. This mechanism may be used when approval can be reliably based on evidence of a drug's effect on a **surrogate endpoint**, or when the **Food and Drug Administration** (FDA) determines an effective drug can be used safely only under restricted distribution or use. Such a surrogate usually can be assessed much sooner than an **end point** such as survival. In accelerated approval, the FDA approves the drug on condition that the **sponsor** studies the actual clinical benefit of the drug.

acceptor sites
A term used to denote sites of drug binding other than those that are directly concerned in the pharmacodynamic response. For example, many drugs are bound to the plasma protein albumin; the binding site on the albumin may be described as an acceptor site. Such binding may affect the rate or duration of drug action, but does not directly produce the drug effect.

access rate
The availability of services and facilities, measured in the rate of discharges and deaths per 1000 **population**.

Accountable Health Partnership (AHP) (US)
An organization of doctors and hospitals which provides care for people structured into large groups of purchasers.

accreditation
A **managed care** term which describes a rigorous on-site review, according to comprehensive standards, by a recognized independent specialized agency that certifies an organization.

accrual
1. (Clinical Trials) The process of getting patients into a trial, or the number of patients in a trial or planned to be in a trial. For example, 'projected accrual 14' means that 14 patients are planned to be treated in the trial. 'Accrual completed' means all the patients planned for the trial have been entered and the trial is closed to new patients.
2. (Health Economics) The amount of money set aside to cover expenses. The accrual is the health plan's best estimate of what those expenses are, and (for medical expenses) is based on a combination of data from the authorization system, the claims system, lag studies and the plan's prior history.

accumulation
The increased concentration of drug in the blood serum, plasma or a tissue following multiple administration (multiple dosing) of a drug. It occurs when drug intake exceeds its **clearance** from the body.

ACDP (UK)
Advisory Committee on Dangerous Pathogens.

ACE Adverse Clinical Event, see **adverse event**.

acetylation
Reaction in which an acetyl radical CH_3CO- is introduced into an organic compound.

ACGM (UK)
Advisory Committee on Genetic Modification.

ACGT (UK)
Advisory Committee on Genetic Testing.

ACHCEW (UK)
Association of Community Health Councils for England and Wales.

ACP (US)
American College of Physicians.

ACPP (ACMIP) (Canada)
Association of Canadian Pharmaceutical Physicians. (ACMIP = *Association Canadienne des Médecins de l'Industrie Pharmaceutique*).

Contact:
PMAC-ACIM
302-111 Prince of Wales Drive
Ottawa, Ontario K2C 3T2, Canada
Tel: +16 13 727 13 80
Fax: +16 13 727 14 07.

ACRA (US)
Associate Commissioner for Regulatory Affairs (**Food and Drug Administration**).

ACRE (UK)
Advisory Committee on Releases to the Environment.

ACRPI see **Association for Clinical Research in the Pharmaceutical Industry.**

ACT
1. Assertive community treatment.
2. (UK) Act of Parliament.

action letter (US)
An official communication from the **Food and Drug Administration** (FDA) informing a **sponsor** whether a drug is **approvable** or **not-approvable**.
See also **approvable, not-approvable**.

activated charcoal
An over-the-counter product that may help relieve intestinal gas. It is also used in various types of filters to remove impurities.
See also **active elimination techniques**.

active elimination techniques
Techniques used in cases of drug poisoning. They include:
1. Repeated oral doses of activated charcoal, which work well to eliminate certain drugs (e.g. aspirin, phenobarbital, and carbamazepine) after they have been absorbed
2. Haemodialysis (for lithium, alcohol)
3. Haemoperfusion (for chloral hydrate and barbiturates).
See also **activated charcoal**.

active implantable medical device (AIMD)
'Any instrument, apparatus, appliance, material or other article, whether used alone or in

combination, together with any accessories or software for its proper functioning, which is intended by the **manufacturer** to be used for human beings' (EEC Council **Directive 90/385/EEC**).

See also **active medical device, custom-made medical device, medical device**.

active ingredient (AI)
The pharmacologically active constituent of a **drug product** which represents an active constituent intended to furnish pharmacological **outcome** or other direct action in the diagnosis, cure, alleviation, treatment, or prevention of disease or to affect the structure or any function of the human or animal body. Many formulations of pharmaceutical products contain **inactive ingredients** that are required to create the particular pharmaceutical formulation. **Placebo** medication may contain all the inactive ingredients but do not contain the AIs.

active medical device
Any **medical device** relying, for its function, on a source of electrical energy or any source of power other than that directly generated by the human body or gravity (**Directive 90/385/EEC**).

See also **active implantable medical device, custom-made medical device, medical device**.

active site-directed design see computer-assisted drug design.

active treatment concurrent control study (Clinical Trials)
When an **investigational product** is compared against a known effective therapy in a **clinical trial**.

activities of daily living (ADL)
An individual's daily habits such as bathing, walking, sitting, standing, dressing and eating. ADLs are often used as an assessment tool to determine an individual's ability to function at home, or in a less restricted environment of care.

acute
A medical experience, a disorder or a condition that occurs suddenly and lasts a short time, as acute pain.

Compare **chronic**.

acute toxicity tests
Animal tests that are required to establish basic data on the **toxicity** of a drug compound with particular objective of identifying the target organs for the toxic effects. The doses, which are used in an escalating fashion, may also give some guidance about the choice of doses or subsequent repeat-dose toxicity studies. The species and routes of administration used in these studies must, therefore, be the same as those intended to be used in repeat-dose toxicity studies. The intravenous route is invariably used as it provides the best estimate of 'intrinsic' acute toxicity, which is uncomplicated by such factors as **absorption**, or effect of the site of administration.

See also **repeat-dose toxicity studies**.

ADAA (US)
Animal Drug Availability Act of 1996.

ADAMHA (US)
Alcohol, Drug Abuse, and Mental Health Administration.

adaptation
The second step in a three-part marketing process (assess–adapt–advocate) for health care

products. It involves adapting to the new health care environment (which has changed in recent years due to health care finance issues) after performing a thorough **SWOT** assessment of internal and external marketing variables. After adaptation, the three-part process requires that the sponsor goes one step further and actually advocates the product among payers, **providers** and **patients**.

See also **advocation, assessment**.

addiction

The compulsive, uncontrolled use, as a result of **dependence**, of habit-forming drugs beyond the period of medical need or under conditions harmful to society to the point that stopping is very difficult and causes severe physical and mental reactions. Defined by the US Drug Addiction Committee of the National Research Council as 'A state of periodic or chronic intoxication, detrimental to the individual and to society, produced by the repeated administration of a drug: its characteristics are a compulsion to continue to take the drug and to increase the dose, with the development of psychological and sometimes physical dependence on the effects of the drug, so that the development of means to continue the administration of the drug becomes an important motive in the addict's existence.'

Compare **dependence, drug abuse, habituation, tolerance**.

additive model

A model in which the combined effect of several factors is the sum of the effects produced by each of the factors. For example, if one factor multiplies risk by a and a second factor by b, the combined effect of the two factors is $a + b$.

address-message concept

Compounds in which part of the molecule is required for binding (address) and part for the biological action (message).

ADE

Adverse drug event (or experience), see **adverse event**.

ADEPT

Antibody-Directed Enzyme Prodrug Therapy.

'adequate and well-controlled clinical trial' (Clinical Trials)

A phrase used to describe trials that have the following:
1. a clear statement of objective(s)
2. proposed method of analysis
3. a valid **comparator**
4. method of selection of subject provides adequate assurances that they have the disease or condition being studied, or evidence of susceptibility and exposure to the condition against which prophylaxis is directed
5. minimization of **bias** and intention to assure comparability of groups
6. well-defined and reliable methods of assessments
7. adequate analysis of the trial results to assess the **efficacy, safety, risk–benefit ratio**, and **compliance** with the **Declaration of Helsinki**, current **good clinical practice** guidelines, the company's **standard operating procedures** and all **applicable regulatory requirements**.

ad hoc review group

A review group that is created for the sole purpose of reviewing a specific application or set of applications. Also referred to as an '*ad hoc* study section', especially if the applications are for grant support.

adiaphoretic
An agent that prevents or reduces perspiration.

adjuvant therapy see **adjuvant treatment**.

adjuvant treatment
Secondary or auxiliary treatment that is given to enhance the effect of a primary therapy or given after all visible disease has been removed by a primary treatment. Adjuvant treatment is given to avert a recurrence of a condition or a disease (e.g. cancer). For example, **chemotherapy** for colon cancer given after surgery or radiation therapy, chemotherapy, or hormone therapy given before or after primary treatment to try to eliminate any cancer cells that may be left.
Compare **neo-adjuvant**.

adjuvant trial
A **clinical trial** of an **adjuvant treatment**. Most adjuvant trials are **randomized**.

ADL see **activities of daily living**.

AdM
Agence du Medicament. The French Medicines Agency.

ADME
Abbreviation for Absorption, Distribution, Metabolism, Excretion.
See also **pharmacokinetics**.

ADME interactions see **drug–drug interaction**.

admission criteria (Clinical Trials) see **inclusion criteria.**

ADP (Statistics)
Automatic/automated data processing.

ADPL
Average daily patient load.

ADQ
Average daily quantity. Average amount of medication prescribed for adults in a defined area.

ADR
1. See **adverse drug reaction**.
2. Adverse Reaction Report.

ADRAC
Adverse Drug Reaction Advisory Committee.

adrenaline (epinephrine) reversal
Refers to the fact that a formerly administered vasopressor dose of adrenaline produces a drop in blood pressure after administration of an α-adrenoceptor antagonist. The drop in blood pressure is the result of unmasking the stimulant action of adrenaline on β-adrenoceptors that mediate vasodilatation.

ADROIT see **Adverse Drug Reactions On-line Information Tracking**.

ADROIT Electronically Generated Information Service (AEGIS) (UK)
An on-line information service, set up by the **Medicines Control Agency** (MCA) and launched in May 1993, that provides a rapid and efficient transfer of **adverse drug reaction** information stored on the MCA's database, **ADROIT (Adverse Drug Reaction On-line Information Tracking)**, to pharmaceutical companies. There are two levels of service: Level One provides on-line access to up-to-date **Drug Analysis Prints, Product Analysis Prints, Anonymized Single Patient Prints** and an electronic mail system; Level Two provides access to all Level One features as well as a variety of analysis reports and an *ad hoc* query service (this is by email request to the MCA and not directly through a database searchable facility).

ADRRS
Adverse Drug Reaction Reporting System.

adsorbent
An agent that binds chemicals to its surface; it is useful in reducing the free availability of toxic chemicals.

adulterated (US)
Made impure by adding an inferior, less valuable, or inert substance. In the US, the **Food and Drug Administration** (FDA) has the right to halt the sale of adulterated products. Generally, these are products which are unsafe or inappropriate for human use. An adulterated product is defined by the **Food, Drug and Cosmetic Act** Section 501[351] as one which 'consists in whole or in part of any filthy, putrid, or decomposed substance; if it has been prepared, packed or held under unsanitary conditions whereby it may have been contaminated with filth, or whereby it may have been rendered injurious to health; when it is not manufactured in compliance with the good manufacturing practice regulation; if its container is composed in whole or in part of any poisonous or deleterious substance which may render the contents injurious to health; it bears or contains, for the purposes of colouring, an unsafe colour additive; or it is an animal feed bearing or containing a new animal drug and such animal feed is unsafe.'

advance payments (Clinical Trials)
Some studies may require the provision of clinical research funds to an investigating centre before a study can begin. The funds may be needed to purchase special equipment, specialist supplies or provide additional staff. Under these circumstances an agreed sum (negotiated between the **investigator** and the **sponsor**) will be provided before the recruitment of any patients. These discussions should also determine whether the advance payment will or will not have to be refunded to the sponsor if the investigator fails to recruit any patients into the study.

adverse drug effect see **adverse event**.

adverse drug reaction (ADR)
A noxious and unintended reaction that occurs at doses normally used in many for **prophylaxis**, diagnosis or therapy of disease or for the modification of physiological function (see the **International Conference on Harmonization** (ICH) Guideline, **E2A guidance document** 'Clinical Safety Data Management: Definitions and Standards for **Expedited Reporting**').

In the pre-**approval** period, where clinical experience may not be established with a new **medicinal product** or its new usages, particularly the therapeutic dose(s), all noxious and unintended responses to a medicinal product related to any dose should be considered ADRs. During a trial, injuries by overdosing, abuse-dependence, an interaction with other medical products should be considered as ADRs. The phrase 'responses to a **medicinal product**' means that a causal relationship between a medicinal product and an **adverse event** (AE) is at least a reasonable possibility, i.e. the relationship cannot be ruled out. ADRs can be classified in different ways, but the simplest from a clinical perspective is where ADRs are divided into two types: **type A reaction** and **type B reaction**. In the US, adverse reactions are defined by 21 **Code of Federal Regulations** (CFR) 314.80 as 'any AE associated with the use of a drug in humans, whether or not considered drug-related', including the following: an AE occurring in the course of the use of a drug product in professional practice; an AE occurring from drug overdose, whether accidental or intentional.

See also **adverse event, serious adverse drug reaction, type A reaction, type B reaction**.

Adverse Drug Reactions On-line Information Tracking (ADROIT) (UK)

The **Medicines Control Agency** (MCA) database for storage and analysis of UK and foreign **adverse drug reactions** (ADRs). It was introduced in June 1991. It was designed by the MCA and Accenture (formerly Andersen Consulting) to become the means of identifying and investigating drug **safety** hazards and provide the basis for improving the safe use of medicines. ADROIT combines an imaging system, which stores documents as images on magnetic tape, with a relational database. Since its launch, it has substantially increased the speed of handling suspected ADR reports (90% of reports are scanned on the database within 48 hours). Detailed information capture is facilitated by comprehensive hierarchical medical and drug dictionaries. This allows flexible data retrieval and analysis at appropriate levels of specificity.

The relational database provides special alert programmes to permit early identification of possible drug safety problems and allows sophisticated analysis of the information to examine risk factors. ADROIT uses a client-server architecture consisting of 56 user workstations linked to a central database server. This allows much of the processing required for data entry and display to be performed on the user workstations. Images and suspected ADR data are then stored centrally and data can be viewed and analysed via any workstation. Access, to selected ADROIT analysis prints, by pharmaceutical companies is provided by **ADROIT Electronically Generated Information Service** (AEGIS).

See also **ADROIT Electronically Generated Information Service, Drug Analysis Print, Product Analysis Print, serious adverse drug reaction**.

adverse effect see adverse event.

adverse event (AE)

Any untoward and undesirable medical experience in a patient or clinical investigation subject administered a **medicinal product** and which does not necessarily have a causal relationship with this treatment. An AE can therefore be any unfavourable and unintended **sign** (including an abnormal laboratory finding), **symptom** or **disease** temporally associated with the use of a medicinal (or investigational) product, whether or not related to the medicinal (or investigational) product. An unexpected AE is an experience that has not previously been reported (in nature, severity or incidence) and not in the current **Summary of Product Characteristics, Investigators Brochure**, the general investigational plan or elsewhere.

When an AE has been assessed and a casual relationship to the investigational drug has been established, then it must be considered an **adverse drug reaction**. Other interchangeable titles for AE include: **adverse effect, adverse clinical event, adverse experience, adverse drug effect**.

According to the US **regulatory authorities**, an adverse experience in the context of a pharmaceutical product is any unexpected or dangerous reaction to a drug. Adverse experiences, which are also referred to as 'adverse events' are defined by 21 **Code of Federal Regulations** (**CFR**) 314.80 as 'any adverse event associated with the use of a drug in humans, whether or not considered drug-related, including the following: an AE occurring in the course of the use of a drug product in professional practice; an AE occurring from drug overdose, whether accidental or intentional; an AE occurring from drug abuse; an AE occurring from drug withdrawal; and any significant failure of expected pharmacological action.'

See also **adverse drug reaction**, **causality assessment**.

adverse experience see **adverse event**.

advertising

As applicable to advertising of medicines, it is normally controlled by a combination of statutory measures the nature of which depends on national law. In the **European Union** (EU), the rules governing such activities are laid down in **Directive 92/28/EEC** which stipulates that advertisements must not be false or misleading or suggest indications for use other than those permitted in the relevant **marketing authorization**. It also emphasizes that advertisements to health professionals must contain the particulars required by the EU **Regulations** in a clear and legible manner. In the EU, advertising to the public is prohibited for medicines indicated for certain conditions and diseases and for all **prescription-only medicines**.

Advisory Committee (US)

A panel of outside experts who convene periodically to advise the **Food and Drug Administration** (FDA) on **safety** and **efficacy** issues about drugs and other FDA-regulated products. The FDA is not bound to take committee recommendations, but usually does.

Advisory Committee on Borderline Substances (ACBS) (UK)

The Committee that can advise on the circumstances in which a product may be regarded as a **borderline product**, a food supplement or a **drug product**.

Advisory Notice (UK)

A notice issued by the **regulatory authorities** to provide information and/or to advise as what action should be taken in the use, modification, disposal or return of a **medical device**.

See also **recall**.

advocation

The final step in a three-part marketing process (assess–adapt–advocate) for health care products. It consists of advocating a product among **payers**, **providers** and **patients**, after first performing a **SWOT** assessment of internal and external marketing variables and adapting to the changing health care environment.

See also **Adaptation**, **Assessment**.

AE see **adverse event**.

AECA see **American European Community Association**.

AEGIS see **ADROIT Electronically Generated Information Service**.

aerosol

A form of drug administration in which atomized particles or a suspension of a liquid in a gas can be packaged under pressure. It is used as inhalation therapy.

AERS (US)

Adverse Event Reporting System (**Food and Drug Administration**).

AESGP

Association Européenne des Specialités Grand Publique. European Proprietary Medicines Manufacturers Association.

aetiological fraction
The reduction in disease when a **risk factor** is removed. If I^* is the number of people that a risk factor is responsible for and I is the total number of cases over the same period, then the aetiological fraction is I^*/I. Equivalently, the aetiological fraction is $(I-Io)/I$, where Io is the number of cases in the absence of the risk factor. Also known as the **attributable fraction**.

aetiology
The science of the causes and modes of operation of diseases.

AFAR
Association Française des Affaires Regulementaire. The French Regulatory Authority.

AFDC
Aid to Families with Dependent Children.

AFDO (US)
Association of Food and Drug Officials (**Food and Drug Administration**).

affiliated provider (US)
A health care **provider** or facility that is part of the **Health Management Organization** (HMO) network usually having formal arrangements to provide services to the HMO member.

affinity
The propensity of a molecule to associate with another. The affinity of a **drug** is its capacity to bind to its biological target (**receptor**, enzyme, transport system, etc.). For pharmacological **receptors** it can be thought of as the frequency with which the drug, when brought into the proximity of a receptor by diffusion, will reside at a position of minimum free energy within the force field of that receptor.

For an **agonist** (or for an **antagonist**), the numerical representation of affinity is the equilibrium constant of the reversible reaction; the reciprocal of the dissociation constant of the ligand-receptor (drug-receptor) complex denoted K_A, calculated as the rate constant for offset (k_{-1}) divided by the rate constant for onset (k_1). Under the most general conditions, where there is a 1:1 binding interaction, at equilibrium the number of receptors engaged by a drug at a given drug concentration is directly proportional to their affinity for each other and inversely related to the tendency of the drug–receptor complex to dissociate. Obviously, affinity depends on the chemical natures of both the drug and the receptor. 'Affinity' is not the same as 'duration of action'.

AFNOR (France)
Association Française de Normalisation. French Standardization Committee.

AFPM
Associate of the Faculty of Pharmaceutical Medicine.

AFR
Annual financial return.

Agency for Health Care Policy and Research (AHCPR) (US)
The AHCPR and its databases were established to enhance the quality, appropriateness, and effectiveness of health care services and access to those services. Focusing on health services research, AHCPR addresses such key issues as the organization, financing, and delivery of health care services and the promotion of improvements in medical practice. The four constituents of the treatment effectiveness programme involve: database development for outcomes research,

research targeted to clinical effectiveness and patient outcomes, the development of clinical practice guidelines, and related dissemination and evaluation.

Agency for Health care Research and Quality (AHRQ) (US)
A part of the US Department of Health and Human Services that is the lead agency charged with supporting research designed to improve the quality of health care, reduce its cost, improve patient safety, decrease medical errors and broaden access to essential services. AHRQ sponsors and conducts research that provides evidence-based information on health care outcomes; quality; and cost, use and access. The information helps health care decision-makers, patients and clinicians, health system leaders, and policy-makers make more informed decisions and improve the quality of health care services. The **Agency for Health Care Policy and Research** was reauthorized by the Health care Research and Quality Act of 1999 and changed its name to AHRQ.

Agency, The (US)
The Agency is health industry jargon for the **Food and Drug Administration**.

age/sex factor (Clinical Trials)
A list of patients sub-divided according to age and sex. It can be used to identify patients meeting particular specified criteria.

age-structured model
A mathematical model which takes into account the division of the host population into different age classes. Such models can be used to consider the consequences of such factors as age-dependent infection, **morbidity** or **mortality** rates or of age-specific vaccination schedules.

agonist
A drug that has affinity for and stimulates physiological activity or a pharmacological response characteristic of that **receptor** (contraction, relaxation, secretion, enzyme activation, etc.) normally stimulated by naturally occurring substances. It can be either an endogenous substance or a **drug**.

agranulocytosis
Also known as severe symptomatic neutropenia. It is the complete absence of granulocytes from the blood which can be drug-induced. Evaluating the risk of severe symptomatic neutropenia from a particular drug is often difficult. Most but not all instances of severe symptomatic neutropenia are drug-induced. Viral infection (e.g. infectious mononucleosis, primary HIV infection), lymphoma and leukaemia are occasional causes. The nature of this idiosyncratic reaction differs for different drugs and possibly for different individuals. In some instances an immune mechanism might be implicated, in others the patient's cells might carry a genetic susceptibility to the drug, while yet other patients might metabolize a drug abnormally.

AHA (UK)
Area Health Authority.

AHCPA (UK)
Association of Health Centre and Practice Administration.

AHCPR see Agency for Health Care Policy and Research.

AICRC
Association of Independent Clinical Research Contractors.

AIII
Association of International Industrial Irradiation.

AIM
1. **Active ingredient** manufacturer.
2. Activity information mapping.
3. Advanced informatics in medicine.
4. Agency information on medicines.

aim of a study (Clinical Trials)
The objective of a **clinical trial**. Each study should only have one main objective. If additional objectives are required then a separate study should be undertaken for each objective.

AIMD see **active implantable medical device**.

AIOPI see **Association of Information Officers in the Pharmaceutical Industry**.

AIP
Approval in principle.

air lock
'An enclosed space with two or more doors, that is interposed between two or more rooms, e.g. of different classes of cleanliness, for the purpose of controlling the air flow between those rooms when they need to be entered. An air lock is designed for either people or goods.' (Crown Copyright).

ALA (UK)
Association of Local (health) Authorities.

alanine aminotransferase (ALT)
A liver enzyme, measured through a blood test, that indicates the health of the liver. Lower counts are better. Levels may go up because of hepatitis and other infections, or because of drug toxicities.

'a lead'
A compound characteristically potent and selective in *in vitro* assay; generally used in the context of **high throughput screening**.

algorithm
Step-by-step procedure, involving a series of alternative decisions, used to solve a mathematical problem; also used to describe step-by-step procedures for making a series of choices among alternative decisions to reach an **outcome**.

allergic response
As applied to **medicinal products**, it is the situation where a drug may act as haptene or allergen in susceptible individuals; re-administration of the haptene to such an individual results in an allergic response which may be sufficiently intense to draw the attention of the patient or the physician. The response may be so severe as to endanger the patient's life. The symptomatology of the allergic response is the result of the complex mechanism that is only 'triggered' by the haptene. Hence, allergic responses to different haptenes are fundamentally alike and qualitatively different from the pharmacological effects the haptene-drugs manifest in normal subjects, i.e. patients not hypersensitive to the drug. Dose–effect curves obtained after administration of antigen to sensitized subjects usually reflect the dose–effect curves of the products of the allergic reaction even though the severity of the effects measured is proportional to the

amount of antigen administered. Positive identification of a response as being allergic in nature depends on the demonstration of an antigen–antibody reaction underlying the response. In the case of specific patients, presumptive diagnoses of an allergic response must sometimes be made since no opportunity exists for formal identification of an antigen–antibody reaction; such diagnoses can be made and justified since the clinical symptomatology of allergic responses is usually characteristic and clear. Obviously, not all untoward effects of drugs are allergic in nature.

Compare **hypersensitivity, hypersensitivity reaction, idiosyncratic response, sensitivity, side-effect.**

allergy

A state of **hypersensitivity** induced by exposure to a particular antigen (allergen) resulting in harmful immunological reactions on subsequent exposures; the term is usually used to refer to hypersensitivity to an environmental antigen (atopic allergy or contact dermatitis) or to drug allergy; the original meaning, now obsolete, included all states of altered immunological reactivity, immunity as well as hypersensitivity.

allocation concealment see **concealment of allocation**.

allocation ratio (Clinical Trials)

Treatment allocation ratio. For example, 1:1 is equal allocation, 3:1 is 75% in one group, and 25% in the other.

allosteric binding sites

These are contained in many enzymes and **receptors**. As a consequence of the binding to allosteric binding sites, the interaction with the normal ligand may be either enhanced or reduced.

allosteric enzyme

An enzyme that contains a region to which small, regulatory molecules ('effectors') may bind in addition to and separate from the substrate binding site and thereby affect the catalytic activity. On binding the effector, the catalytic activity of the enzyme towards the substrate may be enhanced, in which case the effector is an activator; or reduced, in which case it is a de-activator or inhibitor.

allosteric interaction

The interaction caused by the binding of a molecule on an **allosteric binding site** on a macromolecule (e.g. **enzyme**). The binding changes the binding dynamics between another molecule and a different site on the same macromolecule which may in turn result in an increase (positive cooperativity) or a decrease (negative cooperativity of affinity).

allosteric regulation

The regulation of the activity of **allosteric enzymes**.

See also **allosteric binding sites, allosteric enzymes**.

allowable costs (US)

Covered expenses within a given health plan. Items or elements of an institution's costs which are reimbursable under a payment formula. Both **Medicare** and **Medicaid** reimburse hospitals on the basis of only certain costs. Allowable costs may exclude, for example, luxury travel or marketing. **Health Care Finance Administration** (HCFA) publishes an extensive list of rules governing these costs and provides software for determining costs. Normally the costs that are not reasonable expenditures, unnecessary, or are for the efficient delivery of health services to persons covered under the programme in question are not reimbursed. The most common form of cost reimbursement is the 'cost report' methodology used for **diagnosis-related group**-exempt services, such as many out-patient hospital based programmes, long-term care and skilled nursing units, physical rehab, psychiatric and substance abuse inpatient programmes. Some specialty hospitals receive all of their HCFA reimbursement as cost-based reimbursement.

allowed charge (US)

This is the amount **Medicare** approves for payment to a physician, but may not match the amount the physician gets paid by Medicare (due to co-pay or deductibles) and usually does not match what the physician charges patients. Medicare normally pays 80% of the approved charge and the beneficiary pays the remaining 20%. The allowed charge for a non-participating physician is 95% of that for a participating physician. Non-participating physicians may bill beneficiaries for an additional amount above the allowed charge. These rates are published by the **Health Care Finance Administration** intermediary in each State.

all-patient diagnosis-related groups (APDRG) (US)

An enhancement of the original **diagnosis-related groups**, designed to apply to a population broader than that of **Medicare** beneficiaries, who are predominantly older individuals. The APDRG set includes groupings for paediatric and maternity cases as well as of services for HIV-related conditions and other special cases.

all-patient-treated group (Clinical Trials)

All subjects entered into a trial and administered the **investigational product** or who had fluid withdrawn for an *ex-vivo/in-vitro* laboratory test.

ALOS see **average length of stay**.

alpha error see **type I error**.

ALS

Advanced life support.

alternative hypothesis (Statistics)

The **investigator's** initial supposition that the study will demonstrate that 'something is going on', i.e. results observed are more than the outcome of chance. Common examples include situations where there is a difference in outcome measures between groups, correlation between factors of interest, or association between exposure and disease, i.e., observations are the result of real differences or correlations. Alternative hypothesis is the opposite of a **null hypothesis**, i.e. that the treatment has an effect over and above the control.

See **hypothesis**, **null hypothesis**.

am

Ante meridiem (before noon).

AMA

1. see **American Medical Association**.
2. Association of Metropolitan Authorities.

AMAPI

Association of Medical Advisors in the Pharmaceutical Industry.

ambulatory care

Health services provided without the patient being admitted to hospital. The services of ambulatory care centres, hospital outpatient departments, physicians' offices and home health

care services fall under this heading provided that the patient remains at the facility less than 24 hours. No overnight stay in a hospital is required.
Also called outpatient care.

Amendment to an NDA (US)
A submission to change or add information to a **New Drug Application** or supplement not yet approved.

American Academy of Family Physicians (AAFP) (US)
A national, non-profit medical association of more than 88 000 members (family physicians, family practice residents and medical students). The AAFP was founded in 1947 to promote and maintain high quality standards for family doctors who are providing continuing comprehensive health care to the public.

American Academy of Pharmaceutical Physicians (AAPP) (US)
A non-profit association dedicated to:
- Enhancing the proficiency of pharmaceutical physicians
- Promoting the acquisition and dissemination of knowledge concerning the therapeutic action, investigation, and development of medicines and diagnostics
- Protecting the welfare of patients and study subjects.

Physicians, doctors of medicine, dedicated to **pharmaceutical medicine** (PM) research, education, practice and who will uphold the policies of AAPP and subscribe to its by-laws are all eligible to join. To be eligible to join AAPP, a physician must spend more than half of their time working in PM.

American Association of Pharmaceutical Scientists (AAPS) (US)
A professional, scientific society of more than 10 000 members employed in academia, industry, government and other research institutes worldwide. Founded in 1986, AAPS aims to advance science through the open exchange of scientific knowledge, serve as an information resource, serve the pharmaceutical sciences, promote the economic vitality of the pharmaceutical sciences and scientists, represent scientific interests within academia, industry, government, and other private and public institutions and contribute to human health through pharmaceutical research and development. By August of 1997, AAPS membership was more than 7500. Membership is open to any individual who supports the objectives of the association and is willing to contribute to the achievement of these objectives.

American European Community Association (AECA)
Established to encourage and widen cooperation between the US and the **European Community**. It provides a forum for information exchange on political as well as economic issues while remaining non-political.

American Medical Association (AMA) (US)
A professional association for physicians which provides standards, guidelines and education for its members. It is also a strong lobbying force for public health issues.

American National Standards Institute (ANSI) (US)
A national organization founded to develop voluntary business standards in the US.

American Society for Clinical Pharmacology and Therapeutics (ASCPT) (US)
Founded in 1900, the ASCPT comprises over 2200 professionals whose primary interest is to promote and advance the science of human pharmacology and therapeutics. The Society

is the largest scientific and professional organization serving the discipline of clinical pharmacology. Most of the members are physicians (69%) or other doctoral scientists (29%). Pharmacists, nurses, research coordinators, fellows in training and other professionals make up the remaining 2%.

AMG see **German Medicines Act (*Arzneimittelgesetz*)**.

AMIGOS
A computerized case recording system in mental health work.

AMMP (UK)
Association of Manufacturers of Medical Devices.

AMP
Annual Maintenance Plan.

amplification
The amount of change in measured output per unit change in input. The slope of the input–output, or dose–effect, curve.

ampoule
A small glass or plastic container sealed in such a way so as to preserve its contents (a drug, water or **excipient** solution) in a sterile condition; used principally for containing sterile parenteral solutions.
Also called ampule (US).

AMRIC see **Animals in Medicines Research Information Centre**.

ANADA (US)
Abbreviated New Animal Drug Application (**Food and Drug Administration**).

analogous
(Gr. *analogos* according to a due ratio, conformable, proportionate) resembling or similar in some respects, as in function or appearance, but not in origin or development.
Compare **homologous**.

analogue
A **drug** whose structure is related to that of another drug but whose chemical and biological properties may be quite different.
See also **congener**.

Analysis by Intention to Treat see **Intention to Treat (ITT) Analysis**.

Analysis by Treatment Administered see **Intention to Treat (ITT) Analysis**.

anamnesis
1. (Gr. *anamnesis*, a recalling) recollection.
2. A medical or psychiatric patient history, as opposed to catamnesis (follow-up).
3. Immunological memory.

anaphrodisiac (antaphrodisiac)
An agent that represses or diminishes sexual desire.

anaphylactic shock
A severe and **life-threatening** generalized form of **anaphylaxis** which may result in a sudden attack of bronchospasm, collapse, low blood pressure, cardiac arrest and may prove fatal.

anaphylactoid
Resembling **anaphylaxis**, an immediate, transient **allergic reaction**. The underlying **pharmacology** and the involvement of the immune system are poorly understood.

anaphylaxis
(Gr. *Ana* = up, *phulaxis* = guarding). A type of extreme immediate-type **hypersensitivity** reaction, to foreign protein or other substances, which occurs in an individual who has been previously sensitized by contact with an antigen. It involves the cell membrane of mast cells and basophils releasing histamine and other active biochemicals. Anaphylaxis occurs within a few minutes after exposure and characterized by acute systemic reactions. The clinical response depends upon the tissue that is affected. Examples of local anaphylaxis include asthma, hay fever and oedema of the tissues of the throat. Extreme cases are called **anaphylactic shock**.

Anatomical Therapeutic Chemical Classification (ATC)
The coding recommended by the **World Health Organization** for use in drug utilization studies. This is the system used in many drug reference books and formularies such as the **British National Formulary**.

ANC
Ante-natal clinic.

ancillary trial (Clinical Trials)
An investigation, stimulated by and intended to generate information of interest to the main trial, that is designed and carried out by **investigators** from one or more of the study centres and that utilizes resources of the trial (e.g. money, study patients, staff time, etc.), but that is not a required part of the design or data collection procedures of the main trial.

ANCOVA (Statistics)
Analyses of covariance.

ANDA see **Abbreviated New Drug Application**.

androgenic
A term used to describe any substance that produces masculine characteristics.

anhidrotics
Agents that reduce perspiration.

animal pharmacology
The science of the nature and properties of drugs and their actions in various animal species. Animal pharmacology testing is a prerequisite of similar testing in humans.

Animals in Medicines Research Information Centre (AMRIC) (UK)
An information centre, funded by the UK pharmaceutical industry, to provide information to the public about the essential role of laboratory animals in the discovery, development and safety-testing of medicines and vaccines.

Animals (Scientific Procedures) Act, 1986 (UK)
Aims to strike a balance between the needs of research and the welfare of laboratory animals. The main requirements of the Act are that:
- Only competent people can conduct the research
- Research premises must have the staff and facilities to look after the animals properly before, during and after procedures
- The likely benefits of the research must justify any possible distress to the animals.

The law also aims to ensure that studies are well designed so that as few animals as possible are needed and requires that non-animal alternatives are used wherever applicable. Where animals are needed, appropriate steps must be taken to ensure that any distress they may experience is kept to the minimum possible given the nature of the research. Proper veterinary care must be provided at all time.

Home Office approval of each research project must be granted before the work can begin and their **inspectors** regularly visit laboratories, often unannounced, to check that the Act's requirements are being followed.

Animal Test Certificate (ATC) (UK)

The certificate required, in the UK, to conduct research on animals using **medicinal products** or drug substances.

Annual Accountability Agreement (AAA) (UK)

Describes the objectives to be achieved by a **primary care group** and monitored by the health authority.

Annual Report (US)

Every **Investigational New Drug** (IND) is subject to the **Food and Drug Administration's** requirement that an Annual Report be submitted which describes the study's progress during the previous year. The Report generally includes updates on each **protocol** operating under the IND and information on **adverse events** reported during the year.

anodyne

A drug or medicine that relieves pain.

Anonymized Single Patient Print (ASPP) (UK)

A report provided, to the **marketing authorization** (MA) holder, by the UK **competent authority**, the **Medicines Control Agency** (MCA), either as a hard copy upon request or downloaded electronically by the MA holder of the drug (if the MA holder has subscribed for access to the **ADROIT Electronically Generated Information Service** (AEGIS)).

An ASPP provides selected anonymized data for a particular **adverse drug reaction** report which includes:
- age, sex, date of birth and weight of the patient/subject
- details of the drug product
- hospitalization
- company (manufacturer) number [number allocated by the MCA for that company]
- reported reaction details
- past medical history.

An ASPP does not have the patient's or the reporter's details.

anorectic see anorexiant.

anorexiant

A drug or substance that leads to anorexia or diminished appetite; appetite suppressant.

ANOVA (Statistics)

Analysis of **Variance**. This procedure employs the statistic (F) to test the **statistical significance** of the differences among the obtained **means** of two or more **random samples** from a given population. More specifically, using the Central Limit Theorem, one calculates two estimates of a population variance.

1. An estimate in which the s square of the obtained means of the several samples is multiplied by n (the size of the samples).
2. An estimate that is calculated as the average (mean) of the obtained s squares of the several samples.

ANSI
American National Standards Institute.

antacids
Drugs that buffer/neutralize gastric acid and are used in the treatment of dyspepsia, heartburn and reflux. Some antacids also contain agents which reduce flatulence.

antagonism
The joint effect of two or more drugs such that the combined effect is less than the sum of the effects produced by each agent separately. The **agonist** is the agent producing the effect which is diminished by the administration of the **antagonist**. Antagonisms may be any of three general types:

Chemical
Caused by combination of agonist with antagonist, with resulting inactivation of the agonist, e.g. dimercaprol and mercuric ion.

Physiological
Caused by agonist and antagonist acting at two independent sites and inducing independent, but opposite effects.

Pharmacological
1. Pharmacodynamic
   Caused by action of the agonist and antagonist at the same site.
   In the case of pharmacological antagonisms, the terms competitive and non-competitive antagonism are used with meanings **analogous** to competitive and non-competitive enzyme inhibition as used in enzymology. Both types can be reversible or non-reversible.
   a. Non-competitive antagonism: drug A (the antagonist) binds to a binding site other than that of drug B (agonist)
   b. Competitive antagonism: drug A (antagonist) binds to the same binding site as drug B (agonist).
2. Pharmacokinetic
   Where drug A reduces the concentration of drug B at the site of action of drug B.

Compare **affinity, intrinsic activity**.
See also **antagonist**.

antagonist
A drug or a compound that opposes, nullifies, or reverses the action of another chemical substance in the body; one agent that opposes or fights the action of another. For example, insulin lowers the level of glucose (sugar) in the blood, whereas glucagon raises it; therefore, insulin and glucagon are antagonists. At the **receptor** level, it is a chemical entity that opposes **receptor**-associated responses normally induced by another bioactive agent.

antenatal
The period between conception and birth. Same as prenatal.

anthelmintic
An agent that kills or inhibits the development of parasitic worms. Examples include praziquantal, used specifically against helminth or worm infections.

antiandrogen
Antihormonal agents (also called androgen blockers) used to block the production of male hormones.

antiarrhythmic agent
An agent that controls or corrects cardiac arrhythmia.
  Also called cardiac depressant.

antibechic see **antitussive**.

antibiotic resistance
The development by bacteria of the ability to live in the presence of a certain antibiotic, making treatment difficult.

antiblennorrhagic
A remedy for the prophylaxis or treatment of gonorrhoea.

antibromic
A deodorant.

anticonvulsants see **antiepileptics**.

antidiabetic agent
An agent that controls diabetes, usually, by controlling the level of glucose (sugar) in the blood.

antidinic
A remedy that relieves vertigo or prevents its occurrence.

antidipticum
An agent that lessens thirst.

antidiuretic
An agent that suppresses or reduces the formation of urine.

antidote
A remedy to counteract a poison's toxic effects; it may act to eliminate, absorb, or neutralize the poison.

antifebrile see **antipyretic**.

antifilarial
A drug that kills or inhibits pathogenic filarial worms of the superfamily *Filarioidea*, the causative agents of diseases such as loaiasis.

antifolic
An agent antagonistic to the action of folic acid.

antifols
A group of substances used in combination with sulpha drugs or dapsone as antimalarial compounds.

antihypertensives
Drugs used to relieve the symptoms and prevent the damage that can occur from high blood pressure.

anti-infective
A drug used to treat infections caused by bacteria, protozoa and other organisms.

anti-infective, local
A drug that kills a variety of pathogenic micro-organisms and is suitable for sterilizing the skin or wounds.

anti-inflammatory agents (antiphlogistic)
A drug that suppresses or prevents the pain, heat, redness and swelling of inflammation, tissue reaction to irritation, infection, or injury.

antileishmanial
A drug that kills or inhibits pathogenic protozoa of the genus *Leishmania*, the causative agents of diseases such as kala-azar.

antileprotic
An agent that inhibits the growth of *Mycobacterium leprae*, the causative agent of leprosy (Hansen's disease). Examples include dapsone, rifampicin and clofazimine. Other drugs with significant activity against *Mycobacterium leprae* include ofloxacin, minocyclin and clarithromycin but none of these are as active as rifampicin.

antiluetic
Any agent that prevents or cures syphilis.

antimalarial
An antiprotozoal agent used in the prevention or treatment of malaria.

antimetabolite
A structural **analogue** of an intermediate (substrate or **coenzyme**) in a physiologically occurring metabolic pathway (needed by a cell to be incorporated into nucleoproteins of that cell) that acts by replacing the natural substrate thus blocking or diverting the biosynthesis of physiologically important substances. It is used in the treatment of leukaemia.

antimethaemoglobinaemic
A drug that reduces non-functional methaemoglobin (Fe^{+++}) to normal haemoglobin (Fe^{++}).

antimitotic
An agent that prevents reproduction of a cell by mitosis.

antimycotic see **antifungal.**

antineoplastic
An agent that inhibits or prevents the development, maturation, or spread of neoplastic cells.

antineuritic
An agent that prevents neuritis; specially applied to vitamin B complex.

antioxidants
Substances that inhibit oxidation or reactions promoted by oxygen or peroxides. The term also includes substances that protect against cell damage by guarding the cell from oxygen free radicals (highly reactive oxygen compounds) by preventing, reducing or delaying the process of oxidation.

antiparasitic
An agent that prevents or kills parasites.

antiperiodic
A drug that modifies or prevents the return of malarial fever; an **antimalarial**.
See also **antimalarial**.

antiperistaltic
An agent that inhibits intestinal motility, especially for the treatment of diarrhoea. Normally called antidiarrhoeal.

antiphlogistic see **anti-inflammatory**.

antipruritic
An agent that relieves itching.

antipsoriatic
An agent that relieves the symptoms of psoriasis.

antipsychotics
Drugs used to treat severe mental disorders (e.g. schizophrenia) without impairing consciousness. They are capable of inducing a state of calm. Also called neuroleptics, psychoplegics and major tranquillizers. The term minor tranquillizers should not be used to describe an antipsychotic.

antipyretic
An agent that reduces or lessens fever.
Also called **antifebrile**.

antirabic
An agent that prevents or cures rabies.

antirachitic
An agent that prevents or cures rickets.

antirheumatic
A drug that alleviates inflammatory symptoms of arthritis, rheumatism and related connective tissue diseases.

antischitosomal
A drug that kills or inhibits pathogenic flukes of the genus *Schistosoma*, the causative agents of schistosomiasis.

antiscorbutic
An agent that is effective in relieving or preventing scurvy or minor degrees of vitamin C deficiency.

antiseborrhoeic
A drug that aids in the control of seborrhoeic dermatitis (dandruff).

antisense molecule
An oligonucleotide or **analogue** thereof that is complementary to a segment of RNA (ribonucleic acid) or DNA (deoxyribonucleic acid) and that binds to it and inhibits its normal function.

antiseptic
Agent/chemical effective in destroying or inhibiting micro-organisms on living tissues having the effect of limiting or preventing the harmful effects of infection. Normally applied to the skin. Antisepsis is not a synonym for disinfection. Antiseptics are chemical agents used in antisepsis. The original meaning of the term was a substance that opposes sepsis, putrefaction, or decay.

antisialagogue
A saliva inhibitor.

antispasmodic
An agent used to quiet the spasms of voluntary and involuntary muscles, a calmative or antihysteric. It includes medicines that help reduce or stop muscle spasms in the intestines. Examples are dicyclomine (dicycloverine) and atropine.

antithrombotic
An agent (e.g. argatroban) that prevents or interferes with the formation of thrombin.

antithyroid drugs
Drugs that inhibit the synthesis of thyroxine or decrease the activity of the thyroid gland and are used to counteract excessive production of thyroid hormones – classified into four subtypes:
1. Drugs that inhibit organic binding of iodine (e.g. thiocarbamide compounds such as carbimazole and iodothiouracil)
2. Ionic inhibitors that reduce the uptake of iodine (e.g. thiocyanate and perchlorate)
3. Iodine itself, which suppresses the thyroid by an unknown mechanism
4. Radioactive iodine which damages the gland through ionizing radiation.

antitoxin
An antibody produced against the toxic principles of a pathogenic micro-organism, used for passive immunization against the associated disease.

antitreponemal
An agent that is effective against *Treponema*.

antitrichomonal
A drug that kills or inhibits the pathogenic protozoan, *Trichomonas*, the causative agent of trichomonal vaginitis.

antitrypanosomal
A drug that kills or inhibits pathogenic protozoa of the genus *Trypanosoma*, the causative agents of diseases such as West African trypanosomiasis.

antitumour see **antineoplastic**.

antitussive
An agent that prevents or relieves cough.
Also called **antibechic**.

antivenin
A biological drug containing antibodies against the venom of a poisonous animal, and is useful in antidoting the animal's bite.

antiviral
A drug or substance active against viruses.

antitrust (US)
A legal term encompassing a variety of efforts on the part of government to ensure that sellers do not conspire to restrain trade or fix prices for their goods or services in the market.

anxiolytic
A drug that reduces anxiety.

A

APA (US)
1. American Psychiatric Association.
2. American Pharmaceutical Association.

APACHI
Acute Physiology And Chronic Health Evaluation.

APB (Belgium)
Association Pharmaceutique Belge.

APC see **Area Prescribing Committee.**

aperient
A laxative medicine, see **purgative**.

APG
Ambulatory Patient Groups.

Apgar score
A system for evaluating the health of a newborn baby; rated on a scale of 0–10.

APH (UK)
Association of Public Health.

APhA (US)
American Pharmaceutical Association.

API
1. Association of Pharmaceutical Importers.
2. Active pharmaceutical ingredient.

APMA (Australia)
Australian Pharmaceutical Manufacturers Association.

APPA (Australia)
Australian Pharmaceutical Physicians Association.

applicability
The degree to which the results of an observation, study or review hold true in other settings. Also called external **validity**, generalizability, relevance, transferability.

applicable regulatory requirements (Clinical Trials)
Any law(s) and **regulation**(s), issued by the **regulatory authorities**, to address the conduct of **clinical trials** of **investigational products**.

approvable (US)
Recommendation of a **Food and Drug Administration** (FDA) **advisory committee** after review of a **drug product**. Although this opinion is not binding, the Agency will usually follow the advice of its committees and generally grants FDA approval to drugs which are deemed approvable. An 'approvable' letter allows commercial marketing of the product and lists minor issues to be resolved before FDA **approval** can be issued.

approval (Clinical Trials) (US)
The affirmative decision of the **Investigational Review Board** (IRB) that the **clinical trial** has been reviewed and may be conducted at the institution/site within the constraints set forth by the IRB, the institution, **good clinical practice** and **applicable regulatory requirements**.

Approved Training Programme (in Pharmaceutical Medicine) (ATP)
Training that covers all parts of the **Specialist Medical Training** (SMT) and is devised by the Trainee, Supervisor and Educational Adviser and approved by the Specialist Advisory Committee on Pharmaceutical Medicine on Higher Medical Training (SAC-PM). The ATP is recorded in the trainee's training record book and should list the goals or objectives of SMT, and a system of annual reviews provides feedback on their achievement. ATP is the basis of the SMT.

approximation (European Union)
As applied to **European Union** (EU) law, it is the concept of incorporating **Directives** into the national law of the individual **Member State** (MS). Directives are binding only as to the result to be achieved upon each MS. As it is left to the individual MS to create the means of achieving the desired effect, the MS may have to change their national law to bring it in line with the obligations of the Directive; they may need to approximate the wording rather than use the exact wordings. Since **Regulations** are binding *per se*, their implementation does not involve approximation.

See also **Directives**.

AQH see Association for Quality in Health care.

arbitration (European Union)
As applied to the licensing of **medicinal products** in the **European Union** (EU), it is the process adopted to facilitate consensus in **mutual recognition procedure** (MRP) when consensus has not been reached. If a **Member State** (MS) considers that there are grounds for supposing that authorization of a product would present a risk to human health, the MS may refer the matter for arbitration where a scientific evaluation of the matter is undertaken by the **Committee for Proprietary Medicinal Products** (CPMP) at the **European Medicines Evaluation Agency** leading to an **opinion** (that is given to the company) based on which the European Commission would prepare a single **decision** on the area of disagreement, binding on all the MSs. However, any matter dealt with by arbitration in a previous mutual recognition procedure may not be raised again in any subsequent procedure. All members of the CPMP are involved in the arbitration procedure. The MSs where the product is authorized or where an authorizaton is pending shall be required to take action following the **Decision** on arbitration within 30 days.

See also **mutual recognition procedure**.

archiving of clinical trial data
According to **European Union** guidelines, **clinical trial** data should be stored for, at least, 15 years by the **investigator** and for the lifetime of the drug by the pharmaceutical company.

Area Prescribing Committee (APC) (UK)
A health authority-led prescribing committee set up to consider, amongst other issues, the managed entry of new drugs into the **National Health Service**, and the impact of hospital prescribing on **primary care**.

area under the curve (AUC)
The drug plasma concentration versus time following a single dose. It is used as a measure of the comparative **bioavailability** of different **medicinal products'** **formulations** of a drug. AUC calculations are of paramount importance in **bioequivalence** studies.

Compare **availability, bioavailability, clearance**.

ARENA (US)
Applied Research Ethics National Association.

ARR see **absolute risk reduction.**

ARSAC
Administration of Radioactive Substances Advisory Committee.

ART see **WHO-ART.**

ARTG (Australia)
The Australian register (formulary) of therapeutic goods (similar to the **British National Formulary**).

Arzneimittelgesetz **(AMG)** see **German Medicines Act.**

ASA
1. (US) American Society of Anesthesiologists.
2. (UK) Areas of Special Action. It relates to communities within a Health Zone which face particular difficulties.

ascarcide
An agent lethal to roundworms.

ascertainment bias see **detection bias.**

ASCPT see **American Society for Clinical Pharmacology and Therapeutics.**

Aseptic
Free from infection or septic material; sterile. It can also describe a method or means of handling or processing to prevent the introduction of extraneous microbiological or particulate contamination.

ASI
Anxiety Status Inventory.

ASLIB (UK)
Association for Information Management (London).

ASME (UK)
Association for the Study of Medical Education (Dundee).

aspartate aminotransferase
A liver enzyme, measured through a blood test, that indicates the health of the liver. Lower counts are better. Levels may go up because of hepatitis and other infections, or because of drug toxicities.

ASPIRE
Action to Support Practices Implementing Research Evidence.

ASPP see **Anonymized Single Patient Prints.**

ASQC
American Society for Quality Control.

assent (Clinical Trials)
Agreement by an individual not competent to give legally valid informed consent (e.g. a child or cognitively impaired person) to participate in research.

assessment

Assessment is the first step in a three-part marketing process (assess–adapt–advocate) for health care products. It consists of performing a SWOT analysis which provides information regarding the company and its product, as well as information regarding the environment external to the company. After performing a SWOT assessment, the three-part process requires that the company adapts to the external environment and advocates its product among **payers**, **providers** and **patients**.

See also **adaptation**, **advocation**.

Assessment Report (AR) (European Union)

As applied to the **marketing authorization** (MA) procedures in the **European Union** (EU), it is the *key* document which forms the documentary basis for granting a MA. The AR also serves as an audit trail, clearly indicating the reason for requesting supplementary information, how the new information updates the assessment, and the reasons for the draft/final decision.

Article 9.4 of **Directive 75/319/EEC** and Article 9 paragraph 2 of **Regulation (EEC) No. 2309/93** provide for an AR. AR is exchanged between **Member States** (MSs) in the **mutual recognition procedure**, upon which the recognition of other MSs depends. AR also forms part of the scientific opinion in the **centralized procedure**. AR details all of the stages of consideration of the application before the original authorization, and any subsequent major changes to that authorization.

It consists of some or all of the following items:

Part I
1. Cover page
2. Overall conclusion on the medicinal product
   2.1 Executive summary
   2.2 Overall risk/benefit assessment.

Part II Chemical/Pharmaceutical/Biological (Quality Assessment)
1. Critical evaluation
2. Statement on **good manufacturing practice**
3. Conclusion.

Part III Tabular overview of parts III (Pharmaco-toxicological Safety Assessment) and IV (Clinical Efficacy Assessment)
1. Critical evaluation
2. Ecotoxicology/Environmental risk assessment
3. General considerations
4. Conclusion.

Part IV (Clinical Efficacy Assessment)
1. Critical evaluation
2. Human **pharmacology**
3. Clinical pharmacology
4. Clinical experience
5. Post marketing experience
6. Special features on the assessment report for applications in accordance with **Directive 65/65/EEC** Article 4.8 A.
   6.1 Bibliographical applications
   6.2 **Informed consent**
   6.3 Essentially similar

6.4 Other abridged applications
7. Conclusion.

ASSIST (UK)
Association for Information Management and Technology Staff in the **National Health Service**.

'Associated CEECs'
All Central and Eastern European countries that have signed Association Agreements with the European Community.

Association Belge des Médicins de l'Industrie Pharmaceutique see **Belgian Society of Pharmaceutical Physicians.**

Association des Médicins de L'Industrie Pharmaceutique
French **Association of Pharmaceutical Industry Physicians**.

Association for Clinical Research in the Pharmaceutical Industry (ACRPI)
In existence since 1978, ACRPI is open to any person engaged in the design and organization of **clinical trials** within the pharmaceutical industry. Membership is at the discretion of the committee – currently over 4600 members, mostly in the UK, although an increased European outlook has increased overseas membership to 657. ACRPI encourages communication between all its members by supporting the various subcommittees and special interest groups and continues to provide a forum for education and sharing of best practice amongst clinical research professionals.

Association for Quality in Health care (AQH) (UK)
Members of this association have expertise in the field of evidence-linked-practice. The Association can provide information and advice on specific areas.

Association of Independent Contract Research Contractors (AICRC)
An independent association of contract clinical research organizations which aims to ensure the quality of services provided by **Contract Research Organizations**.

Association of Information Officers in the Pharmaceutical Industry (AIOPI)
The professional organizaton for individuals in the pharmaceutical industry involved in the provision and management of information. The Association was formed in 1974 and now represents over 500 members who work in a variety of pharmaceutical information management roles, such as medical information, scientific research information, **pharmacovigilance** and business information. A growing number of members come from pharmaceutical companies outside the UK and from agencies, consultancies and service providers.

Aims
- To provide a forum for the exchange of experience and the advancement of all aspects of medical, scientific, and technical information handling relating to the pharmaceutical industry
- To facilitate friendly communication amongst those who have a special interest in this subject
- To encourage the maintenance and development of professional standards in all aspects of information work in the pharmaceutical industry
- To encourage and facilitate the development of relevant skills and their application to information work in the pharmaceutical industry.

AIOPI organizes a range of different activities to achieve these aims.

AIOPI Newsletter
Published six times a year, the newsletter features relevant articles, AIOPI news and includes advertising from information suppliers and recruitment.

Meetings Programme
AIOPI's current meetings programme covers topics such as: patient information, **evidence based medicine**, internet – information sources, copyright, information technology update, the future information professional, **epidemiology** and health care statistics. AIOPI also holds Information Forum meetings to enable smaller groups of up to 20 members to discuss and debate current issues.

Annual Conference, Exhibition and AGM
Each year in July, AIOPI holds a 3-day conference which also includes the AGM. Alongside the conference is a large exhibition including information service providers and the latest developments in information technology.

Special Interest Groups and Working Parties
AIOPI forms working parties and special interest groups to develop new projects and to focus on specific areas of interest. Current groups include **SIGAR** (the Special Interest Group on Adverse Reactions), Diploma in Pharmacovigilance, Quality Standards in Medical Information, Diploma in Pharmaceutical Information Management, Internet, Records Management, One Person Information Units.

Contact:
Website: http://www.aiopi.org.uk
See also **Medical Information Department, SIGAR**.

Association of Medical Advisors in the Pharmaceutical Industry (AMAPI)
The predecessor of the **British Association of Pharmaceutical Physicians (BrAPP)**. It was founded in 1957 by, initially, 30 medical advisers working in the industry. AMAPI conducted various symposia through the **TERT** which the Association set up.

Association of Pharmaceutical Industry Physicians (France)
(*Association des Médicins de L'Industrie Pharmaceutique*) (AMIP).

Association of the British Pharmaceutical Industry (ABPI) (UK)
The Association of nearly 100 companies in Britain researching, developing and producing prescription medicines, whether branded or generic, as well as other organizations with an interest in the pharmaceutical industry operating in the UK. The Association provides a wide range of services and support for its members. The ABPI represents the views of the pharmaceutical industry to the government, politicians, academia, the media and the general public. As the leading industry association in the pharmaceutical sector, its opinions carry real weight, ensuring a fast track into negotiations between the industry, Government, the **European Union** (EU) and other authorities.

ABPI Structure
The Association's activities are overseen by the Board of Management, consisting of elected, co-opted and *ex officio* representatives from a broad spread of member companies. On a day-to-day basis, it is run by its Executive, headed by the Director-General. Its management departments have a broad range of responsibilities and operate as an integrated team whose prime roles are to generate expertise, develop and implement the policies of ABPI members and represent their interests.

ABPI Departments

1. The International and Commercial Affairs department promotes the interests of the industry and helps to develop regulatory and commercial policies with Government and government bodies, not just in Britain, but in Europe and internationally. It develops and gives advice and assistance on international trade policy and export matters.
2. The Science and Technology department is involved in all aspects of research, development, manufacturing and training. Its current main focus is on innovation in the UK science and manufacturing bases. It helps to coordinate the activities of companies in developing closer links between industry and academia and education, aiming to stimulate an early interest in science in British schools. It provides expert technical advice and guidance on regulations affecting manufacturing, including safety and the environment and generates policy and influence on all matters affecting research and development (R&D). The department also coordinates the activities of the Pharmaceutical Industry National Training Organizaton (PhINTO).
3. The Public Affairs department promotes the image, views and interests of the industry to **opinion leader**s, media, patient groups and the public. It organizes a coordinated programme of events, meetings and publications aimed at a broad range of audiences. It operates an information service for members and the public to provide information about the industry. It is also the unit within the ABPI responsible for government affairs.
4. The Law and Intellectual Property department works closely with Government agencies and other bodies to influence and develop legislation relevant to the pharmaceutical industry, both in the national and international arenas.
5. The Medical department maintains the industry's relations with all the bodies representing the medical professions, including the **British Medical Association** (BMA) and the Royal Colleges. It establishes, monitors and gives guidance on all aspects of medicine, in particular clinical research and good clinical practice, and provides medical advice to the ABPI.
6. The **Office of Health Economics** (OHE) carries out research into the economic aspects of health care, collects data and publishes the results. The Centre for Medicines Research International is an established authority undertaking research on the development and safe use of medicines. The **Animals in Medicines Research Information Centre** provides information to the public about the essential role of animals in the discovery, development and safety testing of medicines and vaccines.
7. The **Prescription Medicines Code of Practice Authority** (PMCPA) administers the Code of Practice for the Pharmaceutical Industry.

The Association is the vehicle through which the Government negotiates the Prescription Pricing Regulation Scheme with the industry. The ABPI represents the industry's views on the development of regulatory standards. It works closely with the UK regulatory authorities, maintaining regular contacts with the **Medicines Control Agency** (MCA) to discuss policy issues at the highest level. On the international level, it also works with **European Federation of Pharmaceutical Industries Association** (EFPIA), European national regulatory authorities, the EC and the **European Medicines Evaluation Agency** in maintaining and monitoring standards in the marketing authorization of products, representing the views of the UK pharmaceutical industry on draft pharmaceutical legislation. The ABPI also works with the Treasury and the Departments of Health and Trade & Industry in formulating policies affecting the pharmaceutical industry, the Government and the **National Health Service** (NHS).

The Association represents the industry's views on computer-based prescribing support systems to the **Department of Health**, so that all parties involved can work together to develop systems that are based on the best interests of patients, the NHS, doctors and industry. The ABPI introduced patient packs for all medicines, working closely with professional bodies in the health care field.

The ABPI Science and Technology Forum held regularly in the European Parliament in Strasbourg, emphasizes the commitment and success of the industry's R&D and its vital role in medical research. The Forum has now become an accepted part of the parliamentary calendar and is supported by Members of the European Parliament from all political parties.

The ABPI has played a key role in representing the industry's views to the government, funding councils and academia about support for the UK science base. The ABPI has been active in identification of the education and training needs, including the development and maintenance of vocational qualifications. It played an active role in the establishment of the new network of NTOs and has represented the industry's views to the OST and DfEE in all consultations on education and training policy. The ABPI continually revises and updates the training syllabus for pharmaceutical sales representatives and administers their examination.

After wide consultation with its members and key professional bodies, the ABPI has set standards on a range of aspects of clinical research and has published guidelines explaining their significance and practical details. The ABPI has regular liaison with the NHS R&D Directorate, which is responsible for the system of multicentre research ethics review in the UK.

The Association is constantly active in the field of intellectual property protection and has been involved in ensuring that the GATT-TRIPS agreement is implemented, to ensure proper standards of intellectual property worldwide.

The ABPI has a regular and formal interaction with the **Japan Pharmaceutical Manufacturers Association** (JPMA) and a regular interface with other pharmaceutical trade associations, notably PhRMA (USA), SNIP (France) and VfA (Germany). The Centre for Medicines Research International's extensive research programme and unique databases have enabled the industry to lobby effectively for changes in a variety of regulations affecting pharmaceuticals.

The ABPI works closely with patient groups to support the industry's case for the effectiveness and value of medicines and the need to encourage future research. Making more information available to patients improves patient health and the public understanding of industry's role in health care.

ABPI members can call on the specialist expertise of the OHE on health economic issues. The OHE/IFPMA health economics database is a unique asset for the international pharmaceutical industry. Equally, CMRI's programme of research into safety evaluation, regulations and innovation/R&D and its unique databases are a further vital resource for the international pharmaceutical industry. The ABPI's parliamentary database provides a new co-ordinated approach to planning contact with political parties, MPs and MEPs. The ABPI maintains close links with other organizations to develop strategy and encourage industry-wide co-ordination. These include other sectors of UK industry, such as the Chemical Industries Association (CIA); other related associations, such as the Proprietary Association of Great Britain (PAGB); and professional organizations such as the BMA and the **Royal Pharmaceutical Society of Great Britian** (RPSGB). The ABPI's participation in EFPIA and IFPMA (the international association of the industry) offers companies an important opportunity to influence decisions at an international level.

Membership

In general terms, membership is for companies that supply prescription medicines for human use, whether branded or generic, or companies engaged in research and/or development with a view to the marketing of medicines for human use. Research Affiliates are essentially contract research and contract development organizations with activities related to those of member companies. In addition to receiving information, Research Affiliates participate in relevant scientific, technical, medical, regulatory and training activities of the Association. General affiliates form a variety of organizations with interests relevant to the activities of the pharmaceutical industry. This covers a wide range of companies including legal and financial service companies as well as recruitment companies, software providers and providers of representative services.

More than 80% of ABPI member companies participate in at least one committee or working group, collectively directing the Association's positions and policies. Companies can therefore participate in sharing information and formulating strategies for the industry on the national and international stages. Affiliates are also able to participate in committees, advising groups and task forces through individuals who may provide a relevant expertise. Members and affiliates receive copies of the extensive series of specialist documents published by the ABPI, keeping them up-to-date in their particular business areas. In addition, information and newsletters on more general issues is circulated to all members and affiliates, offering the latest information on political and health service news and major industry issues.

Strategic objectives
- To safeguard the interests of patients, and enhance the health of the nation, through effective use of medicines
- To promote the growth and success of its members and the international competitiveness and export performance of the industry
- To develop and promote the UK as an attractive **R&D** and manufacturing environment to encourage innovation
- To ensure that the industry is recognized as an integral partner in the provision of health care.

Aims to achieve objectives
- Acting as the leading body in representing the industry view to governments and decision-makers
- Defining, prioritizing and managing, on behalf of and with the participation of its membership, issues of strategic importance to the industry
- Managing, at national level, the interface with the NHS on industry issues
- Managing relationships and effective communication with government, professions, patients and the general public
- Facilitating information exchange among the membership and with related external groups
- Taking a lead role in developing and implementing standards and codes of practice for the industry through self-regulation
- Influencing legislation affecting the industry.

Contact:
ABPI
12 Whitehall
London SW1A 2DY, UK
Tel: +44 207 930 3477
Fax: +44 207 747 1411
Email: abpi@abpi.org.uk
Website: www.abpi.org.com

astringent
An agent that causes constriction of the blood vessels within tissues and arrests secretion or discharge.

ASTRO-PU (UK)
Age Sex Temporary Resident Originated Prescribing Unit. A special, sophisticated prescribing unit.

assurance (US)
A formal written, binding commitment that is submitted to a federal agency in which an institution promises to comply with applicable regulations governing research with human subjects and stipulates the procedures through which compliance will be achieved.

ATC
1. Animal Test Certificate, see **ATC Exemption Scheme**.
2. See **Anatomical Therapeutic Chemical Classification**.

ATC Exemption Scheme (UK)
Animal Trial Certificate. Similar to the **Clinical Trial Exemption** (CTX) scheme but for animal health products.

ATP see **Approved Training Programme**.

attributable fraction
The same as **aetiological fraction**.

attrition bias (Clinical Trials/Statistics)
Systematic differences between comparison groups in withdrawals or exclusions of participants from the results of a study. For example, patients may drop out of a study because of **side-effects** of the intervention. Excluding these patients from the analysis could result in an overestimate of the **effectiveness** of the intervention.

AUC see **area under curve**.

audit
1. A process by which activities can be measured against agreed **protocols** to establish levels of competence, effectiveness and probity. An audit provides reassurance, identifies areas for improvements and investigates actual/suspected problems ('for cause' audits).
2. (Clinical Trials) A systematic and independent comparison of **raw data**, trial-related activities, and associated records with the Interim or **Final Report** to determine whether the raw data have been accurately recorded, analysed and reported. It verifies whether evaluated trial-related activities have been conducted and obtains additional information not provided in the final report. In addition, the purpose of an audit is to determine whether the study was carried out in accordance with the **protocol**, the **sponsor**'s **standard operating procedure**s, **good clinical practice**, the **applicable regulatory requirement**s. It is also carried out to establish whether the practices employed in the development of data that would impair their validity. An audit can be trial-specific or non-trial-specific. It may involve personnel from the **sponsor, trial centre, Contract Research Organization** and/or Health Authority. An **audit certificate** is confirmation that appropriate audit has taken place.
See also **audit certificate**.

audit certificate (Clinical Trials)
A declaration of confirmation by the auditors that a successful audit has taken place at a clinical

research site, an investigative site, a **Contract Research Organization** or within a clinical research department at a pharmaceutical company.

Audit Committee
A committee whose function is to ensure integrity in the control of that body.

audit report (Clinical Trials)
A written evaluation by the **sponsor**'s auditor of the results of the audit.

audit statement (Clinical Trials)
A **sponsor**'s written statement that an **audit** has taken place.

audit trail (Clinical Trials)
The documentation that represents the pathway that is used to allow reconstruction of the course of events and trace the source and the authenticity of **clinical trial** data which appears in the **Final Report**.

Authorized Institutional Official (US)
An officer of an institution with the authority to speak for and legally commit the institution to adherence to the requirements of the federal regulations regarding the involvement of human subjects in biomedical and behavioural research.

authorized representative
In the **European Union** (EU), it is a legal entity, based in Europe, that takes over the responsibilities given by the Medical Devices Directorate, in case neither the **medical device**'s manufacturer nor the distributor is based in the EU.

autoassignment (US)
A term used with **Medicaid** mandatory **managed care** enrolment plans. Medicaid recipients who do not specify their choice for a contracted plan within a specified time frame are assigned to a plan by the state.

automated novel structure generation see computer-assisted drug design.

autoreceptor
A **receptor**, present at a nerve ending, that regulates, via positive or negative feedback processes, the synthesis and/or release of its own physiological ligand.

availability (F)
The fraction of a dose which is absorbed and enters the systemic circulation following administration of a drug by any route other than the intravenous route; the availability of drug to tissues of the body. When the total **clearance** and the **dose** of drug administered are known, F can be determined from the relationship: $(AUC \times Cl_T)/D = F$. When identical doses of a drug have been given by the intravenous and by some other route (x), and the AUCs have been determined, the availability of the drug after administration by route X can be determined: $F = AUC_x/AUC_{iv}$. The amount of free drug recovered in the urine (A_U) after administration of identical doses given intravenously and by route X can also be used to determine availability: $F = A_{U,x}/A_{U,iv}$
Compare **area under the curve, bioavailability, first pass effect**.

average wholesale price (AWP) (US)
Commonly used in pharmacy contracting, the AWP is generally determined through reference to a common source of information. Average cost of a non-discounted item to a pharmacy **provider** by wholesale providers. It is listed in standard price compendia. Published prices

are based primarily on information provided by **manufacturers**, supplemented by other data sources.

AVMA
Action for Victims of Medical Accidents.

avoidable hospital condition
Medical diagnosis for which hospitalization could have been avoided if **ambulatory care** had been provided in a timely and efficient manner.

AWP see **average wholesale price**.

B
Body weight. Sometimes, as a subscript, to indicate 'of, or in, the body'; thus, A_B is the amount of drug in the body.

bacterial toxin
A poison made by a bacteria that kills specific tumour cells without harming normal cells.

bactericide
A chemical agent which, under defined conditions, is capable of killing bacteria but not necessarily bacterial spores.

bacteriostasis
The inhibition of growth or reproduction, but not the killing, of bacteria by various chemotherapeutic agents.

bacteriostatic
Term used to describe a substance that stops the growth of bacteria (such as an antibiotic).

balanced study (Clinical Trials)
A trial in which a particular type of patient is equally represented in each treatment group. For example, each treatment group may contain 75% female and 25% male subjects or there may be the same number of patients receiving each treatment.

BAMM (UK)
British Association of Medical Managers.

BAN see **British Approved Name**.

Bandolier (UK)
A journal produced monthly by the Oxford Anglia **National Health Service** Region in the UK. It contains bullet points of **evidence-based medicine**, hence its title. Access to *Bandolier* on the Internet is free of charge, but it may run several months behind the printed version.
  Website: http://www.jr2.ox.ac.uk:80/Bandolier.

BAPW
British Association of Pharmaceutical Wholesalers.

bar code (Clinical Trials)
A pattern of black vertical lines with information coded in the relative widths of the black lines. Bar codes can be used to identify **clinical trials** supplies and **case record forms** (CRFs) for individual patients. The use of bar codes can improve the tracking of clinical trials supplies and CRFs.

BARDI see **Bayesian Adverse Reaction Diagnostic Instrument**.

BARQA (UK)
British Association of Research Quality Assurance.

base capitation
An established amount (expressed in monetary units, e.g. dollar, pound) covering the cost of basic health care services for an individual, usually excluding pharmacy and administrative costs as well as optional coverages such as mental health/substance abuse service.

baseline assessments (Clinical Trials)
The assessments conducted on **subjects/patients** as they enter a **clinical trial** before they receive any treatment.

batch (or lot)
A group of finished **drug product** units which were all manufactured in the same continuous process, in a unit of time, from start to finish so that it could be expected to be homogenous, having uniform character and quality, within specific limits. Batches are used to separate units of product which differ in some significant way, for example, units which were manufactured at different sites, on different days, or using raw materials from different vendors. In the event of a problem with the product, the use of batches makes it easier to isolate the cause of the problem. Batches are sometimes referred to as 'lots.' For control of the **finished product**, the following definition has been given in **Directive 75/318/EEC**: 'For control of finished product, a batch of a **proprietary medicinal product** comprises all the units of a pharmaceutical form which are made from the same initial mass of material and have undergone a single series of manufacturing operations or a single sterilization operation or, in the case of a continuous production process, all the units manufactured in a given period of time.' (Crown Copyright)

batch certification (US)
The process by which the **Food and Drug Administration** (FDA) reviews and certifies particular **drug products** for market. Generally, **biologicals** must be batch certified by submitting samples of each batch of **finished product** to FDA before the batch can be sold.

batch number (or lot number)
A unique combination of numbers and/or letters which specifically identifies a **batch**.

batch validation
The validation of a set of data that has been entered at the same time (i.e. as a **batch**).

Bayesian Adverse Reaction Diagnostic Instrument (BARDI)
A method for the assessment of the **causality** of an **adverse event/adverse drug reaction**. It is a sensitive, specific method and capable of using most of the information available but not a rapid method for some cases. The method also balances the possibilities of drug cause and non-drug cause for each factor.

Bayesian analysis (Statistics)
An approach that can be used in single studies or **meta-analysis** which incorporates a prior probability distribution based on subjective opinion and objective evidence, such as the results of previous research. Bayesian analysis uses **Bayes' theorem** to update the prior distribution in light of the results of a study, producing a posterior distribution. Statistical inferences (point estimates, confidence intervals, etc.) are based on this posterior distribution. The posterior distribution also acts as the prior distribution for the next study. This approach has many attractive features, but is controversial because it depends on opinions, and frequently they will vary considerably.

Baye's theorem
A probability theorem represented by the mathematical relationship between the probability that an individual has some characteristic (e.g. exposed to an intervention of interest, has the disease, or with a specified result on a diagnostic test) before the test is run to the probability that the individual has the characteristic after the test result is known. This theorem relates to five different probabilities and is crucial to understanding how to optimize the use of imperfect tests

in the diagnostic process. Baye's theorem essentially relates the certainty that the individual has a disease prior to doing the test, the two possible test results, and the certainty that the individual has the disease after doing the test.

BB
Bureau of Biologics (US) (Now **Center for Biologics Evaluation and Review**).

BBSRC (UK)
Biotechnology and Biological Sciences Research Council.

BCDSP see **Boston Collaborative Drug Surveillance Program**.

BCE
Beneficial clinical event.

bd
See BID

bed days
1. The sum of available beds for use for a specified period of time.
2. (US) Number of inpatient hospital days per 1000 health plan members for a specified period, usually annual.

Belgian Society of Pharmaceutical Physicians *(Association Belge des Médicins de l'Industrie Pharmaceutique)* **(ABEMIP** or **BEVAFI)** (Belgium)
Belgian society of physicians in the pharmaceutical industry.

Belmont Report (US) (Clinical Trials)
A statement of basic ethical principles governing research involving human subjects issued by the National Commission for the Protection of Human Subjects in 1978.
See also **beneficence**.

benchmarking
A means of measuring products and services for comparison against industry leaders.

beneficence (US)
An ethical principle discussed in the **Belmont Report** that entails an obligation to protect persons from harm. The principle of beneficence can be expressed in two general rules: (1) do not harm; and (2) protect from harm by maximizing possible benefits and minimizing possible risks of harm.

beneficiary
Individual who is either using or eligible to use insurance benefits, including health insurance benefits, under an insurance contract. Any person eligible as either a subscriber or a dependant for a managed care service in accordance with a contract. An individual who receives benefits from or is covered by an insurance policy or other health care financing programme.
Also called eligible, enrolee, or member.

best evidence (UK)
A database of summaries of articles from the major medical journals, together with expert commentaries. It is the CD-ROM equivalent of the combined American College of Physicians Journal Club and evidence-based medicine output. Details of subscriptions are found at the ***British Medical Journal*** site (http://www.bmjpg.com/data/ebm.htm).

beta error see **type II error**.

between-subject variation see **inter-subject variation**.

BEUC
European Bureau of Consumer Unions.

BEVAFI (Belgium) see **Belgian Society of Pharmaceutical Physicians**.

BfArM (Germany) see **Federal Institute for Drugs and Medical Devices**.

BFG (Germany)
Bundesgesundheitsamt.

BFID (Denmark)
Brancheforeningen af Farmaceutiske Industrivirksomheder i Danmark. Danish Association of Pharmaceutical Industries.

BGA (Germany) see **Instutut für Arzneimittel**.

BGMA (UK)
British Generic Manufacturers Association.

BGVV
Bundesgesundheitsamt (Former German Public Health Authority).

BHF
British Heart Foundation.

BIA (UK)
BioIndustry Association.

bias
Unintentional or intentional effects on a **clinical trial** that result in conclusions that may be incorrect. Examples of bias include those introduced when an **investigator** or patient may know what treatment is being given or received. It is the systematic error (not sampling errors) or deviation in results or inferences. In studies of the effects of health care, bias can arise from systematic differences in the groups that are compared (**selection bias**), the care that is provided, or exposure to other factors apart from the intervention of interest (performance bias), withdrawals or exclusions of people entered into the study (**attrition bias**) or how outcomes are assessed (**detection bias**). Bias does not necessarily carry an imputation of prejudice, such as the investigators' desire for particular results. The occurrence of bias in a clinical trial may give rise to unreliable data. This differs from conventional use of the word in which bias refers to a partisan point of view. Many varieties of bias have been described.
See also **attrition bias, detection bias, reader bias, recall bias, selection bias, validity**.

BID
bis in die. Twice daily dose regimen (lower case version is also commonly used, i.e. bid).

BIDE
Birth, Immigration, Death, Emigration: the four demographic processes which might act on a **population** compartment in a typical **compartmental model**.

BIGRAG (UK)
Biotechnology Industry Government Regulatory Advisory Group.

biliary excretion
The liver secretes 0.25 to 1 litre of bile each day. Some drugs and their metabolites are excreted by the liver into bile. Anions, cations and non-ionized molecules containing both polar and lipophilic groups are excreted into the bile provided that the molecular weight is greater than about 300. Molecular weights around 500 appear optimal for biliary excretion in humans. Lower molecular weight compounds are reabsorbed before being excreted from the bile duct. Conjugates, glucuronides (drug metabolites) are often of sufficient molecular weight for biliary excretion. This can lead to biliary recycling. Indometacin is one compound which undergoes this form of recycling.

binary data see dichotomous data.

bioassay (or biological assay)
A procedure for determining the concentration, purity, **potency**, and/or biological activity of a substance (e.g. vitamin, hormone, antibiotic, enzyme) by measuring its biological indicator (the reactions of living organisms or tissues; its effect on a live animal, an organism, tissue, cell, enzyme or **receptor** preparation compared to a standard preparation).

bioavailability
The rate and extent to which the active drug ingredient or therapeutic moiety is absorbed from a **drug product**, after administration, and becomes available at the site of drug action. More explicitly, the proportion of the active drug in a **formulation** that is absorbed and therefore available to exert its pharmacological effect. Bioavailability is usually estimated from comparison of the concentration of the drug in plasma after intravenous injection to that after administration of the dosage form (e.g. tablet, **capsule**, suppository) from which the drug must be absorbed. The comparison requires pharmacokinetic analysis of the time course of the concentration of the drug in plasma. Bioavailability, therefore, depends on the **formulation**, and consequently on **disintegration time** and dissolution properties of the **dosage form**, and the rate of **biotransformation** relative to rate of **absorption**.

See also **area under the curve, equivalence, first pass metabolism, generic drugs**.

bioavailability study
A study that measures the rate and the extent to which a dose of the test drug reaches the systemic circulation. Most of these studies compare the **bioavailability** of the same drug from two different **formulations**. They usually involve **healthy volunteers**.

biocide
An agent that kills many forms of life.

bioconcentration
The process by which a chemical is passed through the food chain from soil to plants and animals where it accumulates and is ultimately passed to humans.

biodegradable
An organic material's capacity for decomposition as a result of attack by micro-organisms. Sewage-treatment routines are based on this property. Biodegradable materials do not persist in nature.

bioequivalence
Bioequivalence is said to exist when two **drug products** that have different **formulations** but have comparable **bioavailability** (i.e. peak concentration (C_{max}) and **area under the curve**) when administered to the same individuals under similar dosage conditions. If two **active**

ingredients cause identical pharmacological responses in an organism, they are said to be bioequivalent. When testing a new drug product, it is critical to demonstrate that it is bioequivalent to existing products if such claims form the basis of its approval (as in the case of **generic drugs**). Bioequivalence, therefore, forms the scientific basis on which generic and brand-name drugs are compared. Also, bioequivalency must be demonstrated between batches, which indicates a well-controlled manufacturing procedure. To be considered bioequivalent, the bioavailability of two products must not differ significantly when the two products are administered in studies at the same dosage under similar conditions. Some drugs, however, are intended to have a different **absorption** rate. In the US, the **Food and Drug Administration** may consider a product bioequivalent to a second product with a different rate of absorption if the difference is noted in the **labelling** and doesn't affect the drug's **safety** or **effectiveness** or change the drug's effects in any medically significant way.

See also **bioavailability, equivalence**.

bioequivalence requirement (US)

The requirement imposed by the **Food and Drug Administration** (FDA) for the *in vitro* and/or *in vivo* testing of specified **drug products** which must be satisfied as a condition of marketing. The FDA may decide to require **bioavailability** studies for a variety of reasons including:

- Results from clinical studies indicate that different drug products produce different therapeutic results
- Results from bioavailability studies indicate that different products are not bioequivalent
- Drug has a narrow **therapeutic range**
- Low solubility and/or large dose
- **Absorption** is considerably less than 100%.

bioequivalence study

A study conducted using the same drug which has been manufactured by two different companies. The aim of the study is to show that the two drugs have the same **bioavailability** profile (i.e. they are bioequivalent).

bioequivalent drug products

Pharmaceutical equivalents or pharmaceutical alternatives whose rate and extent of **absorption** do not show a significant difference when administered at the same molar dose of the therapeutic moiety under similar experimental conditions, either single dose or multiple dose. Some pharmaceutical equivalents or pharmaceutical alternatives may be equivalent in the extent of their absorption but not in their rate of **absorption** and yet may be considered bioequivalent because such differences in the rate of absorption are intentional and are reflected in the **labelling**, are not essential to the attainment of effective body drug concentrations on chronic use, or are considered medically insignificant for the particular **drug product** studied.

biofeedback

A technique in which patients are trained to gain some voluntary control over certain physiological conditions that are normally automatic, such as blood pressure and muscle tension (to promote relaxation); the function is monitored and relaxation techniques are used to change it to a desired level. Thermal biofeedback helps patients consciously raise hand temperature, which can sometimes reduce the number and intensity of migraines. A way to enhance a body signal so that one is aware of something that usually occurs at a level below consciousness. An electronic device provides information about a body function (such as heart rate) so that the person using biofeedback can learn to control that function. Biofeedback can help people with arthritis learn to relax their muscles. In this case, an electronic device amplifies the sound of a muscle contracting, so the arthritis patient knows that the muscle is not relaxed.

biogenerator
'A contained system, such as a fermenter, into which biological agents are introduced along materials so as to effect their multiplication or their production of other substances by reaction with the other materials. Biogenerators are generally fitted with devices for regulation, control, connection, material addition and material withdrawal.' (Crown Copyright)

bioinformatics
The use by researchers of highly sophisticated computer databases to store, analyse and share biological information, for example, data on genetic markers, genomes, combinatorial libraries, **high throughput screening** results, animal studies, etc.

bioisostere
A compound resulting from the exchange of an atom or of a group of atoms with another, broadly similar, atom or group of atoms. The objective of a bioisosteric replacement is to create a new compound with similar biological properties to the parent compound. The bioisosteric replacement may be physicochemically or topologically based.
See also **isostere**.

biological products
Medicinal products derived from living organisms, and their products or analogous microbial product applicable to the prevention, treatment, or cure of diseases or injuries including antigens, antitoxins, serums, vaccines, etc.
Also called biologic (US).

biological response modifiers (BRMS)
Substances, either natural or synthesized, that boost, direct, or restore normal immune defences. BRMs include interferons, interleukins, thymic hormones and monoclonal antibodies.

Biologicals License Application (BLA) (US)
The formal process by which the **Food and Drug Administration** makes a **biological product** generally available to patients and physicians for specific indications. The BLA supersedes the **Product License Application** (PLA) for biologicals licensing.

biological standardization
The determination of the **potency** of a pharmacologically active preparation by a **bioassay** in which an international biological standard is used for comparison.

Biologicals Subcommittee (UK) see **Committee on Safety of Medicines**

BIOMED (UK)
Biomedicine and Health Research Programme.

biopharmaceutics
The study of the physical and chemical (physicochemical) properties of a drug and the ways in which the pharmaceutical formulation (dosage form) of administered agents can influence their **pharmacodynamic** and **pharmacokinetic** behaviour such as the onset, duration and intensity of drug action. The rate of drug release/dissolution, and the rate of **absorption** determine the **distribution** of the drug in the body. Differences in pharmaceutical properties can cause substantial differences in the biologic properties – and therapeutic usefulness – of

preparations that are identical with respect to their content of **active ingredient**. Pharmaceutical properties known to influence the therapeutic efficacy of drugs include: appearance and taste of the dosage form, solubility of the drug form used in the preparation, the nature of 'fillers', or binders in the dosage form, particle size, stability of the active ingredient, age of the preparation, thickness and type of coating of a dosage form for oral administration, the presence of impurities, etc.

See also **bioavailability, biotransformation, pharmacokinetics**.

biophase
The actual site of action of drugs in the body. It may be the surface of a cell or within the cell, i.e. one of the organelles.

bioprecursor prodrug
A **prodrug** that does not imply the linkage to a carrier group, but results from a molecular modification of the active principle itself. This modification generates a new compound, able to be transformed metabolically or chemically, the resulting compound being the active principle.

BIOSIS
A non-profit organization dedicated to compiling and organizing life sciences information for researchers, students, and information specialists. Based in Philadelphia, PA, USA, it is one of the world's largest life sciences indexing and abstracting service, providing information through online, electronic, and print resources. In 1926, BIOSIS' first issue of the *Biological Abstracts®* index contained only 1878 references. Today, electronic versions of BIOSIS products draw from nearly 13 million unique references dating back to1969. Approximately 550 000 are added annually.

biostatistics
The branch of statistics that deals with the analysis of biological phenomena including error and probability in biological systems.

biotechnology products
Medicinal products produced by rDNA technology controlled gene expression, hybridoma and monoclonal antibody methods. In the context of **European Union** licensing procedures, these products can only obtain a **marketing authorization** via the **centralized procedure** which is coordinated by the **European Medicines Evaluation Agency**.

See also **centralized procedure**.

biotransformation
The chemical change which a drug undergoes *in vivo*. For the majority of drugs, it leads to loss of pharmacological activity. Sometimes, an inactive substance/compound, a **prodrug**, may become pharmacologically active *in vivo*, or an active compound may be converted to one possessing either the same pharmacological activity or to a substance that has a different or no activity. Examples of metabolically activated drugs include the antineoplastic drug, cyclophosphamide and the adrenoceptor antagonist phenoxybenzamine. Almost all drug biotransformations are enzyme catalysed. Biotransformation sometimes is erroneously used to describe detoxification or used interchangeably.

See also **biopharmaceutics, pharmacokinetics**.

BIRA see British Institute of Regulatory Affairs.

BIVDA (UK)
British *In Vitro* Diagnostics Association.

BLA (US)
Biologicals License Application.

black list (US)
The **Food and Drug Administration** (FDA) produces a list of **investigators** who have been 'blacklisted'. This means that studies conducted by these investigators will not be accepted by the FDA. The list of investigators is freely available as a result of the US **Freedom of Information Act**. Black lists do not exist in Europe although **regulatory authorities**, when reviewing **clinical trial** proposals and clinical trials investigators, may well indicate that data from a particular investigator will not be accepted.

black triangle (UK)
In the UK, new drugs are assigned an inverted black triangle (▼) in all product and prescribing literature. The black triangle is intended to alert prescribers to the fact that the product is under intensive surveillance. A drug is considered new if: (a) it contains a new active substance, (b) contains a new combination of active substances, (c) is administered via a new route, which is significantly different from existing routes, or (d) uses a novel drug delivery system. All suspected drug reactions to these new medicines, however minor, should be reported to the **Committee on Safety of Medicines** (CSM). The system was set up to alert prescribers to products where the special reporting requirements apply. These requirements stipulate that prescribers should report ALL the suspected reactions:
- however minor, which could conceivably be attributable to the drug
- even if they are well recognized or if the prescriber is unsure of the causal relationship.

After a minimum of 18 months, the company forwards a safety report which contains data on the product's usage and **adverse drug reactions** (ADRs) reported for that product. When the black triangle is removed, indicating that intensive monitoring is no longer required, only serious ADRs need to be reported.

BLAISE (UK)
British Library Automated Information Service.

blinded medications (Clinical Trials)
Products that appear identical in size, shape, colour, flavour, and other attributes to make it very difficult for **subjects** and **investigators** to determine which medication is being administered.

blinding/masking (Clinical Trials)
A procedure in which one or more parties to the trial are kept unaware of the treatment assignment(s). Single-blinding usually refers to the subject(s) being unaware, and double-blinding usually refers to the **subject**(s), **investigator**(s), or monitor being unaware of the treatment assignment(s).

blinding system (Clinical Trials)
The treatment code for a particular patient may be contained in a tear-off strip which is attached to the **clinical trial** container label. The tear-off strip is removed and attached to the patient's **case record form** as the supplies are dispensed. Alternatively, the treatment code may be contained in an individual envelope. However, if the latter system is used then the **Clinical Research Associate** must ensure that the code cannot be read through the envelope by holding it up to the light or that the envelope used can be opened and re-sealed without detection.

BLIS (UK)
: The **manufacturers**, importers and wholesale dealers licensing system database at the **Medicines Control Agency**. It is an inspection and enforcement database.

blister packaging
: Used to separate individual daily doses, it offers protection to each individual dosage unit with no risk of spilling the rest as one is removed from the pack, and no risk of contamination to the rest of the pack. They also offer the advantage of providing a reminder to the patient to take a dose through the use of calendar-type pack and hence improve **compliance**. Such packaging seems to be less preferable in the US.

  Blister packaging is particularly useful in **clinical trials** with a **double dummy** blinding technique as, for example, the morning and evening doses can be packed in separate blisters to ensure that the patient takes the correct medication at the correct time. This is very important if a once daily treatment (taken at breakfast), is being compared with a twice daily treatment (breakfast and evening), as in the once daily treatment group the evening dose will only contain **placebo** medication. Blister packaging may also be used to pack medication for patients in blocks of one week which may aid treatment **compliance**.

block contract see **contract**.

block randomization (Clinical Trials)
: A **randomization** method where the number of patients assigned to each **investigational product** or treatment is proportional (1:1, 2:1, 3:1) within the **block size** selected.

block size (Clinical Trials)
: In a comparative multicentre study, patients are randomly allocated to their **study medication**. Commonly, the treatments are randomly organized in blocks so that an equal number of patients in each block will receive treatment A and treatment B. The size of the block depends on the number of patients that each **investigator** has to recruit (e.g. if an investigator is asked to recruit 12 patients then the treatments may be randomized in blocks of four so that for every two patients receiving treatment A, two would receive treatment B). The purpose of blocking supplies is to ensure that an approximately equal number of patients receive each of the study treatments even if every **investigator** does not recruit their full quota of patients. The number of patients to be enrolled by each investigator in a multicentre study must be divisible by the block size.

blow/fill/seal technology
: Purpose-built machines in which, in one continuous operation, containers are formed from a thermoplastic granulate, filled and then sealed, all by the one automatic machine. The blow/fill/seal equipment used for aseptic production which is fitted with an effective grade A air shower may be installed in at least grade C environment, provided that grade A/B clothing is used (Crown copyright).

BMJ see *British Medical Journal*.

BN
: Batch number.
  See also **batch**.

BNB (UK)
: British National Bibliography.

board certified
Describes a physician who has passed a written and oral examination given by a medical specialty board and who has been certified as a specialist in that area.

board eligible (US)
Describes a physician who is eligible to take the specialty board examination by virtue of being graduated from an approved medical school, completing a specific type and length of training, and practising for a specified amount of time. Some **Health Management Organizations** and other health facilities accept board eligibility as equivalent to board certification, significant in that many **managed care** companies restrict referrals to physicians without certification.

body surface area (BSA)
A measure used to calculate, normally, paediatric doses. In infants, it is thought to be more accurate than using body weight since many physiological phenomena correlate better to BSA. The calculation assumes a BSA of 1.8 m^2 for a 70-kg human as follows:

$$\text{Approximate paediatric dose} = \frac{\text{surface area of patient (m}^2)}{1.8} \times \text{adult dose}$$

See also **percentage method**.

BOB see **Bureau of Biologics**.

BOE
Board of Examiners of the Faculty of Pharmaceutical Medicine.

bolus
A concentrated mass given as a single dose.

booster
An additional dose of a vaccine taken after the first dose to maintain or renew the first one.

BOPCAS (UK)
British Official Publications Current Awareness Service.

borderline product
A product that falls close to the borderline between a medicine (which needs a licence) and, for example, a food supplement, cosmetics or toilet preparations (which do not need a licence). Classification depends either on the ingredient, or the claim, or both.
See also the **Advisory Committee on Borderline Substances**.

Boston Collaborative Drug Surveillance Program (BCDSP)
An early detection programme using intensive monitoring of **adverse drug reactions**. It involves selected hospitals in several countries. All patients admitted to specially designated general wards are included in the analysis. Specially trained personnel obtain the following information from the patients records:
- Background information (e.g. age, weight, height, etc.)
- Medical history
- Drug exposure
- ADRs
- Treatment outcome
- Laboratory tests during admission.

BP
1. See **British Pharmacopoeia**.
2. Blood Pressure.

BPC see **British Pharmacopoeia Commission**.

bpm
Beats per minute.

BPMF (UK)
British Postgraduate Medical Federation.

BPMRG see **British Pharmaceutical Market Research Group**.

BPRS
Brief Psychiatric Rating Scale.

BPS see **British Pharmacological Society**.

BrAPP see **British Association of Pharmaceutical Physicians**.

brand-name drug
A drug that is sold under the brand name given by the **manufacturer** rather than under its chemical name.

Breast Cancer Fund (BCF) (US)
Founded in 1992 by Andrea Martin to raise awareness and put funding behind cutting-edge projects in research, education, patient support and advocacy. The Fund's mission is to eliminate deaths from breast cancer and make sure women living with breast cancer receive the best available care and support. It works to find ways to reduce breast cancer – through earlier and better detection, more effective, less debilitating treatments and prevention.

Breslow–Day test (Statistics)
A statistical test for the homogeneity of odds ratios.

British Approved Name (BAN) (UK)
The **British Pharmacopoeia Commission** is authorized by the **Medicines Act 1968** to assign generic names to drug substances and to other materials used in the **formulation** of medicines. These names are known as BAN. This work is carried out in close collaboration with other national nomenclature agencies, such as the **US Approved Name** Council. Hence BANs are normally identical to the recommended **International Non-proprietary Name** published by the **World Health Organization**.

British Association for Behavioural and Cognitive Psychotherapies (BABCP)
The BABCP is a multi-disciplinary interest group, founded in 1972, for people involved in the practice and theory of behavioural and cognitive psychotherapy (BCPs). The aims of the Association are to promote the development of the theory and practice of BCP and provide a forum for discussion of matters relevant in all applicable settings in accordance with the Guidelines for Good Practice of BCP.

British Association of Pharmaceutical Physicians (BrAPP) (UK)
The UK association to which **medical advisors** and **medical directors** can belong. It was formerly known as the Association of Medical Advisors in the Pharmaceutical Industry (AMAPI).

Contact:
> British Association of Pharmaceutical Physicians
> C/o Royal Society of Medicine
> 1 Wimpole Street
> London W1M 8AE, UK
> Tel: +44 020 7491 86 10
> Fax: +44 020 7499 24 05.

British Institute of Regulatory Affairs (BIRA) (UK)

The first organization of its kind in Europe, having been established in 1978 and is regarded as a premier professional organization for regulatory professionals.

The objectives of BIRA are:
- to establish a professional identity and standards for **regulatory affairs** personnel
- to promote education and science and promote the professional competency of its members
- to promote cooperative relations with other organizations
- to collect and circulate relevant statistics and information of all kinds.

The permanent staff of the Institute includes the General Manager who reports to the Governing Body; two Meetings Coordinators, the Membership Secretary, the Financial Controller and the Accounts Assistant; the staff also manage the BIRA Business Centre, which offers business facilities for hire within a short walk of the EMEA.

BIRA presents an annual Introductory Course, which has become established as the 'gold standard' in foundation training in the discipline. The Institute also established the first post-graduate qualification in regulatory affairs in 1989, and now offers both a Diploma and MSc in conjunction with the University of Wales. Over 30 events are organized annually by BIRA and its sister organization **ESRA**, taking place across Europe.

BIRA produces a journal, the 'Regulatory Review' available to members and on subscription to non-members. ESRA also publishes the 'Rapporteur', a news digest on all aspects of European regulatory affairs.

Contact:
> Ground Floor,
> No. 7 Heron Quays,
> Marsh Wall,
> London E14 4JB, UK
> Tel: +44 (0) 020 7538 9502
> Fax: +44 (0) 020 7515 7836

British Medical Association (BMA) (UK)

A professional association of doctors, representing their interests and providing services for its 111 000 plus members, including 4500 from overseas and 10 500 who are medical students. More than 80% of British doctors are members.

It is:
- an independent trade union
- a scientific and educational body
- a publishing house
- a limited company, funded largely by its members.

It does not:
- register doctors, that is the responsibility of the General Medical Council (GMC)
- discipline doctors, that is the province of the employer/health authority and/or the GMC
- recommend individual doctors to patients.

The Association was founded, in 1832, as the Provincial Medical and Surgical Association, in Worcester in 1832 by Dr (later Sir) Charles Hastings. The Association lobbied for a regulatory body and this led to the setting up of the **General Medical Council** in 1858. In 1853, it extended its membership to London doctors and became the BMA in 1856. Medical students were first admitted in the late 1970s.

Today the BMA is in continual contact with Ministers, Government Departments, members of both Houses of Parliament and many other influential bodies. The BMA's policies are wide ranging, from public health issues to medical ethics, and include the management and role of the **National Health Service** (NHS), and doctors' contracts. The BMA had produced its own proposals for a NHS long before it was taken up by political parties. A general medical service for the nation was approved by the Representative Body of the BMA in 1930. The BMA is also a limited liability company and its resources are committed to promoting the objectives of the Association.

The Medical Ethics Committee (MEC) of the BMA produces reports, codes of practice and discussion documents on topical, and often controversial, issues. The MEC's staff answer over 4000 queries each year.

Publications

The *British Medical Journal*, *BMA News Review* and books. The BMJ Publishing Group also publishes 24 specialist journals.

British Medical Informatics (BMI)

Formed in 1986 as the equivalent of **Medical Informatics** (MI) societies in North America and other European countries. The broad objectives of the Society are to:
- promote research and the development of information systems to support patient care
- promote the application of information technology in medical education and biomedical research
- assist in the education of MI professionals
- act as an open forum and focal point for professionals from all disciplines and across all sectors
- publish *Biomedical Informatics Today*, a newsletter which aims to keep its membership informed of current issues in Medical Informatics, book and software reviews, and forthcoming events
- arrange open workshops, conferences and other meetings addressing both introductory and research areas
- set up local and special interest groups, electronic bulletin boards and other mechanisms to further the above objectives.

See also **medical informatics**.

British Medical Journal (BMJ) (UK)

A weekly journal that aims to help doctors, everywhere, practise better medicine and to influence the debate on health. The journal publishes original scientific studies, reviews and educational articles, and papers commenting on the clinical, scientific, social, political, and economic factors affecting health from doctors and others. The BMJ publishes only about a sixth of the 4500 articles that it receives each year, but the editors give quick decisions.

British National Formulary (BNF) (UK)

A guide to prescribing in the **National Health Service** of the UK compiled by joint effort of the **Royal Pharmaceutical Society of Great Britain**, the **British Medical Association** and the **Department of Health**. This essential reference provides up-to-date guidance on prescribing, dispensing and administering medicines. It details all medicines on the UK market, with special reference to their uses, cautions, contra-indications, **side-effects**, dosage and costs. The BNF reflects current best practice as well as legal and professional guidelines relating to the use of medicines. It is intended for use by prescribers in the NHS as well as by pharmacists, nurses and other health-care professionals. It is distributed free to all medical students and practising doctors. Updated every 6 months, the BNF is published under the authority of the **Joint Formulary Committee**. Historically, the BNF originally appeared as the National War Formulary which was radically revised in 1981.

British Pharmaceutical Codex (BPC) (UK)

A complementary volume to the **British Pharmacopoeia** (BP) which provides supplementary data including toxicological and therapeutic information on all substances contained in the BP. It also provides information on drugs and medicines not covered in the BP.

British Pharmaceutical Market Research Group (BPMRG) (UK)

An organization whose aim is to promote and enhance the professionalism and status of marketing research within the pharmaceutical industry to create and support standards of practice appropriate for the industry in its marketing research activities. BPMRG offer four educational day meetings per year: an Annual Conference; Ashridge Training Courses for market researchers and Seminars for senior market research personnel on specialist topics. BPMRG offer either corporate or non-transferable personal membership. Personal membership is only available to 'one man band' agencies or freelance researchers.

British Pharmacological Society (BPS) (UK)

The BPS, including its Clinical Pharmacology Section, is the professional association for pharmacologists in the UK. The Society originated in 1931, in Oxford, with a few pharmacologists and now has 2500 members. The object of the Society is to promote and advance pharmacology, including clinical pharmacology. The Society aims are to:
- assist, promote and encourage research and provide a forum for the presentation of pharmacology
- publish the results of research
- promote and encourage the education and training of pharmacologists
- publish material in various forms
- promote and arrange conferences and meetings.

Membership of the Society is by election. Prospective members will normally have published in the Society's journals.

British Pharmacopoeia (BP) (UK)

Produced by staff within the Licensing Division of the **Medicines Control Agency**, in collaboration with the **British Pharmacopoeia Commission**. The Pharmacopoeia staff also make a major contribution to the generation of the **European Pharmacopoeia**. The BP is published for the Health Ministers on the recommendation of the **Medicines Commission** in accordance with section 99(6) of the **Medicines Act 1968**.

British Pharmacopoeia Commission (BPC) (UK)

The BPC is appointed by the Secretary of State concerned with health in England, the Secretaries of State respectively concerned with health and with agriculture in Wales and in Scotland, the Ministry of Agriculture, Fisheries and Food, the Department of Health and Human Services for Northern Ireland, and the Department of Agriculture for Northern Ireland, acting jointly, in exercise of their powers under section 4 of the **Medicines Act 1968**. Members of the BPC are appointed by Ministers, having regard to recommendations made by the **Medicines Commission**. Appointments are usually for a (renewable) term of 4 years.

BRMs see **biological response modifiers**.

BSA see **body surface area**.

BSG (UK)
British Society of Gastroenterology.

BSI (UK)
British Standard Institute.

BTS (UK)
British Thoracic Society.

buffer
A chemical system that prevents change in the acidity or alkalinity of another chemical substance or system by reducing the change in hydrogen ion concentration (pH) otherwise produced by adding acids or bases to a solution. It also refers to anything that slows or inhibits the intermediate action of a chemotherapeutic agent.

bulk product
'Any product which has completed all processing stages up to, but not including, final packaging.' (Crown Copyright)

bulk supplies
Large quantities of unpacked drugs for use in **clinical trials**. Materials obtained from another pharmaceutical company for use in a clinical study will be provided as bulk supplies. Rarely, bulk supplies of trial materials will be provided to a hospital pharmacy. The pharmacy will be responsible for dispensing the individual supplies to study patients. This may be the best course of action when a dose ranging study is being conducted and the dose for each patient is being individually titrated. It would be very difficult to pre-pack trial supplies for every patient in such a study.

Bundesinstitutes für Arzneimittel und Medizinprodukte
The German medicines evaluation agency. See **Federal Institute for Drugs and Medical Devices (BfArM)**.

Bundesinstitut für Arzeneimitte (Austria)
The Austrian medicines evaluation agency (Vienna).

Bundesministerium für Jungend, Familie und Gesundheit
German Ministry of Health.

BUPA (UK)
British United Provident Association. A private health insurance company.

Bureau of Biologics (BOB) (US)
The Bureau of Biologics is the former name of the **Center for Biologics Evaluation and Review** group of **Food and Drug Administration**.

C

C see **concentration**.

C_{max} see **peak plasma concentration**

CA
1. (Clinical Trials) Confidentiality Agreement.
2. see **Competent Authority**.

cachet
A lenticular capsule for enclosing a dose of medicine, usually made of rice paper.

CAD see **computer-assisted drug design**.

CADD see **computer-assisted drug design**.

CADREAC
Collaboration Agreement between Drug Regulatory Authorities in European Union and Associated Countries.

calibration
'The set of operations which establish, under specified conditions, the relationship between values indicated by a measuring instrument or measuring system, or values represented by a material measurement, and the corresponding known values of a reference standard.' (Crown Copyright)

CAMR (UK)
Centre for Applied Microbiology and Research.

Canadian Coordinating Office for Health Technology Assessment (CCOHTA)
Provides information on emerging and existing health care technologies to decision-makers, and facilitates the exchange and coordination of information on health technologies. The CCOHTA Internet site contains some on-line documentation but in general, documents have to be ordered although they are available free of charge. There is free access to full text documents.

Canadian Family Physician Critical Appraisal
An internet site that reviews important articles in the literature relevant to family physicians. Reviews are by family physicians, not experts on the topics. They assess not only the strength of the studies but the bottom line clinical importance for family practice. Also described as 'Family Medicine research reviews with a "bottom line"'.
Website: http://dfcm18.med.utoronto.ca/anthes/evans.htm

Canadian Medical Association (CMA) (Canada)
A national voluntary organization representing the national voice of Canadian physicians. Founded in 1867, CMA's mission is to provide leadership for physicians and to promote the highest standard of health and health care for Canadians. On behalf of its members and the Canadian public, CMA performs a wide variety of functions, such as advocating health promotion and disease/accident prevention policies and strategies, advocating for access to quality health care, facilitating change within the medical profession, and providing leadership and guidance to physicians to help them influence, manage and adapt to changes in health care delivery.

The staff of the CMA is headed by the Secretary General who is the chief executive officer. Association policy is developed by the Board of Directors. A number of councils and committees (whose members are physicians) advise the Board on a range of issues. The CMA also relies on 42 affiliated medical specialty and special-interest organizations (several of which it founded) for contributions to policy development. The various staff directorates of the CMA conduct research, disseminate information and support the policy development process.

Cancer Center (US)
An institution designated by the National Cancer Institute as a comprehensive or clinical cancer centre and is eligible to conduct **Investigational New Drug** drug studies.

CANDA see **Computer-Aided New Drug Application**.

cap see **capitation**.

capital charges (UK)
In 1991, assets within the **National Health Service** became subject to capital charging to more appropriately reflect the costs of managing these capital assets. These consist of two parts: interest on fixed assets which is charged at 6% of the capital worth, and depreciation which is absorbed by the Trust.

capital programme
A plan showing costs and timing of planned capital expenditure. The time period is usually 5 years.

capitation
A method of payment for a group of specified health services (regardless of quantity rendered) in which a physician or hospital is paid a fixed, per capita amount for each person served regardless of the actual number of services provided to each person. Amounts are determined by assessing a payment 'per covered life' or per member. The method of payment in which the provider is paid a fixed amount for each person served no matter what the actual number or nature of services delivered. The cost of providing an individual with a specific set of services over a set period of time, usually a month or a year. A payment system whereby **managed care** plans pay health care providers a fixed amount to care for a patient over a given period. **providers** are not reimbursed for services that exceed the allotted amount. The rate may be fixed for all members or it can be adjusted for the age and gender of the member, based on actuarial projections of medical utilization.

Also called cap, capitate, capped.

CAPLA see **Computer-Aided Product License Application**.

CAPLAR (US)
Computer-Assisted Product License Agreement Review.

CAPRA (Canada)
Canadian Association of Pharmaceutical Regulatory Authorities.

capsule
A soluble container for enclosing a dose of medicine, made from gelatine or other material that can dissolve in the stomach, releasing the contents. The hard gelatine shell disintegrates rapidly and allows the contents to be mixed with the gastrointestinal tract contents. The capsule contents should not be subjected to high compression forces which would tend to reduce the effective surface area, thus a capsule should perform better than a **tablet**. This, however, is not always the case. If a drug is hydrophobic a dispersing agent should be added to the capsule formulation. These diluents will work to disperse the powder, minimize aggregation and maximize the surface area of the powder.

See also **tablet**.

carcinogen
A material that either causes cancer in humans, or, because it causes cancer in animals, is considered capable of causing cancer in humans. A material is considered a carcinogen if the **International Agency for Research on Cancer** has evaluated it and found it to be a carcinogen or a potential carcinogen.

carcinostatic
An agent that inhibits the growth of carcinomas.

cardiac depressant see **antiarrhythmic**.

cardiac stimulant
A drug that increases the contractile force of the myocardium, especially in the weakened conditions such as congestive heart failure.
Also called cardiotonic.

cardiotonic see **cardiac stimulant**.

CARE
Clinical Audit and Research Evidence.

CARM see **Centre for Adverse Reactions Monitoring**.

carminative
A drug or medicine for the relief of flatulence.

carrier-linked prodrug
A **prodrug** that contains a temporary linkage of a given active substance with a transient carrier group that produces improved physicochemical or **pharmacokinetic** properties and that can be easily removed *in vivo*, usually by a hydrolytic cleavage.
Also called carrier prodrug.

carrier substance see **excipient**.

carry-over effect
Effects of treatment that persist beyond the period of treatment, sometimes beyond the time of a medication's known biological activity.

carve-out
To separately purchase specific services, that generally are part of a **managed care** benefits package; i.e. vision, chiropractor benefits. These services are then typically provided by a speciality **Managed Care Organization** (MCO) or **provider** organization. In the US, it is defined as the practice of excluding specific services from a MCO's capitated rate. In some instances, the same provider will still provide the service, but they will be reimbursed on a fee-for-service basis. In other instances, carved out services will be provided by an entirely different provider. A payer strategy in which a payer separates ('carves-out') a portion of the benefit and hires an MCO to provide these benefits. Common carve-outs include such services as psychiatric, rehab, chemical dependency and ambulatory services. Increasingly, oncology and cardiac services are being carved out. This permits the payer to create a separate health benefits package and assume greater control of their costs. Many **Health Management Organizations** and insurance companies adopt this strategy because they do not have in-house expertise related to the service 'carved out.' A 'carve-out' is typically a service provided within a standard benefit package but delivered exclusively by a designated provider or group. This process may or may not seem transparent to the subscriber, but it often means that separate underwriting and pre-

certification entities are involved as well as different payers and providers. Carve-outs are also called sub-contractors, sub-capitators or junior capitation contracts.

See also **capitation**.

CAS
1. Chemical Abstracts Service.
2. See **CAS Number** (CAS Registration Number).
3. Care Assessment Schedule. The Manchester (UK) care assessment schedule that was introduced in 1998 and is used to provide a measurement of assessment and **outcomes** in Mental Health services.

cascade prodrug
A **prodrug** for which the cleavage of the carrier group becomes effective only after unmasking an activating group.

case–control study
Epidemiological investigation/study in which subjects who have the **outcome** of interest (cases) are compared to subjects without the same outcome (disease or **adverse drug reaction**) with regard to a previous exposure to certain **risk factors** (e.g. a particular drug, a surgical procedure, etc.). The advantages of such studies include: low cost, speed, lack of alternative methodology for studying rare disorders and disease with long latency as well as the need for fewer subjects (than that needed in cross-sectional studies). Disadvantages include: the existence of confounders, the potential for **bias** through recall and selection, difficulty in selecting the control group, and the dependence on recall or records to determine exposure status.

case fatality 'rate'
Cumulative **incidence** of death in the group of individuals that develop a disease over a time period (often unstated). It is a proportion, not a rate.

case management
Method designed to accommodate the specific health services needed by an individual through a coordinated effort to achieve the desired health outcome in a cost effective manner. The monitoring and coordination of treatment rendered to patients with specific diagnosis or requiring high-cost or extensive services. It encompasses the whole process by which all health-related matters of a case are managed by a physician or nurse or a designated health professional. Physician case managers coordinate designated components of health care, such as appropriate referral to consultants, specialists, hospitals, ancillary providers and services. Case management is intended to ensure continuity of services and accessibility to overcome rigidity, fragmented services, and the misutilization of facilities and resources. It also attempts to match the appropriate intensity of services with the patient's needs over time.

case mix (US)
The mix of patients treated within a particular institutional setting, such as the hospital. Patient classification systems like **diagnosis-related groups** (DRGs) can be used to measure hospital case mix. Measurement reflecting servicing needs, uses of hospital capabilities, and the general rate of hospital admissions. The types of inpatients a hospital or post-acute facility treats. The more complex the patients' needs, the greater the amount spent for patient care. Case mix is generally established by estimating the relative frequency of various types of patients seen by the provider in question during a given time period and may be measured by factors such as diagnosis, severity of illness, utilization of services, and provider characteristics.

See also **diagnosis-related groups** and **case-mix index**.

case-mix index (CMI) (US)
The average **diagnosis-related group** (DRG) weight for all cases paid under PPS. The CMI is a measure of the relative costliness of the patients treated in each hospital or group of hospitals. A measure of the relative costliness of treating in an inpatient setting. An index of 1.05 means that the facility's patients are 5% more costly than average.
See also **diagnosis-related group**.

case record form (CRF) (Clinical Trials)
The form designed and used to record data (as defined by the **clinical trial protocol** and other information) from a study for an individual **subject**. The form can be a printed, magnetic, optical, or electronic document provided that there is assurance of accurate input and presentation, and allowance for **verification**. There is a CRF for each patient and for each visit, and each study's form is unique to that particular protocol.

case record form correction log (CRFCL) (Clinical Trials)
When **case record forms** (CRFs) are collected from an investigating site they are subjected to internal checks by a **Clinical Research Associate** who has not been involved in monitoring at the study site. In addition, errors and clarification of entries in the CRF may be required during the process of entering data into the computer. Once CRFs have been collected from a site, they are never returned to the **investigator**. All errors and items requiring further clarification are listed on a query log and returned to the investigator with photocopies of the relevant pages of the CRFs where corrections are required. The investigator then clarifies the entries on the photocopied pages of the CRFs and signs and dates the corrections. They are then returned to the sponsor (or **Contract Research Organization**). The corrections are recorded on a CRFCL. The corrected data are entered into the study database and the CRFCLs are stored with the CRFs as they represent a permanent record of changes that were made to the CRF after collection from the investigating site. A copy of the CRFCL is sent to the investigator so that they can be stored with the copies of the CRFs.

case record form sign-off (Clinical Trials)
After each **case record form** (CRF) has been checked and corrected, it has to be signed by the **investigator** to signify that the information contained in the CRF is a true and accurate record of the data for that patient.

case report form see case record form.

case-series (Clinical Trials)
A report on a series of patients with an outcome of interest. No **control group** is involved.

case study form see case record form.

case-surveillance
Studies in patients with diseases for which some cases are likely to be drug-related and to ascertain product exposure. **Marketing authorization** holders who sponsor such studies are expected to liaise particularly closely with the relevant **regulatory authorities** in order to determine the most appropriate arrangement for reporting the cases.

CAS Number (CAS Registration Number)
An assigned number used to identify a chemical. CAS stands for Chemical Abstracts Service, an organization that indexes information published in Chemical Abstracts by the American Chemical Society and that provides index guides by which information about particular

substances may be located in the abstracts. Sequentially assigned CAS numbers identify specific chemicals, except when followed by an asterisk (*) which signifies a compound (often naturally occurring) of variable composition. The numbers have no chemical significance. The CAS number is a concise, unique means of material identification.

Contact
> Chemical Abstracts Service
> Division of American Chemical Society
> Box 3012
> Columbus, OH 43210, USA
> Tel: + 1 614 447-3600.

CASP see **Critical Appraisal Skills Programme**.

CASPE
Clinical Accountability Service Planning and Evaluation.

catalyst
A substance that modifies (slows, or more often quickens) a chemical reaction without being consumed in the reaction.

catalytic model
A (rather misleading name for a) type of **compartmental model** in which the **force of infection** is treated as a parameter to be estimated.

catechol-o-methyltransferase (COMT)
An enzyme that catalyses the transfer of the methyl group from adenosylmethionine to meta- (i.e. 3-) hydroxy group of catecholamine. The 3-methoxy products of dopamine, noradrenaline (norepinephrine) and adrenaline (epinephrine) are 3-methoxytyramine, normetanephrine and metanephrine respectively. COMT is an intracellular cytoplasmic enzyme and is especially abundant in liver and kidneys. It differs in importance at different sites of noradrenergic transmission. At some, it plays a significant role in terminating transmitter action after uptake of the transmitter into the cells containing the enzyme.

catechol-o-methyltransferase inhibitors
Drugs that inhibit COMT. They include catechol, pyrogallol, tropolone derivatives, certain flavenoids, and the compounds 3,5-hydroxy-4-methoxybenzoic acid and dopacitamide.

categorical data
Data which are evaluated by sorting the values into various categories (e.g. mild, moderate and severe).

cathartic see **purgative**.

CAT scan
Abbreviation for computerized axial tomography, an X-ray technique for producing images of internal bodily structures through the assistance of a computer.

causality
The relationship of an **adverse drug reaction** (ADR) to the use of a medication. In assessing causality, the following factors determine the outcome:
- Timing (time interval between taking the drug and the first appearance of the adverse event (AE)/ADR, i.e. plausibility and consistency of time to onset between cases)
- **Dose–response** relationship (positive dose response, known effect in overdose cases)

- Pharmacology (there is a known mechanism, the drug is known to affect the same body system as the AE/ADR, pharmacokinetic evidence, recognized class effect of the drug, similar findings in animals studies, biological plausibility)
- Withdrawal/**rechallenge** (positive **dechallenge** and **rechallenge**)
- Pattern/previous cases (evidence from **clinical trials** and/or PMS studies, similar AEs/ADRs already recognized for the drug, clear-cut easily-evaluated cases, high frequency of reports, recognized consequence of overdose with the drug)
- Reporter's opinion (reports being of high status (credibility))
- Alternative causes (lack of **confounding factors**, lack of obvious alternative explanations, co-medication being unlikely to have played a role).

The likelihood of the event being caused by the drug is classified often as either:
- Unknown (if no evaluation can be made)
- Not related
- Possible
- Probable
- Definite.

Also called imputability.

causality assessment of suspected adverse reactions

Determining whether there is a reasonable possibility that a drug caused or contributed to an **adverse event**. It includes assessing temporal relationships, **dechallenge/rechallenge** information, association (or lack of association) with underlying disease, and the presence (or absence) of a more likely cause. Methods used to assess **causality** include Bayesian method, and **global introspection**. Various **causality** terms are in use but those, below, are used most widely. Some, however, do not use all the terms, for instance many do not believe that a 'certain' classification is possible for a single report and others make no distinction between 'probable' and 'possible'. Where only 'possible' or 'unlikely' are used to describe reactions it must be understood that 'possible' includes those reactions which are called by others 'probable' and 'certain', as well as 'possible'. Whilst 'conditional/unclassified' and 'unassessible/unclassifiable' are not causality terms, they describe the status of adverse reaction reports and therefore allow for practical communication about **adverse drug reaction** (ADR) issues.

Certain

'A clinical event, including laboratory test abnormality, occurring in a plausible time relationship to drug administration, and which cannot be explained by concurrent disease or other drugs or chemicals. The response to withdrawal of the drug (dechallenge) should be clinically plausible. The event must be definitive pharmacologically or phenomenologically, using a satisfactory rechallenge procedure if necessary' (WHO definition, 1991).

It is recognized that this stringent definition will lead to very few reports meeting the criteria, but this is useful because of the special value of such reports. It is considered that time relationships between drug administration and the onset and course of the adverse event are important in causality analysis. So also is the consideration of confounding features, but due weight must be placed on the known pharmacological and other characteristics of the drug product being considered. Sometimes the clinical phenomena described will also be sufficiently specific to allow a confident causality assessment in the absence of confounding features and with appropriate time relationships, e.g. penicillin anaphylaxis.

Probable/likely

'A clinical event, including laboratory test abnormality, with a reasonable time sequence to administration of the drug, unlikely to be attributed to concurrent disease or other drugs or chemicals, and which follows a clinically reasonable response on withdrawal (dechallenge). Rechallenge information is not required to fulfil this definition' (WHO definition, 1991).

This definition has less stringent wording than for 'certain' and does not necessitate prior knowledge of drug characteristics or clinical adverse reaction phenomena. As stated no rechallenge information is needed, but confounding due to drug administration or underlying disease must be absent.

Possible

'A clinical event, including laboratory test abnormality, with a reasonable time sequence to administration of the drug, but which could also be explained by concurrent disease or other drugs or chemicals. Information on drug withdrawal may be lacking or unclear' (WHO definition, 1991).

This is the definition to be used when drug causality is one of other possible causes for the described clinical event.

Unlikely

'A clinical event, including laboratory test abnormality, with a temporal relationship to drug administration which makes a causal relationship improbable, and in which other drugs, chemicals or underlying disease provide plausible explanations' (WHO definition, 1991).

This definition is intended to be used when the exclusion of drug causality of a clinical event seems most plausible.

Conditional/unclassified

'A clinical event, including laboratory test abnormality, reported as an adverse reaction, about which more data is essential for a proper assessment or the additional data are under examination' (WHO definition, 1991).

Unassessible/unclassifiable

'A report suggesting an adverse reaction which cannot be judged because information is insufficient or contradictory, and which cannot be supplemented or verified' (WHO definition, 1991).

In clinical trials, causality assessment is the judgment of either the **Principle Investigator** (PI) or the **sponsor**'s Drug Safety Unit. The final decision of the PI conducting a clinical trial on the causality relationship between the **adverse event** and the investigational product is final and may not, normally, be changed.

causation
US term for causality.

caustic
Any substance that destroys tissue by chemical corrosion or burning and is suitable for removal of abnormal skin growths such as warts.

CBA see **cost–benefit analysis**.

CBCTN
Community Based Clinical Trials Network.

CBER see **Center for Biologics Evaluation and Review**.

CBI (UK)
Confederation of British Industry.

CC
   Coefficient of correlation.

CCC (UK)
   Copyright Clearance Centre.

CCD (Canada)
   Canadian Drugs Directorate.

CCDS see **Company Core Date Sheet**.

CCN see **Community Care Network**.

CCOP see **Community Clinical Oncology Program**.

CCP
   Community Care Plan.

CCRA
   Certified Clinical Research Associate.

CCRC
   Certified Clinical Research Coordinator.

CCSI see **Company Core Safety Information**.

CCST see **Certificate of Completion of Specialist Training** (for junior doctors).

CCT
   1. Compressed and coated tablet.
   2. Compulsory competitive tendering.

CCTA (UK)
   The government centre for information systems.

cd see **controlled drug**.

CD
   Clinical Director, or Clinical Directorate.

CDC see **Centers for Disease Control**.

CDER see **Center for Drugs Evaluation and Review**.

CDM
   Chronic disease management.

CDO
   Chief Dental Officer.

CDP see **clinical development plan**.

CDPH
   Communicable Disease and Public Health.

CDR
   Communicable Disease Report.

CDRH see **Center for Devices and Radiological Health**.

CDS see **Contract Data Set**.

CDSC see **Communicable Disease Surveillance Centre**.

CDSM see **Committee on Dental and Surgical Materials**.

CE
1. Mark signifying compliance with **European Union** harmonized standardization of **medical devices**. All devices other than those for clinical investigation or those which are custom made must bear this mark if they are certified by their manufacturer to meet the adequate quality requirements.
2. Chief Executive.

CEA see **cost-effectiveness analysis**.

CEBP see **Centre for Evidence-Based Pharmacotherapy**.

CEC see **Commission of the European Communities**.

CEE
Communauté Européen Economique (= EEC).

CEEC
Central and Eastern European country.

CEH see **Centre for Health Economics**.

celiac disease
Inability to digest and absorb gliadin, the protein found in wheat. Undigested gliadin causes damage to the lining of the small intestine. This prevents absorption of nutrients from other foods. Celiac disease is also called celiac sprue, gluten intolerance, and non-tropical sprue. People with this disease are intolerant to any medicinal product that has gluten as part of its formulation.
See also **gluten**.

cell bank
'A system whereby successive batches of a product are manufactured by culture in cells derived from the same master cell bank (fully characterized for identity and absence of contamination). A number of containers from the master cell bank are used to prepare a working cell bank. The cell bank system is validated for a passage level or number of population doublings beyond that achieved during routine production.' (Crown Copyright)
See also **master cell bank**.

cell culture
'The results from the *in vitro* growth of cells isolated from multicellular organisms.' (Crown Copyright)

cell tissue toxicity
A measure of the **toxicity** of a drug, **biological**, or **medical device** toward living cells. Measuring this toxicity is often one of the major goals of preclinical studies.

CEMD
Confidential Enquiry into Maternal Deaths.

CEN see **European Standardization Committee**.

CEND see **Clinical Effectiveness Network in Dorset.**

CENELEC see **European Electrotechnical Standardization Committee.**

censoring (Clinical Trials, Statistics)
A term used in survival or time-to-event analyses to denote an individual who has not experienced the event of interest as of a specific point in follow-up, e.g. time of **interim analysis**, end of study, or time at loss to follow-up. The process by which patient outcome data cannot be obtained beyond a specific point in time.

Center for Biologics Evaluation and Review (CBER) (US)
The division of **Food and Drug Administration** responsible for the licensing and regulation of biological **drug products**. These are pharmaceuticals that have biological systems as their origin, such as vaccines, blood products and genetically engineered formulations.
See also **Center for Devices and Radiological Health, Center for Drugs Evaluation and Review.**

Centre for Clinical Effectiveness (Australia)
Opened at Monash Medical Centre in Australia in January 1998. Its objective is to enhance patient outcomes through the clinical application of the best available evidence about treatments.
Website: http://www.med.monash.edu.au/publichealth/cce/

Center for Devices and Radiological Health (CDRH) (US)
A division of the **Food and Drug Administration** responsible for the licensing and regulation of **medical devices** (the equivalent of the **Medical Devices Agency** in the UK). This includes implantables (such as pacemakers) and diagnostic equipment (such as X-ray machines).
Web site: www.fda.gov/cdrh/cdrhhome.html
See also **Center for Biologics Evaluation and Review, Center for Drugs Evaluation and Review.**

Center for Drugs Evaluation and Review (CDER) (US)
The division of the **Food and Drug Administration** that is responsible for the licensing and regulation of **pharmaceuticals** (with the exception of biologics).
See also **Center for Biologics Evaluation and Review, Center for Devices and Radiological Health.**

Center for Small Business (CSB) (US)
Formerly the Device Small Manufacturers Assistance – DSMA
The CSB is a group within **Food and Drug Administration** (FDA)'s **Center for Devices and Radiological Health**. Its goal is to help small businesses understand and operate under the complex, often-overwhelming set of FDA regulations and guidelines.

Center for Veterinary Medicine (CVM)
The **Food and Drug Administration** (FDA) CVM is responsible for ensuring that animal drugs and medicated feeds are safe and effective for their intended uses and that food from treated animals is safe for human consumption. Before a new animal drug can be marketed in the US, it must be approved by the FDA on the basis of **quality**, **safety** and **efficacy**. When the drug is for use in food-producing animals, not only must the safety to the animal be demonstrated, but also the **safety** of food products derived from the treated animals that are intended for human consumption (e.g. elimination of violative residues in meat and milk). Once approved products are on the market, the Center monitors the use of the products through surveillance and **compliance** programmes.
See also **Food and Drug Administration.**

Centers for Disease Control (CDC) (US)
Charged with the tracking and investigation of public health trends and epidemics and publishes weekly and other reports on all deaths and diseases reported in the US.

Central Ethics Committee see **Ethics Committee.**

Central Pharmaceutical Affairs Council (CPAC) (Japan)
An advisory body to the Ministry of Health and Welfare with a responsibility to determine appropriateness of **approval** of manufacture, or import of new drugs. The CPAC consists of over 50 subcommittees who are normally independent experts.

centralized procedure (European Union)
Part of the **European Union** (EU) licensing system which was laid down in Council **Regulation (EEC) No. 2309/93** and Council Directive 93/41/EEC. It became effective in January 1995. This procedure is compulsory for **medicinal products** derived from biotechnological processes, and available at the request of companies for other innovative new products. Council Regulation 2309/93 sets out the types of product which must follow this procedure (Annex A – Biotechnology products), and those which may follow it (Annex B – Innovatory products). This procedure allows the applicants to obtain a **marketing authorization** (MA) that is simultaneously valid in all of the **Member States** (MS) of the EU. Applications are submitted directly to the **European Medicines Evaluation Agency** (EMEA), in London, for scientific evaluation to be assessed by the **Committee for Proprietary Medicinal Products** (CPMP) or the **Committee for Veterinary Medicinal Products** (CVMP) as applicable. The CPMP or CVMP appoints (usually following the receipt of the letter of intention to submit an application) one of its members as a **rapporteur** and another member as **co-rapporteur** who coordinate the evaluation of an application. The comments or objections of the CPMP or CVMP are communicated to the applicant for comments. The rapporteur and co-rapporteur then assess the applicant's comments and submit them to the CPMP or CVMP for discussion. The time limit for the evaluation, by the EMEA, is 210 days. The Agency then has 30 days to forward its opinion to the Commission.

The Commission has 30 days to prepare a draft **decision.** The draft decision is then sent to the Standing Committee on Medicinal Products for Human Use, or the Standing Committee on Veterinary Medicinal Products (MSs have one representative each in both of these committees) for their **opinions.** The procedure ultimately results in a Commission decision, which is binding on all MSs of the EU to authorize the product. The decision is published in the official journal of the EC.

The authorizaton is valid for 5 years and renewable for 5 years upon application by the holder, to the EMEA, as stipulated in Article 13.1 of Council Regulation (EEC) No. 2377/93.
See also **mutual recognition procedure.**

Centre for Adverse Reactions Monitoring (CARM) (New Zealand)
Located in the Dunedin School of Medicine at the University of Otago, the centre is part of the National Toxicology Group which includes the National Poisons & Hazardous Chemicals Information Centre. CARM acts as an advisory body to the Ministry of Health but has no regulatory powers. **The Intensive Medicines Monitoring Programme** is part of CARM.
See also **Intensive Medicines Monitoring Programme.**

Centre for Evidence-Based Child Health (UK)
An educational resource offering training and support to clinicians. The Centre aims to promote

the skills required to integrate research evidence and clinical expertise. Courses run by the Centre introduce health care professionals to the skills required to practise evidence-based child health.

Centre for Evidence Based Dentistry (UK)

The main objective of the Centre, based at the Institute of Health Sciences in Oxford, is to promote the teaching, learning, practice and evaluation of evidence-based dentistry throughout the UK.

Website: http://www.ihs.ox.ac.uk/cebd/index.htm.

Centre for Evidence-Based Medicine (CEBM) (UK)

Established in Oxford as the first of several centres in the UK whose aim broadly is to promote evidence-based health care (EBHC) and provide support and resources to anyone who wants to make use of them. The Centre's web site contains the EBM Toolbox with numerous aids to the practice and teaching of EBHC, including: pre-test probabilities, likelihood ratios, **SpPins** and **SnNouts**, numbers needed to treat and other measures of **effectiveness** for diagnostic tests, therapy and prognosis; teaching materials for public health, **primary care**, hospital medicine, child health, neonatology, mental health, surgery, obstetrics and gynaecology; a glossary of terms; hints, tips and worksheets on asking clinical questions, searching and critical appraisal; slide presentations on the background to EBM; and much more.

Website: http://cebm.jr2.ox.ac.uk/

Centre for Evidence-Based Nursing (UK)

The Centre works with nurses in practice, other researchers, nurse educators and managers to identify evidence-based practice through primary research and systematic reviews. It also promotes the uptake of evidence into practice through education and implementation activities in areas of nursing where good evidence is available.

Centre for Evidence-Based Pharmacotherapy (CEBP) (UK)

Initiated in July 1995 to undertake research in the methodology of medicines assessment, **pharmacoepidemiology** and **pharmacoeconomics** and to undertake such studies. The Centre is active within the **Cochrane Collaboration** with membership of the editorial team of the Menstrual Disorders Review Group and coordination of the Pharmaceuticals Field as well as membership of the Statistical Methods Working Group. The Centre also has close links with the Consumers Association.

Website: http://www.aston.ac.uk/pharmacy/cebp/

Centre for Health Economics (CEH) (UK)

A specialist **health economics** research unit within the University of York, whose mission is to undertake and disseminate high quality research in the field of health economics. CHE was established in 1983 and has continually expanded since its inception. Providing research of worldwide repute, its principal areas of activity include economic evaluation of health technologies, measurement and valuation of **outcomes, primary care**, the economics of addiction and health promotion, health economics in low and middle income countries, resource allocation and health policy.

Centre for Medicines Research International (CMRI)

An independent scientific unit, established in 1981, aiming to be the centre of excellence for addressing strategic issues in the discovery, development, regulation and safe use of medicines for the benefit of society. The centre also aims to facilitate international knowledge exchange, contribute to increased productivity and efficiency, and to improve the global environment for research and development.

Centres of excellence
Hospitals or other delivery sites that have demonstrated the ability to provide top-notch health care within a certain field.

CEO
Chief Executive Officer.

CER
Control event rate, see **event rate**.

certainty
The condition of an event in which the probability of occurrence is equal to 1 (e.g. death).

Certificate of Authority (COA) (US)
Issued by State governments, it gives a **Health Maintenance Organization** or insurance company its licence to operate within the State.

Certificate of Completion of Specialist Training (CCST) (UK)
A certificate awarded by the **Specialist Training Authority** (STA) in the UK on completion of a nationally recognized training programme in a listed medical speciality. The CCST-UK denotes specialist status of the holder and is mutually recognized by **Member States** for those specialties that are listed throughout the **European Union**.

Certificate of Coverage (COC) (US)
Outlines the terms of coverage and benefits available in a carrier's health plan.

Certificate of Destruction (Clinical Trials)
All returned and unused medication has to be destroyed at the end of the study. Normally this material is returned to the **sponsor** together with the appropriate inventory and the supplies are destroyed. A Certificate of Destruction is issued which lists the drugs and the quantity destroyed on a given date. This certificate is filed in the **Clinical Trial Master File**.

CESDI (UK)
Confidential Enquiry into Stillbirths and Deaths in Infancy.

CF see **conversion factor**.

CFC
Chlorofluorocarbon; used in aerosols as propellants but are being phased out due to their association with damage to the Earth's ozone layer.

CFR see **Code of Federal Regulations (Food and Drug Administration)**.

CFR 29 Section 1910.1200 (US)
The **Occupational Safety Health Administration** regulation known as the Hazard Communication Standard.

CFSAN (US)
Center for Food Safety and Applied Nutrition (**Food and Drug Administration**).

CGMP (US)
Current good manufacturing practices.

C

CGRDU see **Clinical Governance Research and Development Unit**.

CHAIN see **Contact Help Advice Information Network for Effective Health Care**.

CHAMPUS (US)
Civilian Health and Medical Program of the Uniformed Services.

chance (Statistics)
The unknown and the unpredictable elements which leads to an event having one **outcome** as opposed to another.

ChB
Basic surgical medical degree. It does not usually appear by itself without the MB.

CHC
1. see **Community Health Centre**.
2. see **Community Health Council**.

CHDGP (UK)
Collection of Health Data from General Practice project.

cheese reaction
A phrase used to describe the potentiation by monoamine oxidase (MAO) inhibitors of the vasopressor actions of indirectly acting sympathomimetic amines, notably tyramine, in certain foods, including some cheeses) but also yeast and meat extracts, pickled herrings and certain wines). A serious hypertensive crisis may arise when patients being treated with MAO inhibitors ingest such foods, and they are strongly warned against them by doctors, pharmacists and the drug **manufacturer** (via the **patient information leaflet**).

chemical inventory
List of hazardous materials in a workplace.

chemical name
The name used by chemists to indicate the chemical structure of the drug.

chemical pathology
The study of the changes that occur in disease in the chemical constitution and biochemical mechanisms of the body. Clinical chemistry is a branch of chemical pathology. It involves undertaking and interpreting biochemical tests performed on patients.

chemical-protective clothing (CPC)
Personal protective clothing; suit, apron, gloves, etc. that is manufactured to be resistant to penetration by specific chemicals for a certain period of time.

Chemistry, Manufacturing and Controls Section (CMC Section) (US)
The section of a **New Drug Application** or **Investigational New Drug** that describes the composition, manufacture and specifications of a **drug product**, as well as the ingredients that make up the product. The CMC section is divided into four major sections:
1. Drug substance
2. **Drug product**
3. Method's validation
4. Environmental assessment

Chemistry, Pharmacy and Standards Subcommittee (CPS) see **Committee on Safety of Medicines**

chemobiotic
The combination of a chemotherapeutic agent with an antibiotic.

chemopharmacodynamic
Denoting the relationship between chemical constitution and pharmacological activity.

chemoprophylaxis
The use of a chemotherapeutic agent as a means of preventing development or future occurrences of a specific disease. Treatment may be **chemotherapy** as far as an individual is concerned but chemoprophylactic for the population as a whole.

chemoreceptor
A molecular structure on the surface of a cell that is sensitive to chemical substances, such as epinephrine released by nerve cells.

chemotaxis
The movement of an organism or an individual cell in response to a chemical concentration gradient.

chemotherapy
A therapy that is chemical in nature. The term is sometimes restricted to antibiotics and cancer chemotherapy.

chemotic
An agent that increases the production of lymph in the ocular conjunctiva.

CHI
1. (UK) see **Commission for Health Improvement Programme**, aka CHImP.
2. Community Health Index.

CHImP see **Commission for Health Improvement Programme**.

CHIN see **Community Health Information Network**.

CHINA (UK)
Citizen Health Information Network and Alliance.

chi squared test (Statistics)
A **hypothesis** test which can be used to analyse the relationship between two categorized variables. Rather than measuring the value of each of a set of items, a calculated value of chi square compares the frequencies of various kinds (or categories) of items in a random sample to the frequencies that are expected if the population frequencies are as hypothesized by the **investigator**.

Chi square is often used to assess the 'goodness of fit' between an obtained set of frequencies in a random sample and what is expected under a given statistical **hypothesis**. For example, chi square can be used to determine if there is reason to reject the statistical hypothesis that the frequencies in a random sample are as expected when the items are from a **normal distribution**.

CHMU
Central Health Monitoring Unit.

cholagogue
A drug that stmulates the flow of bile from the gall bladder and bile ducts into the duodenum.
Compare **cholerectic**.

cholerectic
A drug that increases the production and secretion of bile by the liver.
Compare **cholagogue**.

cholinergic crisis
Muscle weakness consequent upon excessive use of anticholinergic drugs by patients with myasthenia gravis. Temporary withdrawal of the anticholinesterase drug and subsequent readjustment of dose restores the expected beneficial effects.

CHOU
Central Health Outcomes Unit.

chronic
Present over a long period of time. Diabetes is an example of chronic disease.
Compare **acute**.

chronic toxicity
Adverse health effects resulting from long-term exposure to a chemical (e.g. months, years, decades).

chronopharmacokinetics
The study of **pharmacokinetic** drug parameters as affected by circadian rhythm or diurnal variation.

chronotrophic effect
The effect of a drug on the force of heart beat.

CHS
Community Health Services.

CI
1. Clinical indicator.
2. (Statistics) See **confidence interval**.

C/I see **contraindication**.

CIOMS see **Council for the International Organization of Medical Sciences**.

CIOMS form see **Council for the International Organization of Medical Sciences**.

CIOMS Reportable Case Histories (CIOMS Reports)
Serious, medically substantiated, unlabelled **adverse drug reactions** about which there is sufficient information. Four pieces of information constitute a minimum report: an identifiable source of the information, a patient (even if not precisely identified by name and date of birth), a suspect drug and a suspect reaction.
See also **reportable adverse reaction**.

CIP
Cost Improvement Programme.

CIPG
Community Investment Partnership Group.

CIS
Clinical Information System.
CISH
Confidential Inquiry into Suicide and mental Health.
CISP
Community Information System Project.
CITAC
The Cooperation on International Traceability in Analytical Chemistry.
CJEC
Court of Justice of the European Communities, see **European Court of Justice**.
Cl, Clx see clearance.
CLA (UK)
Copyright Licensing Agency.
class
A collection of individuals or values sharing common characteristics.
Class I, II, III Devices (US)
Classification by the **Food and Drug Administration** of **medical devices** according to potential risks or hazards.
classical epidemiology
A term that describes the varieties of **epidemiology** primarily concerned with the statistical relationships between disease agents, both infectious and non-infectious; for example a study to establish the relative risk of lung cancer associated with smoking.
Compare **ecological epidemiology**.
clastogenic
An agent that causes damage to genetic material (i.e. breakage or disruption of chromosomes). Also called aneugenic.
clean area
'An area with defined environmental control of particulate and microbial contamination constructed and used in such a way as to reduce the introduction, generation and retention of contaminants within the area.' (Crown Copyright)
See also **clean/contained area, contained area**.
clean/contained area
'An area constructed and operated in such a way that will achieve the aims of both a clean area and a contained area at the same time.' (Crown Copyright)
See also **clean area, contained area**.
clean database (Clinical Trials)
A database from which all errors, relating to a particular trial, have been eliminated and in which measurements and other values are provided in the same units.
cleaning data (Statistics)
The process of dealing with errors and omissions in a set of data and ensuring that measurements are given in the same units and to the same degree of accuracy.

clearance (Cl or Cl_x)
The rate at which a drug substance is eliminated from blood. It depends mostly on the efficiency with which the liver and/or the kidneys can eliminate the drug. It is calculated, mathematically by the division of the dose rate by the average plasma concentration at steady state. Since dose rate units of amount/time, e.g. mg/h and the average plasma concentration has units of amount/volume, e.g. mg/l, clearance has units of volume/time, e.g. l/h.

CLIA
Clinical Laboratory Improvements Amendments.

Clinical Brochure (Clinical Trials)
The US term for **Investigator's Brochure**. This document contains all relevant information about the drug, including animal screening, preclinical **toxicology** and detailed pharmaceutical data. Also included, if available, is a summary of current knowledge about **pharmacology** and mechanism of action and a full description of the clinical toxicities.

Compare **Investigator's Brochure**.

clinical budgeting
The allocation of financial resources to specific consultant clinical staff, for which they have responsibility.

clinical data repository
That component of a computer-based patient record (CPR) which accepts, files and stores clinical data over time from a variety of supplemental treatment and intervention systems for such purposes as practice guidelines, outcomes management, and clinical research.

Also called data warehouse.

clinical decision support see decision support systems.

clinical development plan (CDP)
The plan containing the total framework and activities for global clinical development of an **investigational product's** registration and marketing. It encompasses finding out whether there is a dose range and schedule at which the drug can be shown to be simultaneously effective and safe, to the extent that the risk–benefit relationship is acceptable, the particular patients who might benefit from the drug and the specific indications for its use and so on.

Satisfying these broad aims usually requires an ordered programme of **clinical trials**, each with its own specific objectives. This should be specified in a clinical plan, or a series of plans, with appropriate decision points and flexibility to allow modification as knowledge accumulates. A licence application should clearly describe the main content of such plans and the contribution made by each trial. Interpretation and assessment of the evidence from the total programme of trials involves synthesis of the evidence from the individual trials. This is facilitated by ensuring that common standards are adopted for a number of features of the trials such as dictionaries of medical terms, definition and timing of the main measurements, handling of **protocol** deviations and so on. A formal statistical overview or meta-analysis may be informative when medical questions are addressed in more than one trial. Where possible this should be envisaged in the plan so that the relevant trials are clearly identified and any required common features of their designs are specified in advance. Other major statistical issues (if any) which are expected to affect a number of trials in a common plan should be addressed in that plan.

Clinical Directorate (UK)
A management unit in a **National Health Service** Trust which focuses on a specific

clinical care group. Usually, led by a consultant medical officer with business management support.

Clinical Effectiveness Network in Dorset (CEND) (UK)
A collaborative project between the Health Authority, Dorset Research & Development Support Unit, the **National Health Service** Trusts and **Primary Care** Teams in Dorset; working together to ensure that clinical practice is based on the most up-to-date, well-validated research.
Website: http://www.cend.org.uk/index.htm

Clinical Effectiveness Strategy Group (UK)
Established by **Clinical Resources and Audit Group** to link their work with that of the Chief Scientist Office.

Clinical Effectiveness Unit (CEU) (UK)
Formerly the Surgical Epidemiology & Audit Unit but, following an external review in 1996, its council endorsed the recommendation to create an academic partnership with a local university. As a result, the CEU was re-established, in 1990, as a collaboration between the College and the Health Services Research Unit at the London School of Hygiene & Tropical Medicine (LSHTM). The CEU is assisted and advised by the Clinical Effectiveness Committee which comprises members of Council, surgeons representing the main subspecialties, and senior academics with relevant expertise. The committee has the task of developing strategies for implementing the government's quality assurance agenda for the **National Health Service** described in the consultation document 'A First Class Service'.

Clinical Evidence 99 (UK)
A compendium of the best available research findings on common and important clinical questions, updated and expanded every 6 months. Sample pages are available as Acrobat files on the website: http://www.evidence.org.

clinical governance (UK)
An initiative detailed in the 1997 White Paper 'The New **National Health Service** (NHS): Modern and Dependable' to ensure and improve clinical standards at local level throughout the NHS. It is a system or a framework through which NHS organizations are accountable for continuously improving the **quality** of their services and safeguarding high standards of care by creating an environment in which excellence in clinical care will flourish. Quality and good practice are brought together under the heading of 'Quality Organizations', with the aim being to develop leadership skills, identify poor clinical performance at an early stage and ensure evidence-based practice is in place. In practice, this means clinical **audit**, postgraduate education, peer review. Professionals would be accountable for their own individual professional development, continuing professional development (CPD), would develop programmes for their practice team which are based on national initiatives but sensitive to local issues.

The national initiatives are **National Institute for Clinical Excellence** (NICE) and the **Commission for Health Improvement** (CHImP).

Clinical Governance Research and Development Unit (CGRDU) (UK)
The CGRDU came into existence on 1 April 1999 as a successor of the Eli Lilly National Clinical Audit Centre. Since 1992, the Lilly Audit Centre was a national resource in the field of clinical audit, particularly in the setting of **primary care** and at the interface of primary and secondary care. It is now an independent resource to Audit or **Primary Care Groups** (PCGs), Health Authorities (HAs) and others involved in **clinical governance**. The CGRDU is an integral part

of the department of General Practice and Primary Health Care, at the University of Leicester and has access to all necessary facilities. It is funded by Leicestershire Health Authority, with substantial pump priming funds from Eli Lilly and Company Ltd. In June 1999, the CGRDU launched the *Journal of Clinical Governance*, which succeeded *Audit Trends*.

clinical guidelines

Systematically developed statements to assist practitioner and patient decisions about appropriate health care for specific clinical circumstances. Guidelines provide recommendations for effective practice in the management of clinical conditions where variations in practice are known to occur and where effective care may not be delivered uniformly throughout.

clinical hold (US)

If the **Food and Drug Administration** (FDA) has a question or concern during a **clinical trial** of a **drug product** or **medical device**, it can temporarily halt the trial. This is known as a clinical hold. If the issue is resolved, the FDA may lift the hold and the trial may resume.

clinical indicator (CI) (UK)

An indicator that provides information about the **quality**, **efficacy**, and **outcomes** of the **National Health Service** services. It is used in conjunction with the **high level performance indicator**.

clinical investigation see clinical trial.

Clinical Investigation Brochure see Investigator's Brochure.

clinical observations

The observation of clinical **signs** and **symptoms** in a patient. Any measurements made as a result of these form part of the record of the clinical observations.

clinical pathways

A 'map' of preferred treatment/intervention activities, which outlines the types of information needed to make decisions, the timelines for applying that information, and what action needs to be taken by whom. Clinical pathways provide a way to monitor care 'in real time'. These pathways are developed by clinicians for specific diseases or events. Proactive providers are working now to develop these pathways for the majority of their interventions and developing the software capacity to distribute and store this information.

Also called critical pathways.

clinical pharmacology

The scientific study of drugs in man. It therefore embraces all studies in human subjects, with or without **therapeutic intent**, and includes studies performed both early and late in a drug's history. Types of study can be broadly differentiated into **pharmacokinetic** (what the body does to the drug), which includes **absorption, distribution, metabolism** and **excretion**; **Pharmacodynamic** (what the drug does to the body), which includes the effect on metabolism and biological action; and therapeutic (what the drug does to the disease). For convenience and traditional reasons, therapeutic studies are referred to as **clinical trials**.

See also **pharmacology**.

clinical phase

The phase of **drug product** or device development that encompasses all human testing. It follows the research and development phase (laboratory testing) and preclinical (animal testing) phase. In the US, it is the final step before the regulator's **approval** is sought via a **Product Licence Application**, **Premarket Approval Application** or **New Drug Application**.

Clinical Practice Guideline
A systematically developed written statement designed to assist and guide the practitioner (in the diagnosis and treatment) and the patient to make decisions about appropriate health care for specific clinical circumstances, disease or condition. Ideally, they are based on clinical data which demonstrate the optimum course of therapy for a given set of symptoms or disease state. For example, if an emergency room patient presents with chest pain, there are several options available to the treating physician. Should a muscle relaxant be prescribed? Should an electrocardiogram be performed? If a clinical guideline were available, it would guide the physician through a fixed diagnostic procedure, which would allow him or her to prescribe the most appropriate treatment (based on past clinical experience). The intent of clinical guidelines is to make possible the delivery of consistently good health care with high cost-effectiveness. Therefore, they are rapidly gaining favour with **Managed Care Organizations**, which are attempting to manage the delivery of health care to control costs.

Clinical Practice Guideline Infobase (Canada)
A database within the **Canadian Medical Association** (CMA) website which was produced by a national or provincial medical or health organization, professional society, government agency or expert panel. This new product is being developed in three stages. During the first stage, CMA is providing access to guidelines previously published in the *Canadian Medical Association Journal* (CMAJ); the guidelines to which CMAJ does not hold copyright are listed and the full text will be added when the developers have granted permission. Other guidelines are to be added as they become available.
    Website: http://www.mls.cps.bc.ca/mlsbkmk.htm

Clinical Research Associate (CRA) (Clinical Trials)
Person employed by a **sponsor**, or by a **Contract Research Organization** acting on a sponsor's behalf, who has responsibility for recruiting investigators, initiating studies, monitoring the progress of **investigator** sites participating in a clinical study and closing down clinical sites at the end of studies. At some (primarily academic) sites, clinical research coordinators are called CRAs. In addition, CRAs are expected to be able to write protocols, design **case record forms** and write **Final Reports** when studies are completed.
    See also **monitor**.

Clinical Research Coordinator see **Clinical Trial Coordinator**.

clinical research site see **clinical trial site**.

Clinical Resources and Audit Group (CRAG) (UK)
A health group that works closely with **SIGN** (Scotland). It is chaired by the Chief Medical Officer.

Clinical Safety Data Management: Definitions and Standards for Expedited Reporting see **E2A guidance document**.

clinical significance (Clinical Trials)
Change in a **subject**'s or a **patient**'s clinical condition regarded as important whether or not due to the investigational product. Some statistically significant changes (in blood tests, for example) have no clinical significance. The criterion or criteria for clinical significance should be stated in the **protocol**.
    Compare **statistical significance**.

clinical study see **clinical trial**.

clinical study report see **clinical trial/study report**.

Clinical Therapeutic Index see **Therapeutic Index**.

clinical trial
A scientifically and systematically controlled study of a **medicinal product**, a technology or a procedure to test the effectiveness or verify the effects (pharmacological and/or other **pharmacodynamic**) of and/or identify any adverse reaction to and/or to study their **absorption, distribution, metabolism** and **excretion** with the object of ascertaining its safety and/or efficacy. A clinical trial is carried out in human population (patients with a particular disease or class of diseases or **healthy volunteers**) in a clinic or hospital setting. Most drugs are first studied in non-patient healthy volunteers. Limited studies are then undertaken in patients with the disease for which the drug is being developed. After this, clinical trials involving a much larger number of patients are completed. Further trials may be required after marketing. Following American practice these stages have become known as phase I–IV. Clinical trials are normally only allowed by **ethics committees** after the product has undergone chemical and animal testing. For a new pharmaceutical, the entire process typically takes 10 years and $200–250 million. In the US, the **Food and Drug Administration approval** process can take from 6 months to 10 years after the licence application is filed; the average time now stands at about 30 months. **Medical devices** tend to take a shorter time and, therefore have a somewhat lower development cost.

See also **Clinical Trial Team, phase I clinical trial, phase II clinical trial, phase III clinical trial, phase IV clinical trial**.

clinical trial budget
The amount of money that is available to pay for all the external services required to complete a clinical study (e.g. **investigator** payments, laboratory services, **contract research organizations**, packaging of clinical supplies, statistical analysis, writing services for the final report and the paper for publication).

Clinical Trial Certificate (CTC) (UK)
The older of two licences granted by the Licensing Division of the UK's **Medicines Control Agency** to permit the administration of new medicinal products to patients. Securing such a licence involves the submission of comprehensive exploratory data. The scheme involves full assessment of all data with the intention of demonstrating adequacy of quality and **safety** for the intended use applied. **Efficacy** data are not required for CTCs. To apply, the applicant company submits an MLA 202 form.

See also **Clinical Trial Exemption**.

clinical trial coordinator (CTC) (Clinical Trials)
Person (usually a nurse, medical assistant, etc.) who handles most of the administrative responsibilities (the required paperwork for a study) of a **clinical trial**, acts as liaison between investigative site and **sponsor**, and reviews all data and records before a monitor's visit.

Also called trial coordinator, study coordinator, research coordinator, clinical coordinator, research nurse, or protocol nurse.

clinical trial end date
The date the last subject has completed the last assessment (including post-treatment, if applicable).

Clinical Trial Exemption (CTX) (UK, Australia)
A scheme created by the **Medicines Control Agency** (MCA) of the UK which allows **sponsors** (companies) to apply for **approval** (licence) for each clinical study. It came into operation in March 1981 and was welcomed by companies as it provided a rapid alternative to the **Clinical**

Trial Certificate (CTC) scheme. It can be used for clinical trials on existing as well as new products. The data requirements, however, depend on the status of the **active ingredients** (i.e. pharmacopoeial, previously licensed, or novel), the frequency and route of administration, trial duration, dosage, inclusion of novel **excipients** or the inclusion of an established excipient but for a new route of administration. Whether the application can be considered to be suitable for the CTX scheme is decided when an application is made for the CTX (not before). If the MCA deems a certain application to be unsuitable for the CTX scheme due to insufficient information, the company can either resubmit the application with the required data or apply for a CTC. If, however, the MCA having considered the CTX application, believes that advisory committee advice is necessary or full data assessment is needed, companies have to submit an application for a CTC. Companies are not allowed to simultaneously apply for both schemes and there is no appeal procedure against the MCA's refusal to grant a CTX. The data supporting the application is submitted to the MCA and approval or rejection is received within 35 working days unless the MCA requests an extension (further 28 days). Approval means that the company is exempt from the need to hold a CTC. While the CTX application involves negative vetting of the summary of data supplied (by the company), the CTC scheme involves full positive assessment of complete data. CTX approval is valid for three years but can be renewed. The CTX application has to be signed on behalf of the company by a UK registered medically qualified doctor. This may be an employee of the company or a medical consultant acting on behalf of the company. By far, it is the more commonly employed licence used by pharmaceutical companies. When a company changes the name of an **investigational product**, a notification of change must be submitted with an updated Usage Guideline. Every **adverse drug reaction** reported to the authorities must have the CTX number on the report. When a CTX is to be terminated or a company does not intend to renew it, a notification should be sent to the Clinical Trials Unit, at the MCA, so that the file can be archived.

The CTX system was implemented in Australia on 1 August 1987 as a result of the recommendation by the **APMA**. The Commonwealth Department of Health then proposed to implement the scheme with a checklist for the pharmaceutical chemistry data and an exemption period for 60 days, rather than 35 calendar days (UK version), as a realistic initial time frame.

See also **Clinical Trial Certificate**.

clinical trial facilities

The facilities that are available to an **investigator** at a **clinical site**. **Clinical trial** centres must have the equipment to undertake a particular test and staff at the site must have the expertise to use the equipment properly. The investigator should also have adequate human resources (both clinical and non-clinical) to undertake a clinical trial. These should be inspected and the findings recorded in a Pre-Study Visit Report.

clinical trial master file (TMF) (Clinical Trials)

A hard copy, file or archive of all the documentation relating to a **clinical trial** as defined by **good clinical practice** guidelines.

See also **documentation**.

clinical trial materials

Complete set of supplies provided to an **investigator** by the trial **sponsor**.

clinical trial payments

The payments made to **investigators**, **contract research organizations**, contract laboratories and the providers of any other services required in connection with a clinical study. Investigators are usually paid a fee for the number of visits that were completed by each patient in the trial. An agreed amount of money is payable for each type of visit. Contract laboratories are paid by the number of tests that are undertaken for each particular trial. The payments for other services are negotiated prior to the work being undertaken.

clinical trial report see **clinical trial/study report**.

clinical trial site
The physical place where patients are seen and research data is gathered. Research sites are usually doctor's offices or hospitals.

clinical trial status report
A report giving the current status of a particular trial which usually provides information on the following:
- number of patients that have been recruited into the study
- number of patients that have completed the study
- number of patients currently ongoing (i.e. still being treated or followed up)
- number of patients who have dropped out of the study
- number of **serious adverse events** to date
- total amount of research funds that have been paid to the **investigator** to date.

If the study is multicentre then this information is provided for each investigator and then combined to provide the overall status of the study.

clinical trial/study report (Clinical Trials)
A complete and comprehensive written description of the trial of any therapeutic, prophylactic, or diagnostic agent after its completion including a description of experimental (including statistics) methods and materials, a presentation and evaluation of results, statistical analyses and a critical statistical and clinical appraisal (as directed by the **International Conference on Harmonization** Guideline for Structure and Content of Clinical Trial/study Report).

Also called **final report**.

clinical trial supplies
The **drug** supplies that are required to undertake a particular **clinical trial**. They include the test drug and the comparator (which may be **placebo**, or a competitive drug). For a **double-blind study**, the test drug and the comparator drug are visibly indistinguishable. If the two drugs look different, the study can be made into a double blind study using the **double dummy technique**.

See also **clinical trial materials**.

clinical trial team
The team responsible for an individual clinical trial or a group of trials in a project. This team is set up at the protocol-writing stage and usually consists of:
1. Medical research/project manager
2. Medical advisor
3. Drug safety surveillance representative
4. Clinical research associate
5. Data manager
6. Regulatory affairs department representative
7. Statistician
8. Case record form designer
9. Depending on the protocol, a representative from other departments, such as Department of Drug Metabolism and Kinetics, may also be a member of the team.

clinical trial update
Information on the current status of a study. It may be provided on a global basis or for each **investigator** participating in a study. It is important to provide investigators (particularly in a multicentre trial) with current information on the status of a clinical study in which they are involved.
See also **clinical trial status report**.

clinical trial variables
The parameters that are being observed, measured or assessed during the course of a **clinical trial**.

clinic without walls (CWW) (US)
Similar to an independent practice association and identical to a practice without walls (PWW). Practitioners who form CWWs and PWWs want the economies of scale and bargaining power offered by centralizing some administrative functions, but still choose to practise separately. Many of these were formed to allow practitioners the ability to effectively contract with managed care.
Also called Group Practice without Walls (GPWW).

ClinTrial
A data storage and retrieval system for clinical trial data. It is a trademark of BBN Software Products Corporation.

clone
A **population** of genetically identical copies of cells, genes or organisms produced from a common ancestor. Sometimes, 'clone' is also used for a number of recombinant DNA molecules all carrying the same inserted sequence.

close down (Clinical Trials)
The act of terminating a clinical study. Sites may be closed down because the study has been completed at that site. Sometimes the trial has to be terminated due to the high incidence of **adverse events** or high drop out, or maybe because the drug proved to be ineffective. Rarely, studies are terminated because additional animal work has revealed the possibility of a toxic effect if the drug is taken for long-term treatment.

CM
Community Midwife.

CMA see **Canadian Medical Association**.

CMC Section see **Chemistry, Manufacturing and Controls Section**.

CMDS
Core Minimum Data Set.

CME see **Continuing Medical Education**.

CMEA see **Council of Mutual Economic Assistance**.

CMO
Chief Medical Officer.

CMRI see **Centre for Medicines Research International**.

C

CMS see **Concerned Member State**.

CNM
Clinical Nurse Manager.

CNO
Chief Nurse Officer.

CNS
1. Clinical nurse specialist.
2. Central nervous system.
3. Community Nurse Service.

coagulant
A drug that aids the process of coagulation.

COBRA see **Consolidated Omnibus Budget Reconciliation Act**.

co-carcinogen
A substance that does not cause cancer by itself, but increases the effect of a substance that does cause cancer.

Cochrane Collaboration
An organization which aims to facilitate the creation, review, maintenance and dissemination of systematic overviews of the effects of health care (i.e. **evidence-based medicine**).
See also **Cochrane Library**.

Cochrane Library
An electronic library which consists of Database of Systematic Reviews (CDSR), the Database of Abstracts of Reviews of Effectiveness (DARE), and the Cochrane Controlled Trials Register (CCTR). The format of a Cochrane Review has several objectives. It helps readers to find the results of research quickly and to assess the validity, applicability and implications of those results. It guides reviewers to report their work explicitly and concisely, and minimizes the effort required to do this. The format is also suited to electronic publication and updating, and it generates reports that are informative and readable when viewed on a computer monitor or printed. The format of a Cochrane Review is flexible enough to fit different types of reviews, including those making a single comparison, those making multiple comparisons and those prepared by collaborative trialists' groups using individual patient data. Each review consists of:
- a cover sheet – giving the title, citation details and contact addresses
- an abstract – using a structured format
- the text of the review – consisting of an introduction (background and objective), materials (selection criteria and search strategy) and methods, results (description of studies, methodological quality, and results), discussion and conclusions
- standard tables and figures – showing characteristics of the included studies, specification of the interventions that were compared, the results of the included studies, and a log of the studies that were excluded
- references.

COCIR
Coordination Committee of Radiological and Electrochemical Equipment.

Code of Federal Regulations (CFR) (US)
The official set of regulations in the US. Of particular interest to **drug**, **biological** and **medical device** manufacturers is Title 21 of the CFR (often written as '21 CFR'), which governs the manufacturing, licensing, and sale of foods, drugs and cosmetics. Generally, new federal regulations are published in the federal register for comment some time before they are actually enacted.

Code of Practice (Clinical Trials) (UK)
There are a number of Codes of Practice in the UK which are related to the conduct of **clinical trials**. Most of these have been produced by the **Association of British Pharmaceutical Industry** (ABPI) and are accepted by the majority of the UK and foreign companies conducting studies in the UK. However, it should be noted that these codes of practice are not legally binding. The codes of practice are:
- Good Clinical Practice (GCP)
- Medical Experiments in Non-Patient Human Volunteers
- Clinical Trial Compensation Guidelines
- Code of Practice for the Clinical Assessment of Licensed Medicinal Products in General Practice.

Codex
An authorized medicinal formulary.

coding (US)
A mechanism for identifying and defining physicians' and hospitals' services. Coding provides universal definition and recognition of diagnoses, procedures and level of care. Coders usually work in medical records departments and coding is also a function of billing. **Medicare** fraud **investigators** look closely at the medical record documentation which supports codes and look for consistency. Lack of consistency of documentation can earmark a record as 'upcoded' which is considered fraud. A national certification exists for coding professionals and many compliance programmes are raising standards of quality for their coding procedures.

coding of clinical trial data
Data from **case record forms** are often coded before being entered into a computer database (e.g. **adverse events** may be coded using the **COSTART** coding system). **Coding** is used to provide consistency in the way in which data are entered into a computer system.

cognitively impaired (Clinical Trials)
Having either a psychiatric disorder (e.g. psychosis, neurosis, personality or behaviour disorders, or dementia) or a developmental disorder (e.g. mental retardation) that affects cognitive or emotional functions to the extent that capacity for judgment and reasoning is significantly diminished. Others, including persons under the influence of or dependent on drugs or alcohol; those suffering from degenerative diseases affecting the brain; terminally ill patients; and persons with severely disabling physical handicaps, may also be compromised in their ability to make decisions in their best interests (i.e. consent).
See also **informed consent**.

cohort
A cohort is a group of patients or subjects involved in a **clinical trial** who are identified as having one or more characteristics in common (i.e. are alike enough), usually age (e.g. all those individuals in the UK born in 1963 form a birth cohort) to be considered useful for study and analysis.

cohort study
An epidemiological investigational study that involves identification of two groups (**cohorts**) of patients, one which was exposed to a **risk factor** (e.g. drug, surgical procedure) and usually another group not exposed to that risk factor. Following and comparing these cohorts forward, is then carried out, taking into account the emergent patterns of disease or the outcome of interest. The advantages of such studies include the ease with which the inclusion criteria and outcome assessment can be standardized, matching of the subjects, cost, ease compared to **randomized clinical trials** and, most importantly, safety. The disadvantages, however, include difficulty in identifying and blinding patients, lack of **randomization**, possibility of an unseen link between the confounder and exposure and if the disease is rare then large sample sizes or long follow-up is required.

co-investigator (Clinical Trials)
A doctor who is part of the team at a particular centre and is involved in recruiting patients into the study but is not the senior member of that team.

College Ter Beoordeling Van Geneesmiddelen (Holland)
Medicines Evaluation Board.

combination drug
A **drug product** which contains two or more pharmacologically **active ingredients** in the same pharmaceutical preparation.
Compare **combination product**.

combination product
A product that has the characteristics of at least two of the product types, for instance, one which fits the definition of both a drug and a device.
Compare **combination drug**.

combinatorial chemistry/synthesis
The use of parallel or matrix synthetic methods to rapidly generate libraries of potential new drug compounds, i.e. to prepare large sets of organic compounds by combining sets of building blocks. The technology used is various but dominated mainly by robots designed to greatly accelerate the rate at which compounds can be produced.

combinatorial library
A set of compounds prepared by combinatorial synthesis.

COMECON
Council for Mutual Economic Assistance.

CoMFA see Comparative Molecular Field Analysis.

Comité Permanent see Standing Committee of European Doctors.

Commissioner
1. A person involved in purchasing health care. The term Commissioner is somehow distinct from the term '**purchaser**' as the role of a commissioner includes evaluating population needs and buying or encouraging development of appropriate care provision.
    See also **commissioning, contracts, purchasing intelligence**.
    Compare **purchaser**.
2. As applied to the EC institution, The European Commission, a Commissioner is a member

of the Commission appointed by the **Member States** (MSs) for a 4-year renewable term. The Commissioners act as the policy-making body of the Community and are obliged to act in the Community's interest independently of their governments.

See also **European Commission**.

Commission for Health Improvement (CHI, CHImP) (UK)

A national body which was introduced in a government White Paper to support and oversee the quality of **clinical governance** and of clinical services.

commissioning

The process of gathering and analysing the requests and needs of the population, identifying the services required to meet those needs, and monitoring the services as they are delivered. **Purchasers** negotiate contracts with **providers** for the provision of health care for the coming year.

Also called **contracting**.

See also **Commissioner, contracts, purchaser, purchasing intelligence**.

Commission, The see Commission of the European Communities.

Committee for Proprietary Medicinal Products (CPMP) (European Union)

One of the main **European Union** (EU) bodies dealing with pharmaceutical matters. It is based at the **European Medicines Evaluation Agency** premises (in London). It was established in 1975 in accordance with Council **Directive 75/319/EEC,** which was adopted on 20 May 1975 and brought into effect on 20 November 1977 (as amended by **Directive 83/570/EEC**). The Directive defines the purpose of the Committee as: 'to facilitate the adoption of a common position by the **Member States** (MSs) with regard to decisions on the issuing of **marketing authorizations** (MAs) and to promote thereby the free movement of proprietary medicinal products.' As dictated by Council **Regulation 2309/93**, it consists of two representatives, from each MS, who are appointed for a term of 3 years which is renewable.

The main role of the CPMP is to consider:

- Questions concerning the refusal, suspension or revocation of MA at the request of an MS or the Commission and in accordance with Articles 9 to 14 of Directive 75/319/EEC.
- Applications relating to it under Article 12 of 75/319/EEC as being of Community interest.
- Questions relating to the **pharmacovigilance** of already authorized products.
- Policy questions raised by the MSs in considering MA applications.
- Proposals for harmonizing requirements for testing of products.
- Guidance on procedures and technical requirements.

The CPMP appoints a **rapporteur** and a **co-rapporteur** from its membership, to coordinate the evaluation of each MA application going through the **centralized procedure**. It also appoints a rapporteur for cases referred to it due to differences in national decisions, where the interest of the Community is involved and arbitration procedures required within the **mutual recognition procedure**. The actual evaluation is performed by experts, chosen by the rapporteur, who may be selected from national agency staff or by external experts, but failing this, an opinion may be reached by a majority vote.

To assist the CPMP to prepare guidelines and make recommendations, the following permanent working parties have been formed: Biotechnology, **Efficacy**, **Safety**, **Pharmacovigilance** (PhVWP), Quality and Inspection. In addition, *ad hoc* working parties such as the 'Notice to applicants' and 'Anti-retroviral medicinal products' are also convened when necessary.

Contact:
7 Westferry Circus, Canary Wharf
London E14 4HB, UK
Tel: +44 (0)20 7418 8400
Fax: +44 (0)20 7418 8416

Committee for Veterinary Medicinal Products (CVMP) (European Union)
One of the main **European Union** (EU) bodies dealing with veterinary matters. It is the veterinary equivalent to **Committee for Proprietary Medicinal Products (CPMP)**. Both the CVMP and the CPMP were created as the scientific committees responsible for formulating the **European Medicines Evaluation Agency's** (EMEA) opinion on any question relating to the evaluation of medicines for human use (the CPMP) and veterinary use (the CVMP). The CVMP was set up under **Directive 81/851/EEC** and has functions similar to those of the CPMP. It has a number of working parties (e.g. Residues, **Efficacy** and Hormones). Both committees meet every month and have two representatives from each **Member State**, appointed to give independent scientific advice to the EMEA.

Committee on Dental and Surgical Materials (CDSM) (UK)
The official committee set up by the Licensing Authority under section 4 of the **Medicines Act**, to provide advice on a range of products which fell outside the expertise of the **Committee on Safety of Medicines**. It has been disbanded.

Committee on Radiation from Radioactive Medicinal Products (CRRMP) (UK)
The official committee whose function is to provide advice with respect to **safety**, **quality** and **efficacy** in relation to such products.

Committee on Review of Medicines (CRM) (UK)
A committee which provided advice on **Product Licences of Right** (PLRs). It no longer exists.

Committee on Safety of Drugs (CSD)
A group formed prior to the Committee on Safety of Medicines that was involved in the approval and safety monitoring of medicines.
See also **Committee on Safety of Medicines**.

Committee on Safety of Medicines (CSM) (UK)
One of the expert independent advisory committees established under Section 4 of the **Medicines Act (1968)**. It advises the UK Licensing Authority (Government Health Ministers) on the **quality**, **efficacy** and **safety** of medicines (excluding instruments, apparatus or appliances) for human use to which any provision of the Medicines Act is applicable. It also monitors adverse reactions to medicines already on the market in order to ensure that appropriate public health standards are met and maintained.

The Committee's responsibilities are, broadly, two-fold:
- To provide advice to the Licensing Authority on whether new products (new active substances) submitted to the UK **Medicines Control Agency** (MCA) should be granted a **marketing authorization** (MA). These responsibilities require close collaboration with the MCA's Licensing Division.
- To monitor the safety of marketed medicines, in close association with the MCA's Post-Licensing Division to ensure that medicines meet acceptable standards of safety and efficacy.

The CSM comprises 34 members who are appointed by the UK's Health Ministers. Members include pharmacists, pharmacologists, toxicologists, two lay members, and physicians from a wide range of disciplines working in general practice, hospitals and universities across the UK. The Committee meets fortnightly (except in August) and its Secretariat is provided by the staff of the MCA.

The CSM is supported in its work by three subcommittees:
- Subcommittee on Chemistry, Pharmacy & Standards (CPS).
To advise the main Committee on the quality in relation to safety and efficacy of medicinal products which are the subject of marketing authorization applications; and to advise on other matters referred to it. It meets once a month.
- Subcommittee on Biologicals & Biotechnology (BIOLS).
To advise the main committee on the quality (in relation to safety and efficacy) of medicines of biological origin including vaccines, blood products, and products derived from biotechnological sources. It meets at 6-week intervals.
- Sub-Committee on Pharmacovigilance (SCOP).
To advise the main Committee on the safety and risk–benefit considerations relating to marketed medicines and has particular responsibilities for oversight of the **Yellow Card Scheme**. It meets every 2 months.

The CSM has established jointly with the MCA an External Advisory Panel who may be called upon to provide additional expertise in areas not represented on the main Committee. The Committee and MCA, on occasions, establish Working Parties to undertake detailed assessments of specific issues relating to the quality, efficacy or safety of medicines. Working Parties are usually established where concerns have arisen over classes of medicines rather than individual products (e.g. safety of pancreatic supplements, safety of calcium channel blockers, oral contraceptives and breast cancer).

'common name'

As applicable to **European Community** Directives, it is 'the international non-proprietary name recommended by the WHO, or, if it does not exist, the usual common name'. (**Directive 92/27/EEC**)

Common Rule see Federal Policy (The).

Commonwealth Department of Health and Aged Care (Australia)

The Australian medicines evaluation agency.
See also **Therapeutic Goods Administration**.

Commonwealth Pharmaceutical Association (CPA)

One of a number of Commonwealth professional associations founded as a result of initiatives following the Commonwealth Prime Ministers' Meeting in 1965. The CPA was officially founded in 1970. The objectives of the Association are to encourage the highest possible standards of pharmaceutical education, practice and professional conduct in all Commonwealth countries. The overall objective is to ensure that those who are prescribed or who buy medicines receive the best possible therapeutic care.

The main members of the Association are the national professional bodies in the Commonwealth countries, together with individual Commonwealth pharmacists who join as 'personal members'. Of the 39 member associations, some 32 are in less developed or developing countries (according to the UN classification). This membership is reflected in the emphasis given to the activities of the Association. The CPA is constantly striving to develop further the basic pharmaceutical services in the majority of its member countries.

With the support of the **Royal Pharmaceutical Society of Great Britain** a regular quarterly newsletter, occasional regional activity, the 4-yearly Council meetings and conferences, the biannual meetings of the Executive Committee and a number of projects are all supported. Once a year for the past 13 years the CPA has coordinated the collection and distribution of copies of the previous year's **British National Formulary** to developing countries. It has also produced several policy documents and international surveys and 'twinned' a number of pharmaceutical manufacturing companies with schools of pharmacy so that unwanted reference materials from the companies' libraries can be redistributed. More recently, the CPA has organized a number of influential 'expert' visits to developing countries to advise on service development, carried out several 'train the trainer' workshops in a number of developing countries, and commissioned a major distance learning package on 'the management of drug supplies'.

communicable disease
A disease that can be passed from one individual to another.

Communicable Disease Surveillance Centre (CDSC) (UK)
Established in 1977 to undertake national surveillance of **communicable disease** and to provide epidemiological assistance and coordination in the investigation and control of infection in England and Wales. Mathematical models to predict the future incidence of vaccine preventable diseases have been developed at CDSC. The models can be used to determine the need for and the potential impact of future vaccination policies. A system of assessing **adverse events** attributable to vaccination has also been developed.

Communications
As applicable to the **European Union** (EU) law, unlike the legal instruments (**Decisions**, **Directives**, **Regulations**) but like **Opinions** and **Recommendations**, have only persuasive but no legally binding power. For example, the **Commission of the European Communities** (CEC) issued the text of a Communication on **parallel imports** on 6 May 1982 setting out guidance for the **Member States** as to how to regulate this trade. The Communication took into account the precedents set by the various European Court judgments.
See also **Decisions**, **Directives**, **Regulations**.

Community Care
The assessment and commissioning of health and social care for people who require services outside of hospital care.

Community Care Network (CCN) (US)
A vehicle that provides coordinated, organized, and comprehensive care to a community's population. Hospitals, **primary care** physicians and specialists link preventive and treatment services through contractual and financial arrangements, producing a network which provides coordinated care with continuous monitoring of quality and accountability to the public. While the term CCN often is used interchangeably with **Integrated Delivery System** (IDS), the CCN tends to be community-based and non-profit-making.

Community Clinical Oncology Program (CCOP) (US)
A cooperative agreement–supported programme which provides support to community-based oncologists to participate in clinical trials sponsored by the clinical cooperative groups and/or cancer centres. Each CCOP is expected to enter a minimum of 50 patients per year in **National Cancer Institute** approved research protocols.

Community Health Centre (CHC)
1. A community general practitioner practice.
2. (US) Refers to an ambulatory health care programme (defined under section 330 of the Public Health Service Act) usually serving a catchment area which has scarce or nonexistent health services or a population with special health needs; sometimes known as the neighbourhood health centre. Community Health Centers attempt to coordinate federal, State and local resources into a single organization capable of delivering both health and related social services to a defined **population**. While such a centre may not directly provide all types of health care, it usually takes responsibility to arrange all medical services needed by its patient population.

Community Health Councils (CHC) (UK)
Statutory **National Health Service** public patient watchdog organizations which were established by **Regional Health Authority**. The role of CHCs is to represent the public's interest in the local provision of health services and to be the channel for consumer concerns. They also monitor the health services and assist patients and carers in complaints. As a general rule, there is one CHC for every **District Health Authority**. CHCs normally have 18 or 24 members nominated by voluntary organizations, local authorities.

Community Health Information Network (CHIN) (US)
An integrated collection of computer and telecommunication capabilities that permit multiple **providers**, **payers**, employers, and related health care entities within a geographic area to share and communicate client, clinical and payment information.

Also known as Community Health Management Information System.

Community Health Management Information System see Community Health Information Network (CHIN).

Community Health Service
Care and treatment that is provided outside of hospital services, and also for health promotion, screening and immunization.

co-morbid condition see co-morbidities.

co-morbidities
Symptoms or conditions, existing at diagnosis or admission to a clinic, hospital, or enrolment into a clinical study, which are concurrent with a particular disease state. For example, cancer patients undergoing **chemotherapy** may have nausea and vomiting as comorbidities to their cancer.

Company Core Data Sheet (CCDS)
A document prepared by the **marketing authorization** (MA) holder containing, in addition to safety information, material relating to **indications**, dosing, **pharmacology** and other information concerning the product.

Company Core Safety Information (CCSI)
All relevant safety information contained in the **Company Core Data Sheet** prepared by the **marketing authorization** (MA) holder and which the MA holder requires to be listed in all countries where the company markets the drug, except when the local regulatory authority specifically requires a modification. The CCSI is the reference information by which listed and unlisted are determined for the purpose of periodic reporting for marketed products, but not by which expected and unexpected are determined for **expedited reporting**. Whenever

possible, an estimate of frequency should be provided, expressed in standard category of frequency.

It is always difficult to estimate incidence on the basis of spontaneous reports, owing to the uncertainty inherent in estimating the denominator and degree of under-reporting. However, the **CIOMS** Working Group III, Geneva 1999, felt that, whenever possible, an estimate of frequency should be provided and in a standard form. The following standard categories of frequency are recommended:

Very common*	≥1/10	(≥ 10%)
Common (frequent)	≥ 1/100 and < 1/10	(≥ 1% and < 10%)
Uncommon (infrequent)	≥ 1/1000 and < 1/100	(≥ 0.1% and < 1 %)
Rare	≥ 1/10 000 and < 1/1000	(≥ 0.01% and < 0.1%)
Very rare*	< 1/10 000	(< 0.01%)

* Optional categories

Precise rates will inevitably be based on studies and limited to the more common reactions. For reactions that are fewer than 'common', estimates of frequency will inevitably be based on spontaneous reports or on very large post-marketing studies or other special studies, and the numbers will be less precise; therefore, the source of the estimates (spontaneous or clinical) should be indicated. Stating the absolute numbers of cases reported may be misleading since they inevitably will become outdated (CIOMS, Chapter 5, Good Safety Information Practices).

comparative advertising
An advertisement that compares the subject drug with a competitive product for convenience, effectiveness and/or safety.

Comparative Molecular Field Analysis (CoMFA)
A **3D-QSAR** method that uses statistical correlation techniques for the analysis of the quantitative relationship between the biological activity of a set of compounds with a specified alignment, and their three-dimensional electronic and steric properties. Other properties such as hydrophobicity and hydrogen bonding can also be incorporated into the analysis.
See also **Three-dimensional Quantitative Structure–Activity Relationship**.

comparative study see comparative trial.

comparative trial (Clinical Trials)
A study in which the **investigational product**/drug is compared against another which may be an active drug or **placebo**.

comparator drug (Clinical Trials)
In a **comparative trial**, the **investigational product** or marketed product is compared against a standard drug (or **placebo**). The standard (or reference) or placebo medication is called the comparator drug.

comparator (product) see comparator drug.

compartmental model
A mathematical model which divides hosts into different compartments according to their infectious state. A typical model for microparasites might be a SEIR model. Sometimes referred to as a **prevalence** model.

COMPASS (US)
Computerized On-line **Medicaid** Pharmaceutical Analysis and Surveillance System.

compassionate or open arm (Clinical Trials)
A branch of a **clinical trial** (or during any phase of a trial) which allows people who do not participate in the research study (because they do not satisfy **inclusion criteria**, the trial is not available in their geographic region or for other good reasons) to have access to the drug or treatment being tested if it is considered necessary and ethical. It is an uncontrolled trial (or branch of) in subjects with a serious or immediately **life-threatening** disease(s) or medical condition(s) for whom no comparable or satisfactory alternative drug or other therapy is available. It may also be a special clinical trial enrolling subjects who previously participated in a clinical trial because withdrawal of the unregistered drug product would be unethical.

Since 1987, the US **Food and Drug Administration** (FDA) has permitted an investigational drug to be used for treatment under a treatment protocol or treatment (**Investigational New Drug** (IND)) if the drug is intended to treat a serious or immediately life-threatening disease, for which no comparable alternatives exist. The FDA has an emergency IND procedure which allows for the clinical use of an unlicensed product in a single patient.

See also **named patient basis**.

compensation for drug-induced injury (Clinical Trials)
Patients taking part in **clinical trials** (with unlicensed products) who suffer a drug-induced injury as a result should get immediate no-fault compensation payments from pharmaceutical companies. The payment of monetary awards to patients does not require the company to admit or accept liability for the injury. In the UK, the **Association of the British Pharmaceutical Industry** has published a code of practice dealing with compensation.

See also **Codes of Practice**.

Competent Authority (CA)
The regulatory body charged with monitoring compliance with the national statutes and regulations of European **Member States** (MSs). In the UK, this is the **Medicines Control Agency**. 'The authorities of the MSs are the Competent Authorities for **medicinal products** authorized nationally through national procedures, including **mutual recognition procedure**.' 'The responsibilities for **pharmacovigilance** rest with the competent authorities of all the MSs in which the authorizations are held' (CPMP/PhVWP/108/99 corr.).

completed subject letter (Clinical Trials)
The collection of data clarification queries asked after the **case report form** booklet has been passed to Data Quality Control/Clinical Data Management.

compliance (Clinical Trials)
Adherence to all the trial-related, **good clinical practice**, and the **applicable regulatory requirements**. In simple terms, it is a measure of how well subjects/patients have taken their study medication. The number of **tablets** returned at each follow-up visit are counted and this is taken as a measure of compliance. Unfortunately, this does not prove that the patient has taken all the tablets which are missing. They could have been thrown away.

Sometimes, blood samples are taken from patients in studies to determine the level of drug in the blood. Another method of checking compliance is to add a small amount of isoniazid to the medication. Its presence in urine can be determined by simple colourimetric test. These are some of the techniques that can be used to show that patients have, at least, taken some of their study medication.

complications
Developments of a disease which adversely affect some patients and can lead to changes in the length or the cause of the disease. The term is also used to describe a medical condition that arises during a course of treatment and is expected to increase the length of stay by at least 1 day for most patients.

composite rate
Group rate billed to all subscribers of a given group in a health plan.

computational chemistry
A discipline that uses mathematical methods, computer modelling, and computer-based algorithms to examine the molecular structure of compounds and their interaction with biological targets and for the calculation of molecular properties or for the simulation of molecular behaviour.

computational science see computational chemistry.

computed axial tomography (CAT) scan see computed tomography (CT) scan.

Computer-Aided New Drug Application (CANDA) (US)
An electronic version of a traditional **New Drug Application**. In the US, the **Food and Drug Administration** (FDA) is encouraging manufacturers to move toward all-electronic submissions, and hopes to eliminate the paper-based variety. The FDA believes CANDAs will allow for more comprehensive reviews of submissions and may actually speed up the **FDA approval** process.
See also **Computer-Aided New Product License Application**.

Computer-Aided Product License Application (CAPLA)
An electronic version of a traditional Product License Application. It is the **PL** version of CANDA.
See also **Computer-Aided New Drug Application**.

computer-assisted drug design (CADD)
CADD involves all computer-assisted techniques used to discover, design and optimize biologically active compounds with a putative use as **drugs**. A few methodologies exist to accomplish CADD including:
1. Active site-directed design.
   This involves the recognition of the important areas controlling vital ligand/receptor binding interactions. A prerequisite for such recognition is knowledge of the three-dimensional structure of the active site involved in the drug–receptor complex which normally comes from **X-ray crystallography** or nuclear magnetic resonance spectroscopic studies.
2. Automated novel structure generation.
   Like active site-directed design, the automated structure generation would require the knowledge of three-dimensional structure of the active site. It is accomplished with the help of programmes which incorporate the active site structure to provide sterically and electrostatically appropriate templates.

computer-based patient record (CPR)
A term for the process of replacing the traditional paper-based chart through automated electronic means; generally includes the collection of patient-specific information from various supplemental treatment systems, i.e. a day programme and a personal care provider; its display in graphical format; and its storage for individual and aggregate purposes.

COMT see **catechol-O-methyltransferase**.

concept approval (Clinical Trials)
Occasionally, a study may need to be conducted which is not part of the original clinical plan. Under these circumstances, the study concept and the financial cost of undertaking the study will have to be approved by the Project Team and Senior Management. An abbreviated **protocol** (or concept protocol) rather than a complete protocol may be sufficient for this purpose.

concept document (Clinical Trials)
A document containing the outline of a study (and possibly an abbreviated **protocol**) and the financial costs which are presented to a project team with a request that the study be added to the clinical plan for the development of the drug. If approved by the project team, the concept document will be forwarded to senior management for approval.

Concerned Member States (CMS) (European Union)
Member States, within the **European Union**, who are involved with the licensing process of **medicinal products** but who are not the State doing the assessment.

concertation procedure
Old procedure whereby **European Community Member States** jointly consider high-technology medicines before national licensing decisions are made. It was superseded by the **centralized procedure**.

concomitant medication (Clinical Trials)
Medication (excluding the trial drugs) taken by a patient in addition to the study medication during a trial. They may have been prescribed for a different condition prescribed by the investigator for the patient or it may be an **over-the-counter** (OTC) preparation that is bought by the patient and taken during the trial period. A concomitant medication is only allowed if it does not interfere with the study assessments that are needed to evaluate the study medication. Sometimes, study groups are stratified into those who receive concomitant treatment and those who do not.

concomitant treatment see **concomitant medication**.

concordance
The concept that the work of the prescriber and patient in the consultation is a negotiation between equals and that the aim is a therapeutic alliance between them.

concurrent review
Review of a procedure or hospital admission done by a health care professional (usually a nurse) other than the one providing the care, during the same time frame that the care is provided. Usually conducted during a hospital confinement to determine the appropriateness of the confinement and the medical necessity for continued stay.
See also **utilization review, medical necessity**.

confidence interval (CI) (Statistics)
This defines a range of values within which the population mean is likely to lie with a given degree of certainty. Usually 95% confidence limits are quoted which means that there is 95% probability that the true population mean will lie somewhere between the upper and lower confidence limits. CI is the most common form of **interval estimates**. The 95% confidence interval for the population mean is approximated by:
Sample mean +/− 1.96 × standard error.

Confidential Disclosure Agreement (CDA)
A document between two parties which ensures the **confidentiality** of information provided by one party to the other. The recipient of the information agrees to keep the information confidential for a fixed period of time or until the information becomes available in the public domain. CDAs are used by companies before providing information on new drugs to potential investigators, external consultants or contractors.

confidentiality
1. (General) Pertains to the treatment of information that an individual has disclosed in a relationship of trust and with the expectation that it will not be divulged to others without permission in ways that are inconsistent with the understanding of the original disclosure.
2. (Clinical Trials) Prevention of disclosure, to other than authorized individuals, of a **sponsor's** proprietary information or of a subject's identity. The aim is maintenance of the privacy of trial subjects including their personal identity and all personal medical information. If data verification procedures demand inspection of such details, this may only be done by a properly authorized person. Identifiable personal details must always be kept in confidence. The trial subject's consent to the use of records for data verification purposes should be obtained prior to the trials and assurance should be given that confidentiality will be maintained. When reporting **adverse events** or any other information to the sponsor and/or the relevant authorities, the investigator should assure that the subject's privacy is not violated.

confirmatory studies (Clinical Trials)
Confirmatory studies are necessary for the definitive proof of **efficacy**. In such trials the key hypothesis of interest is always pre-defined, and corresponds to the hypothesis which is subsequently tested when the trial is complete. However, in a confirmatory trial it is equally important to estimate with due precision the size of the effects attributable to the treatment of interest and to relate these effects to their clinical significance.

Confirmatory trials are the cornerstone of decision making and hence adherence to their planned design and procedures is particularly important; unavoidable changes must be explained and documented, and their effect examined. A detailed and justified account of the design of each such trial, and all other statistical aspects such as the planned analysis, should be set out in the **protocol**. Each trial should address only a limited number of questions.

Firm evidence of **efficacy** requires that the results of the pivotal trials demonstrate that the medical product under test has unequivocal clinical benefits. The number of pivotal trials should therefore be sufficient to answer each key clinical question relevant to the efficacy claim clearly and definitively. In addition, it is important that the basis for generalization to the intended patient population is understood and explained; this may also influence the number of pivotal trials required. Replication of important studies is of great value during the interpretation of results. Two of the many situations requiring replication are when unforeseen problems have arisen during conduct or analysis or when earlier studies provide an insecure basis for the main hypothesis to be tested.

See also **exploratory studies**.

conflict of interest
A person has a conflict of interest when the person is in a position of trust which requires them to exercise judgment on behalf of others (people, institutions, etc.) and also has interests or obligations of the sort that might interfere with the exercise of their judgment, and which the

person is morally required to either avoid or openly acknowledge. The lesser requirement of open acknowledgement is usually adopted when it seems too burdensome to require that the person in a position of trust divest themselves of the interest that conflicts with their position of responsibility. For example, some journals require that authors disclose any substantial financial interests that might have biased their research assessment. Requiring investigators to divest themselves of investments that they may have made on the basis of their scientific judgment would be too burdensome, and might even suppress publication.

conformity assessment
The process by which compliance with the **essential requirements** is assessed.

confounding factor (CF) (Statistics)
A variable other than the **risk factor** under study which is associated independently with exposure and outcome. It may create an association or mask a real association. Confounding can be by:
- indication – where the indication for the drug is the CF
- association – for example smoking is the association between lung cancer and anti-ulcer drugs.

A CF represents the variable affecting the patient's disease or condition and is associated statistically with the **investigational product** or treatment being evaluated. CFs include:
- underlying disease
- tolerance
- transient event
- chance
- drug–drug interaction, or food–drug interaction
- drug withdrawal.

In a well designed experiment an **investigator** will randomly assign subjects to two or more groups and except for differences in the experimental procedure applied to each group, the groups will be treated exactly alike. Under these circumstances any differences between the groups that are statistically significant are attributed to differences in the treatment conditions. This, of course, assumes that except for the various treatment conditions the groups were, in fact, treated exactly alike. Unfortunately, however, it is always possible that despite an experimenter's best intentions there was some unsuspected systematic differences in the way the groups were treated in addition to the intended treatment conditions. Statisticians describe systematic differences of this sort as CFs or confounding variables.

confounding variable see **confounding factor**.

congener
A congener is a substance generated or synthesized by essentially the same synthetic chemical reactions and the same procedures. **Analogues** are substances that are analogous in some respect to the prototype agent in chemical structure. Clearly, congeners may be analogues or vice versa but not necessarily. The term congener, while most often a synonym for homologue, has become somewhat more diffuse in meaning so that the terms congener and analogue are frequently used interchangeably in the literature.

congenital
Present or existing at the time of birth.

congenital defects
Problems or conditions that are present at birth.

CONQUEST (US)
*CO*mputerized *N*eeds-*O*riented *QU*ality *M*easurement *E*valuation Sys*T*em. It is a prototype system for collecting and evaluating clinical performance measures from the **Agency for Health Care Policy Research**.

consent see **informed consent**.

consent form (Clinical Trials)
The document which is signed by the patient when written **informed consent** is obtained. If oral consent is obtained, the consent form is signed by the **investigator** and the person who witnessed the consent procedure.

CONSORT (Clinical Trials)
*CON*solidated *S*tandards of *R*eporting *T*rials.

consumer product
When used in the context of the pharmaceutical industry, this term refers to a non-prescription, **over-the-counter** drug.

Consumer Safety Officer (CSO) (US)
Food and Drug Administration official who coordinates the review process of various applications.

Contact Help Advice Information Network for Effective Health Care (CHAIN) (UK)
A reference database for clinical effectiveness and evidence-based health care activities in the North Thames Region, and beyond.
Website: http://www.nthames-health.tpmde.ac.uk/chain/chain.htm.

contagious distribution
Same as an aggregated distribution.

contained area
An area built and operated in such a way (and equipped with suitable air handling and filtration) so as to prevent contamination of the external environment by biological agents from within the area.
See also **clean/contained area, containment, primary containment**.

containment
The act of confining a biological agent or other entity inside a defined area.
See also **clean/contained area, contained area, primary containment**.

continuation protocol (Clinical Trials)
A **protocol** which allows a patient to continue on study medication after the completion of the original study. The information collected during this additional treatment period is provided to the company on a set of specially prepared **case record forms**.

continuing care eligibility criteria
Criteria to determine whether an individual is eligible for continuing care and the responsibilities of the statutory agencies for funding individual packages.

continuing medical education (CME)
CME programmes are those which help physicians and other medical professionals maintain their technical proficiency. In the past, these were often used by the pharmaceutical industry as a means of product promotion. A series of abuses led to guidelines being issued which placed limits on how industry-sponsored CME programmes could be run.

contract
1. (Clinical Trials) A written, dated and signed agreement between two or more involved parties that sets out any arrangements on delegation and distribution of tasks and obligations and, if appropriate, on financial matters. The **protocol** may serve as the basis of a contract.

   In the US, it is defined as the agreement that a specific research activity will be performed at the request, and under the direction of, The Agency (i.e. the **Food and Drug Administration**) providing the funds. Research performed under contract is more closely controlled by the agency than research performed under a grant.
   Compare **grant**.
2. (UK) The agreement between **purchasers** and **providers** about the level and quality of services that are to be delivered. Now superseded by long-term **service agreements**. Types used include:
   (i) Block Contract – where an agreed sum of money was given to a provider in return for a loosely defined service, e.g. a number of bed days and community contract for each specific care group.
   (ii) Cost and Volume – where levels of service were more clearly defined and often linked funding to more specific service delivery, e.g. finished consultant episodes (FCEs) for inpatient episodes.

Contract Data Set (CDS) (UK)
A collection of information recorded by the **National Health Service provider** and relayed to the commissioner of care.

contract house see contract research organization.

contracting see commissioning.

contract research organization (CRO) (Clinical Trials)
An institution, scientific body (commercial, academic or other) or company to which a **sponsor** (drug company) may transfer some tasks, responsibilities and obligations (e.g. trial monitoring, data analysis) of the drug development process. Any such transfer should be defined in writing.

contraindication (C/I)
A situation where a treatment (or **investigational product** in a **clinical trial**) should not be used in certain individuals or conditions due to risks outweighing the benefits due to an aspect of the patient's condition or the presence of modifying condition or disease (e.g. a drug may be contraindicated for pregnant women and persons with high blood pressure).

control (Clinical Trials)
Material or preparation used in preclinical or **clinical trials** for comparison purposes with the study intervention or drug. Often the control is a **placebo** or inert material.

control group (Clinical Trials)
In **clinical trials**, a group of patients (arm of a **randomized trial**) used for comparison, that receives the standard treatment, a treatment or intervention currently being used and considered to be of proved effectiveness on the basis of past studies. Results in patients receiving newly developed treatments may then be compared to the control group. In cases where no standard treatment yet exists for a particular condition, the control group would receive no treatment. No patient is placed in a control group without treatment if there is any beneficial treatment known for that patient. In some randomized trials, both of the treatments are standard

treatments, or both equally well known new treatments, and in such cases it is not appropriate to use the term 'a control group'.

controlled area
'An area constructed and operated in such a manner that some attempt is made to control the introduction of potential contamination and the consequences of accidental release of living organisms. The level of control exercised should reflect the nature of the organism employed in the process. At a minimum, the area should be maintained at a pressure negative to the immediate external environment and allow for the efficient removal of small quantities of airborne containments.' (Crown Copyright)
See also **clean/contained area, containment.**

controlled clinical trial
A **clinical trial** that utilizes a **control group** and in which the effects of the **investigational product** are being compared with a treatment whose effects are known. The objective of the methodology is to minimize **bias**. The control group may be receiving a **placebo** or a standard treatment or even no treatment at all. Sometimes the control group is randomized, while occasionally it is concurrent, that is, a group that does not consist of study participants but are followed simultaneously. Both groups of patients are managed in an identical manner with the exception of treatment received. An **'adequate & well-controlled clinical trial'** utilizes such methodology.
See also **observation arm.**

controlled drug (cd)
Designated substances/drugs for which many countries have legislations designed to minimize their social and medical misuse by controlling the manufacture, distribution, prescription, and dispensing of such substances/drugs, e.g. opioid analgesics, amfetamines, etc.

In the US, the preferred name is **'controlled substance'** and it is defined as any substance listed in any schedule of the Controlled Substance Act 21 USC 801; 21 **Code of Federal Regulations** (CFR) Part 1308 of the US.
See also **Misuse of Drugs Act.**

controlled study see controlled clinical trial.

controlled substance
US preferred term for **controlled drug (cd)**.

control (subjects) or controls see control group.

cooperativity
The interaction process by which binding of a ligand to one site on a macromolecule (enzyme, **receptor**, etc.) influences binding at a second site, e.g. between the substrate binding sites of an **allosteric enzyme**. Cooperative enzymes typically display a sigmoid (S-shaped) plot of the reaction rate against substrate concentration.
See also **allosteric binding sites.**

Coordinating Centre (Clinical Trials)
Headquarters for a multi-site/**multicentre trial** that collects all data.

Coordinating Committee (Clinical Trials)
A committee that a **sponsor** may organize to coordinate the conduct of a **multicentre trial.**

Coordinating Investigator (Clinical Trials)
An **investigator** assigned the responsibility for the coordination of investigators at different centres participating in a **multicentre trial**.

co-rapporteur
A member of the **Committee for Proprietary Medicine Products** appointed by the Committee itself in addition to a **rapporteur**, for each application for a **marketing authorization** (**centralized procedure**) submitted to the **European Medicines Evaluation Agency**.
See also **rapporteur**.

CORE
Cardiovascular Outcome and Risk Evaluations Study.

core data sheet see **core safety data sheet**.

core safety data sheet (CSDS)
A reference document (prepared by the pharmaceutical manufacturer) required to judge whether an **adverse event** or reaction is expected (labelled) or unexpected (unlabelled) and is therefore always included in a **Periodic Safety Update Report**. In many countries involved in **International Conference on Harmonization** as members or observers, this kind of document is similar to the **labelling** approved as part of the **marketing authorization** but often there are differences, due to differences in the scope of the document, principles for inclusion, indications and/or recommended dosage of the drug, experience drawn from pre-registration studies and from the market, local habits for concomitant drugs and local or ethnic sensitivity. The classification 'labelled' or 'unlabelled' has many more consequences for expedited reporting than for periodic reporting. The CSDS must be dated, including the date of last revision (or all revision dates).

COREPEPER
Committee of Permanent Representatives of the EEC Ambassadors.

corporate governance (UK)
Collective term to describe measures put in place by a health authority to ensure that it is acting within the **National Health Service** regulatory framework and observing the codes of conduct and accountability.

correlation (Statistics)
The relationship of one variable to another, not to be confused with causality. Given a pair of related measures (X and Y) on each of a set of items, the correlation coefficient (r) provides an index of the degree to which the paired measures co-vary in a linear fashion. In general, r will be positive when items with large values of X also tend to have large values of Y whereas items with small values of X tend to have small values of Y. Correspondingly, r will be negative when items with large values of X tend to have small values of Y, whereas items with small values of X tend to have large values of Y. The value of r is calculated by first converting the Xs and Ys into their respective Z scores and, keeping track of which Z score goes with which item, determining the value of the mean Z score product. Numerically, r can assume any value between -1 and $+1$ depending upon the degree of the relationship. Plus and minus one indicate perfect positive and negative relationships whereas 0 indicates that the X and Y values do not co-vary in any linear fashion.

C

correlation coefficient (r) (Statistics)
The Pearson's correlation coefficient is the extent to which the association between two variables can be described by a straight line. Plus one is a straight line with a positive slope and all data points being on the line, 0 being no linear association (completely random), and −1 being a straight line with a negative slope and all data points being on the line. Values in between −1 and +1 indicate that the data points are scattered around the line with values closer to 0 indicating wider scatter. Depending on how the points are distributed, the correlation coefficient can be a very misleading indicator of the relationship between the two variables so looking at a plot of the data points is recommended.

corrugant
The name applied to any drug that stops secretion.

corticoid
Possessing or exhibiting an action similar to that of a steroid hormone of the adrenal gland.

COSHH (UK)
Control of Substances Hazardous to Health (1994).

COSLA (UK)
Convention of Scottish Local Authorities.

cosmetic
A beautifying substance or preparation. As defined by the US **Food, Drug and Cosmetic Act**, it is 'An article which is intended to be rubbed, poured, sprinkled, or sprayed on, introduced into, or otherwise applied to the human body or any part thereof for cleansing, beautifying, promoting attractiveness, or altering the appearance; and any article that is intended for use as a component of any such articles; except that such term shall not include soap.'

cost
In general, a measure of the resources consumed by the illness or by providing treatment. The resources used in the course of managing any disease are considered to be the costs of an illness. These costs include direct medical and non-medical costs, indirect costs and intangible costs. *Direct medical costs* are those related to providing medical services, such as hospital care, physician fees and drug costs. *Direct non-medical costs* are expenses, such as transportation costs, that are a direct result of the illness. *Indirect costs* are associated with changes of individual productivity and include such costs as those related to loss of work and unpaid caregivers' time. *Intangible costs* are hard to quantify as they include such things as pain and suffering. Direct medical costs are always a part of **pharmacoeconomic** analyses.
Other costs may be included, but they are more difficult to value. Humanistic benefits, which represent the optimal goal of any health care goods and services, may be evaluated to assign a value to indirect and intangible costs.
See also **pharmacoeconomics, pharmacoeconomic analysis**.

cost and volume contract see **contract**.

COSTART (US)
*C*oding *S*ymbols for a *T*hesaurus of *A*dverse *R*eactions *T*erms. A coding system devised by the **Food and Drug Administration**.

cost–benefit analysis (CBA)
A type of economic analysis of medical interventions (e.g. a particular medicine or surgical

procedure) in which the **cost** of treatment is compared with the **cost** of the **outcome** (benefit) for a period of time to quantify, in monetary terms, the benefits associated with the use of the intervention where no direct savings are immediately apparent. In this analysis, therefore, results are valued monetarily as an aid in determining the best investment of resources. For example, the cost of establishing an immunization service might be compared with the total cost of medical care and lost productivity which will be eliminated as a result of more persons being immunized. CBA can also be applied to specific medical tests and treatments. The CBA is strictly a comparison of the monetary value of alternative uses of resources. The decision to proceed depends on the benefits being greater than the costs incurred.

Also referred to as cost–benefit evaluation.

cost–benefit evaluation see cost–benefit analysis.

cost-containment

A term used freely in health care to illustrate the majority of **cost** cutback activities by **providers**. Control of inefficiencies in the consumption, allocation, or production of health care services that contribute to higher than necessary costs and is a critical objective of all **Managed Care Organizations** (MCOs) in countries where they exist. Inefficiencies are thought to exist in consumption when health services are inappropriately utilized; inefficiencies in allocation exist when health services could be delivered in less costly settings without loss of quality; and, inefficiencies in production exist when the costs of producing health services could be reduced by using a different combination of resources. Cost containment can be performed in many different ways, including the following:

1. Incentive on the use of generic drugs
2. Use of a drug **formulary**
3. Caps on reimbursement for certain drugs
4. Contracts with **PPO**s and **EPO**s in the US
5. Drug Utilization Review (DUR) in the US.

Also referred to as cost minimization.

See also **cost containment analysis**.

cost-containment analysis (CCA)

A very simplistic type of economic analysis of medical interventions. It compares costs when consequences have similar safety and efficacy profiles and the only comparison is based on cost of treatment. Cost-effectiveness analysis and cost-utility analysis are most frequently used in comparing alternative drug therapies.

Also called cost identification analysis and cost minimization analysis.

See also **cost containment, cost-utility analysis, cost-effectiveness analysis, cost–benefit analysis**.

cost contract (US)

An arrangement between a managed health care plan and **Health Care Finance Administration** under Section 1876 or 1833 of the Social Security Act, under which the health plan provides health services and is reimbursed its costs. The **beneficiary** can use **providers** outside the plan's provider network.

cost-effectiveness

The inherent measure of a therapy's worth in relation to its cost. In mathematical terms, cost-effectiveness = worth/cost. It is one of a range of comparative measures of economic appraisal techniques.

cost-effectiveness analysis (CEA)
One of four types of the most commonly used **pharmacoeconomic** analyses. It is the inherent measure of a therapy's worth in relation to its **cost**. CEA compares the costs of alternatives in terms of a natural unit or health outcome such as the number of cases successfully treated, life-years gained or reduction in blood pressure and describes the costs for some additional health gain (e.g. cost per additional myocardial infarction prevented). There are several ways to define and measure both 'worth' and 'cost.' (For example, if a cancer patient has his or her tumour size reduced, yet can't walk or eat without assistance, what is the worth of the therapy? How can it be quantified?). For cost-effectiveness comparisons among therapeutic regimens to be useful, therefore, 'cost' and 'worth' must be measured the same way for each course of therapy. As health care monitory unit (pound, dollar) becomes more scarce, payers are increasingly reliant on cost-effectiveness data for making coverage decisions. In the absence of these data, they often make decisions based on cost alone. It is becoming increasingly crucial for health care manufacturers to measure, understand and promote the cost-effectiveness of their products.

See also **cost–benefit analysis, cost–utility analysis**.

cost-effectiveness evaluation see cost-effectiveness analysis.

cost-identification analysis see cost-containment analysis.

cost-minimization see cost containment.

cost-minimization analysis see cost-containment analysis.

cost outlier
A case which is more costly to treat compared with other patients in a particular diagnosis related group. Outliers also refer to any unusual occurrence of cost, cases which skew average costs or unusual procedures.

cost–utility analysis (CUA)
One of four types of the most commonly used **pharmacoeconomic** analyses of medical interventions. It measures consequences in terms of life-years gained or lost adjusted by a quality factor based on patient preference or on the quality of the health care **outcome**. In other words it converts effects into personal preferences (or utilities) and describes how much it costs for some additional quality gain (e.g. cost per additional **quality-adjusted life-year** (QALY)). Essential to this analysis, therefore, is the valuation of utility of outcome. A statement resulting from this type of analysis might be: 'Drug A costs £10 000 for every QALY gained.'

Council for the International Organization of Medical Sciences (CIOMS)
Founded in 1949 as the non-governmental, non-political arm of the **World Health Organization**. The organization provides a platform for discussions between representatives of international pharmaceutical companies and regulatory authorities.

CIOMS provides informed opinion on developments in biology and medicine, and explores related social, ethical, moral, legal and administrative issues and their implications. Since 1977, it has also acted as an independent, neutral forum for policy matter discussions between pharmaceutical companies and national regulatory authorities. CIOMS has completed a number of projects in drug safety monitoring:

CIOMS I: International regulatory reporting of individual serious unexpected (unlabelled) **adverse drug reaction** (ADR) cases (1990). The corresponding **International Conference on Harmonization** (ICH) report was ICH E2A. CIOMS I was the first step to harmonizing international differences in ADR reporting, the CIOMS I working party devised a form that might be used by all countries for expedited reporting of individual case reports. The guidelines for the standardized reporting form specify about 20 items of information that should be given for each case, e.g. patient age and sex, drug(s) implicated, dosage and duration of treatment, indication for therapy and patient **outcome**. CIOMS I reporting guidelines are exclusively for drugs that are available on the market.

CIOMS Ia: Harmonization of data elements and data fields for electronic reporting of individual ADRs. The corresponding ICH report is ICH E2B. CIOMS Ia provide strategy for such reports. The CIOMS Ia working party also suggest that:
- Internationally agreed standards should be used where appropriate
- A case-numbering system should be used that identifies the first custodian, their case reference number and the drug in question
- A short (500 character) field for comment/narrative should be available
- According to the recommendations, whoever first receives the case report of an ADR is the first custodian who becomes responsible for following up the report with the notifier.

The first custodian may be the **regulatory authority** or the drug company and they have the responsibility of putting the data in the shared area.

CIOMS II: International reporting of periodic drug safety updated summaries (1992). The corresponding ICH report is ICH E2C. CIOMS II outlines the information to be included in the report as well as the format the information should take.

CIOMS III: Guidelines for preparing core clinical safety information on drugs. It provides guidelines on how to organize the safety information for prescribers for whom pharmaceutical companies have a legal duty to warn about ADRs and also a duty not to dilute warnings.

CIOMS IV: Risk–benefit assessments. This CIOMS focuses on the basic principles of risk-benefit assessments for drugs. The document contains sections on such evaluations and how to do the two together and how to assess the impact of such a combined evaluation and also actual examples.

CIOMS V: Good Case Management and Reporting Practices.

Council of Ministers

European Community institution whose members directly represent the government of each of the **Member States** (MSs). The relevant Ministers attend the relevant Council meeting. So for trade issues, the trade Ministers meet, for health issues, the Health Ministers meet and so on. The role of the Council of Ministers is to agree and rectify policies and legislations brought forward by the **Commission**. The meeting is chaired by the Head of State of the host country (who is holding the presidency of the **European Union** (EU) at the time), who for 6 months assumes a position as the senior elected political head of Europe. The **Commission of the European Communities** (CEC) can propose a legal instrument (a **Regulation**, **Directive** or **Decision**) to the relevant Council of Ministers, and, after consultations with the Economic and Social Committee and the European Parliament, may agree to the proposals and may adopt them. The decisions are made if members of the Council are unanimous on the proposals, however, decisions can still be made by a qualified majority vote. Votes are weighed according to the population of each MS. The draft measure is examined firstly by the expert Working groups, then by the Committee of Permanent Representatives of the EEC Ambassadors (COREPER).

The General Secretariat assists the Council by carrying out all the necessary work for the activities of the council, its permanent representatives, and working parties.

See also **European Commission** (EC).

Council of Mutual Economic Assistance (CMEA)
The Eastern European equivalent of **European Free Trade Association** and EEC. The members were Bulgaria, Czechoslovakia, German Democratic Republic, Hungary, Poland, Romania, USSR, Cuba, Mongolia, Yugoslavia. The CMEA members cooperate with each other to establish mutually acceptable standards on the assessment of drugs.

Council Recommendations 83/571/EEC
The first series of **Committee for Proprietary Medicinal Products** Notes for Guidance. These related to repeated dose toxicity, reproduction studies, carcinogenic potential, pharmacokinetic and metabolic studies in the safety evaluation of new drugs in animals, and to fixed combination products. They were adopted by the **Council of Ministers** on 26 October 1983.

counterirritant
An agent, such as methyl salicylate or a liniment, that produces irritation or mild inflammation of the skin with the object of relieving a more deep-seated irritation, inflammation, pain or discomfort.

CP
1. Calendar pack of a **drug product**.
2. *Comité Permanent*, see **Standing Committee of European Doctors**.

CPA
Critical path analysis.

CPAC see Central Pharmaceutical Affairs Council.

CPC/EPC (European Union)
Community Convention on Patent Protection.

CPEP
Clinical Practice Evaluation Programme.

CPHL
Central Public Health Laboratory.

CPHVA (UK)
Community Practitioners and Health Visitors Association.

CPMP see Committee for Proprietary Medicinal Products.

CPN
Community Psychiatric Nurse.

CPNA (UK)
Community Psychiatric Nurse Association.

CPR
Cardiopulmonary resuscitation.

CPS see Chemistry, Pharmacy and Standards Subcommittee.

CPSC (US)
Consumer Product Safety Commission.

CPSM
Council for Professions Supplementary to Medicine.

CPT see **current procedural terminology**.

CPU see **Contracts and Purchasing Unit**.

CQI
Continual Quality Improvement.

CRA see **Clinical Research Associate**.

CRADA
Cooperative Research and Development Agreement.

CRAG see **Clinical Resources and Audit Group**.

CRC
Clinical Research Co-ordinator, see **Clinical Trial Coordinator**.

CRD
1. Clinical Research Department.
2. (UK) see **NHS Centre for Reviews and Dissemination**.

cream
Name applied to any semi-solid preparation in pharmacy; less greasy than an ointment, water miscible or dispersible and possessing 'vanishing' properties when rubbed into the skin.

credentialing
Review procedure where a potential or existing provider must meet certain standards in order to begin or continue participation in a given health care plan, on a panel, in a group, or in a hospital medical staff organization. The process of reviewing a practitioner's credentials, i.e. training, experience, or demonstrated ability, for the purpose of determining if criteria for clinical privileging are met. The recognition of professional or technical competence. The credentialing process may include registration, certification, licensing, professional association membership, or the award of a degree in the field. Certification and licensing affect the supply of health personnel by controlling entry into practice and influence the stability of the labour force by affecting geographic distribution, mobility and retention of workers. Credentialing also determines the quality of personnel by providing standards for evaluating competence and by defining the scope of functions and how personnel may be used. In **managed care** arenas, one hears of a new basis for credentialing, referred to as financial credentialing. This refers to an organization's evaluation of a **provider** based on that provider's ability to provide value, or high quality care at a reasonable **cost**.

CRF see **case record form**.

CRFCL see **case record form correction log**.

crisis management
A process used at a point of conflict between an organization and its market place and is a dynamic activity that is used best and most successfully when the crisis is anticipated.

Critical Appraisal Skills Programme (CASP) (UK)
A UK project that aims to help health service decision-makers and those that seek to influence the decision-makers develop skills to find, critically appraise and change practice in line with evidence of effectiveness. These skills promote the delivery of evidence-based health care. At the heart of CASP's work is a cascade of half-day workshops where participants learn through going on an interactive journey.

CASP introduces people to the ideas of evidence-based health care and, through critical appraisal of systematic reviews, introduces people to the related ideas of the **Cochrane Collaboration**. CASP is developing an interactive CD-ROM, to be used in conjunction with workshops, video conferencing, as a stand alone package or to reinforce learning, thereby taking these skills to a wider audience and giving opportunities for independent practice or learning.

Website: http://www.phru.org/casp/

critical instrument
Instruments necessary to ensure safe equipment operation or used to control or evaluate product quality.

critical path (Clinical Trials)
The shortest time from planning the study to the production of a **Final Report**.

critical region (Statistics)
The region which leads to the rejection of the **null hypothesis**. The critical region will depend upon the significance levels at which the test is conducted.

critical step
A step that is difficult to control, usually because one or more critical variables cannot be sufficiently engineered out of the process. When a process is poorly developed and undercharacterized, as in the development of a new process, all variables can be critical. Process development and scale-up is largely an activity of removing critical variables, or at least understanding them so they can be controlled and the process made robust. Similarly, a new step can be critical because of unreliable equipment, insufficient training, or improper application of equipment. Through well-characterized process development, such variables can be identified and adjusted to produce a process that will not be difficult to control for equipment or instrumentation reasons. Remaining critical variables will cause a particular unit operation to be labelled as a critical step.

critical value
The value of a test **statistic** that is borderline between acceptance and rejection of the **null hypothesis**. The actual value depends on the level of significance chosen and whether the test is one-tailed or two-tailed.

critical variable
A variable is considered critical if its operating range is near the edge of failure. If there is some scientific basis or observation to suggest that $17°C$ or $23°C$ will affect step performance or product quality, then an extensive investigation will be made and corrective action will be taken.

CRM see **Committee on the Review of Medicines**.
CRO see **Contract Research Organization**.

cross-contamination
Contamination of a material or a product with another material or product.

cross-over clinical trial
In cross-over trials, each subject receives both treatments being compared or the treatment and control. Such trials are used for patients who have a stable, usually chronic, condition during both treatment periods. The advantages of such designs include:
- reduction in the error of variance and hence the sample size needed since all subjects serve as own control

- all patients receive treatment (at least some of the time)
- statistical tests assuming **randomization** can be used
- blinding can be maintained.

Disadvantages of such designs, however, are just as many including the facts that:
- all subjects receive **placebo** or alternative treatment at some point
- washout period lengthy or unknown
- cannot be used for treatments with permanent effects
- even for the **investigator** with the best knowledge and intentions, the economics and logistics of experimentation may prevent carrying out a complete and perfect cross-over experiment.

Such designs are not widely used nowadays due to the carry over effects as patients change from one medication to the other.

cross-sectional study see **horizontal study**.

cross-sectional survey see **horizontal study**.

CRRMP see **Committee on Radiation from Radioactive Medicinal Products**.

crude birth rate
The number of live births in a year divided by the **population** size.

crude death rate
The number of deaths in a year divided by the **population** size.

cryogenic vessel
A container designed to contain liquefied gas at extremely low temperature.

CSAG
Clinical Standards Advisory Group.

CSD see **Committee on Safety of Drugs**.

CSI (US)
Consumer Safety Inspector (**Food and Drug Administration**).

CSM see **Committee on Safety of Medicines**.

CSO
1. (US) Consumer Safety Officer (**Food and Drug Administration**).
2. Central Statistical Office.

CSP
Comité de Specialités Pharmaceutiques.

CTC
1. see **Clinical Trial Certificate**.
2. see **Clinical Trial Coordinator**.

CTD
Common Technical Document.

CTEB (US)
Cancer Therapy Evaluation Program.

CTEP
Clinical Therapeutics Evaluation Programme.

CT scanning
Computerized tomography scanning. A procedure that uses X-rays and computers to create cross-sectional images of the body to diagnose and monitor disease.

CTX see **Clinical Trial Exemption**.

CUA see **cost-utility analysis**.

culture
The artificial growth of cells, tissue, or micro-organisms such as bacteria in a laboratory.

cumulative action
The condition in which repeated administration of a drug may produce effects (normally toxic effects) that are more pronounced than the effect(s) produced by the first **dose**. It happens when the dosing intervals are not long enough for it to be either metabolized or excreted by the body.

curie
Unit of measure for radioactivity. Equal to 3.7×10^{10} disintegrations per second.

Current Problems in Pharmacovigilance (UK)
The drug safety bulletin of the **Medicines Control Agency** and **Committee on Safety of Medicines**. The bulletin is produced three or four times a year and is mailed to all doctors, dentists, pharmacists and coroners in the UK. It alerts them to problems with medicines and provides advice on the ways medicines may be used more safely. It includes information on newly identified drug problems, reminders of known problems, changes in the risk/benefit profiles of drugs, advice on minimizing risk, and an overview of the side-effect profiles of drugs particularly at the time of removal from intensive monitoring. The bulletin is also available on the Internet at the website.

http://www.open.gov.uk/mca/cuprblms.htm.

current procedural terminology (CPT-4-Physicians) (US)
A standardized mechanism (**coding** system) of reporting services using numeric codes as established (in 1966) and updated annually by the CPT Editorial Panel of the **American Medical Association** to provide a uniform language to accurately describe medical, surgical and diagnostic services. It allocates five digit codes to medical services and procedures to standardize claims processing and **data** analysis. The CPT is the basis of the **Medicare** coding system for physicians services.
See also **coding**.

curriculum vitae **(CV)** (Clinical Trials)
A statement of qualifications of the investigators showing the education, training and experience that qualifies them as an expert for conducting the **clinical trial**.

customary charge (US)
One of the factors determining a physician's payment for a service under **Medicare**. Calculated as the physician's median charge for that service over a prior 12-month period.

customary, prevailing and reasonable (CPR) (US)
Current method of paying physicians under **Medicare**. Payment for a service is limited to the

lowest of (1) the physician's billed charge for the service, (2) the physician's customary charge for the service, or (3) the prevailing charge for that service in the community. Similar to the Usual, Customary, and Reasonable system used by private insurers.

custom-made medical device
An **active implantable medical device** specifically made in accordance with a medical specialist's written prescription which gives, under the specialist's responsibility, specific design characteristics and is intended to be used only for an individual named patient (EEC Council **Directive 90/385/EEC**).

cut-off date see **data lock-point**.

CV see *curriculum vitae*.

CVM (US)
Center for Veterinary Medicine (**Food and Drug Administration**).

CVMP see **Committee for Veterinary Medicinal Products**.

CXMP
Committee for Proprietary and/or Veterinary Products.

cycloplegic
A drug that causes paralysis of the ciliary muscle of the eye. This causes inability to alter the focus of the eye and is usually accompanied by paralysis of the muscles of the pupil, resulting in fixed dilation of the pupil (mydriasis) and loss of accommodation. Such drugs include atropine which is used to rest the muscle in cases of inflammation of the iris and ciliary body.

cytochrome P450
Liver enzymes involved in oxidative metabolism of several endogenous and exogenous compounds. These enzymes are divided into families (1, 2, 3 etc.), and families are further subdivided into subfamilies (1A2, 2A6 etc.). The P450 3A4 isoform is believed to be involved in the majority of oxidative drug metabolism.
See also **enzyme-inducing drugs**

cytotoxic
Destructive to cells.

3D-QSAR see **three-dimensional quantitative structure–activity relationship**.

D* see **loading dose**.

D
Dose (q.v.); also the 'maintenance doses' administered after a **loading dose** (q.v.).

DAB
Deutsches Arzneibuch.

DAL (US)
Defect Action Level (**Food and Drug Administration**).

DAP see **Drug Analysis Print**.

DAT see **Drugs Action Team-Inter-Agency-Group**.

data (Clinical Trials)
An observation or a measurement that is recorded in a **case record form**. A collection of data values is referred to as data.

Data and Safety Monitoring Board (DSMB) (Clinical Trials)
A committee of scientists, physicians, statisticians and others that collects and analyses data during the course of a **clinical trial** to monitor for **adverse effects** and other trends (such as an indication that one treatment is significantly better than another, particularly when one arm of the trial involves a **placebo** control) that would warrant modification or termination of the trial or notification of subjects about new information that might affect their willingness to continue in the trial. A DSMB can stop a trial if toxicities are found or if treatment is proved beneficial.
See also **Independent Data Monitoring Committee**.

Data Archive, The (UK)
A national resource centre which acquires, stores and disseminates computer-readable copies of social science and humanities datasets for further analysis by the research community. It is a multidisciplinary facility and is the largest UK collection of accessible computer-readable data relating to contemporary and historical social and economic affairs. By bringing together data which would otherwise be scattered, destroyed or become unreadable over time, the Data Archive offers those wanting to analyse sets of data, quick, easy and cheap access to a rich resource of materials. The wide scope of the data encourage 'secondary' analyses of data for purposes often quite different from those for which the data have originally been obtained.

Data are acquired from academic, commercial and public sector sources and the Archive now holds over 4000 datasets. Most relate to post-war Britain, although an increasing number of historical studies pertaining to earlier periods are now becoming available through the Archive.

The Data Archive was founded at the University of Essex in Colchester in 1967 and is jointly funded by the Economic and Social Research Council (ESRC), the Joint Information Systems Committee (JISC) of the Higher Education Funding Councils (HEFCs) and the University of Essex. The data extend across the full range of the social sciences and humanities and contain information about most areas of social and economic life. In addition to British cross-sectional studies from academic, government and commercial sources, the Archive holds time-series data, major longitudinal studies, panel and cohort surveys and major cross-sectional studies. Typical of the larger data holdings include:
- Census Data

- General Household Surveys
- **Office for National Statistics** (ONS) Databank
- National Child Development Study
- British Household Panel Study
- British and N. Ireland Social Attitudes Surveys
- Health Surveys for England.

The Data Archive's main functions are:
- Establishing user needs particularly within the UK social science and historical academic community
- Negotiation and acquisition of data from a variety of sources (primarily government and academic)
- **Validation** of data and documentation
- Improving and supplementing documentation
- Preservation of data and documentation so that they continue to be accessible over time
- Cataloguing and indexing of the data in a catalogue accessible on the Web
- Reformatting and delivery to users according to users' specifications
- Promoting use and supporting users through workshops and user groups.

Access to the Archive's data holdings is available to all social, economic and historical researchers subject only to restrictions required by the owner of the data. Direct online access to the Archive is available via Manchester Computing's MIMAS service. The access is administered by the Archive but users log directly into the Manchester service when clearance has been given. The Data Archive is also working on a project to provide web-based modular training material for researchers, including those in the field of social policy.

data audit trail (Clinical Trials)

The hard copy documentation that tracks the changes that have been made to a **clinical trial** database. It provides a paper trail which explains the differences that exist between the original data contained in the **case record forms** and that which is entered into the final version of the clinical trial database.

data clarification form (Clinical Trials)

A collection of data clarification queries asked before the **case record form** booklet is sent to Data Quality Control/Clinical Data Management.

data cleaning see **cleaning data**.

data dredging (Clinical Trials)

In general, it is a term used to characterize analyses that are done on an *ad hoc* basis, without benefit of pre-stated hypotheses. It is the exhaustive statistical analysis of **clinical trial** data until a significant result is found. In any clinical study where no statistical difference is found between two different treatments, the continued analysis of sub-sets of the data will eventually yield a statistically significant result. Data dredging is less common nowadays as the statistical analysis that will be undertaken at the end of the study is clearly defined in the study **protocol**. The reason for conducting any additional analysis has to be clearly explained in the statistical report.

data editing (Clinical Trials)

1. The process of reviewing data for the purpose of detecting deficiencies or errors in the way they are collected or recorded.
2. The process of validating and detecting deficient or erroneous values on completed data forms.

Data Elements for Transmission of Individual Case Safety Reports see **E2B** guidance document.

data entry
1. The process of keying (transcribing) data, as contained on completed data forms [**case record forms (clinical trials)** or **adverse event (pharmacovigilance)**], in order to render information into an arrangement more suitable for storage, especially on a computer database, for subsequent retrieval and/or analysis.
2. The process of filling out a data form.

data integrity
The accuracy and **validity** of **data**.

data lock-point (cut-off date)
The date designated as the cut-off date for data to be included into a particular **safety** update such as the **Periodic Safety Update Report**. On this date, the data available to the author of the safety report are extracted for review and stored.

data monitoring (Clinical Trials)
Process by which **case report forms** are examined for completeness, consistency and accuracy.

Data Monitoring Committee see **Independent Data Monitoring Committee**.

Data Sheet see **Summary of Product Characteristics**.

DataStar

An online literature research tool for up-to-date business and technical information owned by the Dialog Corporation. It has a comprehensive European coverage and is a primary source for biomedical, pharmaceutical, and health care information. The database's search capabilities offer high speed access to over 350 databases categorized into ten meticulously indexed subject areas. DataStar Web enables searchers to have the ease of a web browser.

data validation see **validation of data**.

data warehouse see **Clinical Data Repository**.

DAW see **dispense as written**.

DAWN
Drug Abuse Warning Network.

day outlier
A patient with a typically long length of hospital stay compared with other patients in a particular **diagnosis-related group**.

15-day report
A term used to describe a rule regarding **adverse drug reactions** (ADRs) reporting **regulations**. The single case documentation of a serious ADR, interaction is reportable within 15 days of receipt, by the **manufacturer**, to the **competent authorities**.
See also **expedited reporting**.

DBMS
Database Management System.

DD (Sweden)
Department of Drugs (Swedish Regulatory Agency).

DDD see **defined daily dose**.

DDRB
Doctors' and Dentists' Review Body.

DDX see **Doctors' and Dentists' Exemption Scheme**.

DEA (US)
Drug Enforcement Administration.

death rate see **mortality rate**.

debriefing (Clinical Trials)
Giving subjects previously undisclosed information about the research project following completion of their participation in research. (Note that this usage, which occurs within the behavioural sciences, departs from standard English, in which debriefing is obtaining rather than imparting information.)

decentralized procedure see **mutual recognition procedure**.

dechallenge
The withdrawal of a drug after a possible **adverse drug reaction** has occurred. The response to dechallenge is a major factor used in the evaluation of **causality assessment**. A dechallenge is 'positive' or 'suggestive' if the reaction abates when the drug is withdrawn, and is considered to be 'negative' or 'against' if the reaction does not abate when the treatment is withdrawn. A dechallenge, however, can be inconclusive due to the spontaneous evolution of the disease, or specific treatment being not evaluable (death), or irreversible.

decisions (European Union)
As applicable to **European Union** (EU) law, these are issued by the **Council of Ministers** or the **Commission of European Communities** (CEC). It is legally binding in its entirety on those to whom it is addressed. It may be addressed to **Member States**, to individuals, or to companies. It must be notified to whom it is directed, and it takes effect on such a notification.

In 1975, in accordance with Council **Directive 75/319/EEC**, which was adopted on 20 May 1975 and brought into effect on 20 November 1977 (as amended by **Directive 83/570/EEC**), a scientific committee (the **Committee for Proprietary Medicinal Products** (CPMP)) was established. It was also proposed as part of the future system proposals, that the CEC would have powers to issue Decisions on individual **marketing authorization** applications after receiving the **Opinion** of the **CPMP** for human pharmaceutical products, or the **CVMP** for veterinary products. These Decisions would be addressed to both the applicant company and the Member States.

See also **Communications, Directives, Opinions, Recommendations, Regulations**.

decision analysis
A technique used to aid decision-making under conditions of uncertainty by systematically representing and examining all of the relevant information for a decision and the uncertainty around that information. The available choices are plotted on a decision tree. At each branch, or decision node, the probabilities of each outcome that can be predicted are estimated. The relative worth or preferences of decision-makers for the various possible outcomes for a decision can also be estimated and incorporated in a decision analysis.

decision support systems
Computer technologies used in health care which allow **providers** to collect, offer relevant key information at all points of prescribing to allow the most rational, safe and effective prescribing decision to be made, and analyse data in more sophisticated and complex ways. Activities supported include **case mix**, budgeting, cost accounting, clinical **protocol**s and pathways, **outcome**s, and **actuarial** analysis. Also a key functional requirement to support clinical or critical pathways.

Declaration of Helsinki
A set of recommendations or basic principles that guide medical doctors in the conduct and ethics of biomedical research involving human subjects to safeguard their health. It was adopted by the 18th World Medical Assembly (Helsinki, Finland, 1964) and revised by the 29th (Tokyo, 1975) and 35th (Venice, Italy, 1983) World Medical Assemblies. The South Africa version was published in 1996.

decongestant
An agent that relieves congestion, especially a **vasoconstrictor agent**, used to shrink the inflamed and oedematous nasal mucosa of patients suffering from the common cold and allergies.

defective medicinal product see Defective Medicines Report Centre.

Defective Medicines Report Centre (DMRC) (UK)
A body, operated by the **Medicines Control Agency** (MCA)'s Inspection and Enforcement Division, that deals with defective **medicinal products**. It assists with the investigation of problems arising from products that are thought to be defective and organizes any essential protective action. The DMRC aims to minimize the hazard to patients arising from the distribution of defective products for human use by providing an emergency assessment and communications system between the supplier (**manufacturer** and distributors), the **regulatory authorities** and the users. The DMRC defines a 'defective medicinal product' as 'One whose quality does not conform to the requirements of its **marketing authorization** or in some other way is not of the quality intended.' Manufacturers and importers are obliged to report to the Licensing Authority any quality defect in a medicinal product which could result in a recall or restriction on supply. The DMRC does not deal with **adverse drug reactions**, defective **medical devices**, or defective veterinary medicinal products. The Veterinary Medicines Directorate operates a comparable system.

See also **Medical Devices Agency**

defensive medicine
Doctors in recent years have admitted to and have been accused of prescribing additional tests or procedures to justify their care, strengthen support for their decisions or simply to corroborate their diagnosis. This defensiveness is a result of lawsuits, malpractice claims and the onslaught of external entities questioning care decisions. Defensive medicine is said to be one of the primary causes of the increasing cost of health care. In the US many physicians and the **American Medical Association** fight for reform to reduce the need for defensive medicine.

defined daily dose (DDD)
Amount of a drug representing the internationally agreed estimate of the daily maintenance dose for an adult. The term is usually used in drug consumption/utilization studies.

degrees of freedom (Statistics)
The number of independent comparisons that can be made between the members of a sample.

It is the number of independent contributions to a sampling distribution (such as **chi-square** distribution). In a contingency table it is one less than the number of row categories multiplied by one less than the number of column categories; e.g. a 2 × 2 table comparing two groups for a dichotomous **outcome**, such as death, has one degree of freedom.

deliquescent
A water-soluble salt (usually powdered) that tends to absorb moisture from the air and to soften or dissolve as a result.

delivery system (US)
The mechanism by which health care is delivered to a patient. Examples of delivery systems are hospitals, physicians' offices and home health care.

DEMAND
Database service for global **incidence**, **prevalence**, **mortality**, hospital discharges, unitary **costs**, **outcomes**, key cost drivers, available from Pharmametrics (Germany).

demographic data (Clinical Trials)
Characteristics of subjects or study **populations**, which include such information as age, sex, family history of the disease or condition for which they are being treated, and other characteristics relevant to the study in which they are participating.

demography (Clinical Trials)
A description of the features of the **clinical trial population**: their racial and physical characteristics, age patterns, disease history, etc.

demulcent
A material capable of soothing or protecting inflamed, irritated mucous membranes.

de novo design
The design of bioactive compounds by incremental construction of a ligand model within a model of the **receptor** or enzyme active site, the structure of which is known from X-ray or nuclear magnetic resonance (NMR) data.

deodorant
An agent that corrects, masks, or removes unpleasant body odours.

Department of Health (DoH) (UK)
The UK governmental health body whose overall aim is to improve the health and well-being of the people, through the resources available, by:
- supporting activity at national level to protect, promote and improve the nation's health
- securing the provision of comprehensive, high quality health care for all those who need it
- securing responsive social care and child protection for those who lack the support they need
- setting policy framework for the **National Health Service** (NHS)
- negotiating with the Treasury on the level of funding for the NHS
- monitoring the performance of health authorities and trusts.

The Department is organized into three areas:
- the NHS Executive
- the public health group
- the social care group.

The Department also has responsibility for a number of non-departmental public bodies including:

- English National Board for Nursing Midwifery and Health Visiting
- **Public Health Laboratory Service** (PHLS)
- National Biological Standards Board
- **Medicines Control Agency** (MCA)
- Human Fertilization and Embryology Authority Body
- National Radiology Protection Board
- **Medical Devices Agency** (MDA).

Department of Health and Human Services (HHS or DHHS) (US)
A department of the US government that has jurisdiction over public health, welfare and civil rights issues and is the highest level government body with such jurisdiction. The legal authority given to the Secretary of the DHHS is provided by the legislative acts issued by the US Congress (US Senate and the House of Representatives). The federal **regulations** are prepared and issued under direction of the Secretary and reflect the DHHS interpretation of the meaning and intent of the congressional acts. The Congress has given authority to the Secretary of the DHHS to enforce compliance with the **Food, Drug and Cosmetic Act** and to prosecute violators of this act when such action is required to protect the health and **safety** of the public. Reporting into the DHHS are several agencies, including **Health Care Finance Administration**, the PHS and the Social Security Administration.

Website: www.os.dhhs.gov.

dependence
A state in which a person experiences a physical state of withdrawal symptoms (abstinence syndrome) which can be alleviated by taking the same drug that they are dependent on. It occurs mostly with central nervous system (CNS) depressants as they produce more far-reaching adaptive changes. The **metabolism** of the CNS is apparently affected to such an extent that normal functioning can only continue in the presence of the drug. It was this condition of physical dependence that was originally defined as '**addiction**'. 'Drug dependence' has been recommended as a term to be substituted for such words as 'addiction' and '**habituation**' since it is frequently difficult to classify specific agents as being only addictive, habituating, or non-addicting or non-habituating. It has been suggested that the general term be used and modified, appropriately, in specific instances, e.g. drug dependence of the barbiturate type.

Compare **addiction**, **drug abuse**, **habituation**.

dependant
Person covered by someone else's health plan. In a payer's policy of insurance, a person other than the subscriber eligible to receive care because of a subscriber's contract.

dependent variables
The **outcome**s that are measured in an experiment. Dependent variables are expected to change as a result of an experimental manipulation of the independent variable(s).

depilatory agents
(Latin: *de*, away; *pilus*, hair). Chemical hair removers that normally act by the softening action on keratin allowing hair to be be gently scraped away. Examples of these agents include thioglycolic acid and barium sulphide.

depot injection
Injection of a drug into a muscle; the drug is designed to diffuse slowly into the body.

depot phase
The portion of a prolonged release dosage form which liberates the drug at a slower rate than its unrestricted activity.

descriptive study
Any study that is not truly experimental (e.g. **quasi-experimental** studies, correlational studies, record reviews, case histories, and **observational studies**).

desensitization
A method of making a person less allergic to a substance by injecting, gradually increasing, amounts of the substance. For instance, if a person with diabetes has a bad reaction to taking a full dose of beef insulin, the doctor gives the person a very small amount of the insulin at first. Over a period of time, larger doses are given until the person is taking the full dose. This is one way to help the body get used to the full dose and to avoid having an allergic reaction or **anaphylactic shock**.

DESI (US)
Drug Efficacy Study Implementation Notice/Programme (**Food and Drug Administration**).

designated mental health provider (US)
Person or place authorized by a health plan to provide or suggest appropriate mental health and substance abuse care.

detection bias (Statistics)
Systematic differences between comparison groups in how **outcomes** are ascertained, diagnosed or verified.
Also called ascertainment bias.

detergent
An emulsifying agent useful for cleansing wounds and ulcers as well as the skin.

deterministic model
A mathematical model in which the parameters and variables are not subject to **random** fluctuations, so that the system is at any time entirely defined by the initial conditions chosen.
Compare **stochastic model**.

detoxification
Treatment given either to fight a person's **dependence** on alcohol or other drugs or to rid the body of a poisonous substance and its effects.
See also **dependence**.

deviation (Clinical Trials)
Also known as a discrepancy or variation and is a test result or observation that is not in agreement with the predetermined acceptance criteria as listed in the **protocol**, or a **validation** challenge conducted outside of the challenge description provided in the protocol.

device see **medical device**.

device classification (US)
A system of categories for devices defined by the **Food and Drug Administration**. These categories are based on the intended use of a device and determine the type of submission necessary to market it. The categories are Class I, Class II and Class III.
See also **medical device**.

Device Master Record (DMR) (US)
A file that the **manufacturer** of a **medical device** must prepare and maintain. The file describes in detail the various aspects of manufacturing the device. The **manufacturer** is not expected to submit a copy of the DMR to the **Food and Drug Administration** (FDA) but must make the file available to any FDA inspector visiting the manufacturing facility.

DG see **Directorate General** (of the European Commission).

DGH
District General Hospital.

DGSF (Italy)
Italian Drugs directorate.

DHA see **District Health Authority**.

DHAEMAE
Disposable Hypodermic and Allied Equipment Manufacturers' Association of Europe.

DHEW (US)
Department of Health, Education and Welfare.

DHHS see **Department of Health and Human Services**.

DHSS (UK)
Department of Health and Social Security. Now split into the **Department of Health** (DoH) and the Department of Social Security.

DIA see **Drug Information Association**.

diagnosis-related group (DRG) (US)
An inpatient or hospital classification system used for reimbursement purposes to pay a hospital or other **provider** for their services and to categorize illness by diagnosis and treatment. Used under **Medicare's** prospective payment system to reimburse inpatient hospitals, regardless of the cost to the hospital to provide services. Patients are first classified by 23 Major Diagnostic Categories (MDCs), then they are classified further by more specific diagnoses. There are 468 DRGs in the system. Patients in the same DRG will use roughly the same amount of health care resources. Groupings of diagnostic categories drawn from the **International Classification of Diseases** and modified by the presence of a surgical procedure, patient age, presence or absence of significant comorbidities or complications, and other relevant criteria.

diagnostic aid
1. A drug used to determine the functional state of a body organ or the presence of a disease.
2. (Procedure) Tests used to identify a disorder or disease in a living person.

Diagnostic and Statistical Manual of Mental Disorders, Fourth Edition (DSM-IV)
This is the first manual of mental disorders created specifically for use by **primary care** physicians, i.e. the 'Primary Care Version'. Developed as a collaborative effort between the **American Psychiatric Association** and **primary care groups**, this concise, user-friendly manual is a resource for every primary care physician. Unlike other versions of DSM-IV, this manual is compatible with how the physician manages the primary care visit.

diaphoretic (sudorific)
An agent that stimulates the secretion of sweat.

dichotomous data (Statistics)
Observations with two possible categories such as dead/alive, smoker/non-smoker, present/not present.
Also called binary data.

difference equation (Statistics)
The mathematical formulation corresponding to a **discrete time model**.

differential equation (Statistics)
The mathematical formulation corresponding to a **continuous model**; an equation involving derivatives.

digestants
Medicines that aid or stimulate digestion. An example is a digestive enzyme such as Lactaid for people with lactase deficiency.

diluent
An agent that dilutes or renders a drug less potent or irritant.

Diploma in Pharmaceutical Information Management (UK)
Run jointly by the **Association of Information Officers in the Pharmaceutical Industry** and City University, this modular course covers all aspects of information management within the pharmaceutical industry and is applicable to both medical information and research information scientists.

Diploma in Pharmaceutical Medicine (Dip. Pharm. Med.) (UK)
A degree obtainable upon successful completion of a course run by the Faculty of Pharmaceutical Medicine (PM) of the Royal Colleges of Physicians of the UK. The purpose of the course is to ensure that standards in PM are maintained. Candidates who are successful are entitled to apply for the Associateship of the Faculty of PM (AFPM).

Dip. Pharm. Med. see **Diploma in Pharmaceutical Medicine**.

DIP Reports
Disease **incidence** and **prevalence** estimates based on best available evidence. Also contains key outcome measures. Ranges from specific cancers to atherosclerosis.

direct access (Clinical Trials)
Permission to examine, analyse, verify and reproduce any records and reports that are important to the evaluation of a **clinical trial**. Any party (e.g. domestic and foreign **regulatory authorities**, **sponsor**'s **monitors** and auditors) with direct access should take all reasonable precautions within the constraints of the **applicable regulatory requirement(s)** to maintain the **confidentiality** of subject's identities and **sponsor's** proprietary information.

Directive
As applicable to **European Union** (EU) law, it is a legal instrument issued by the **Council of Ministers** or the **Commission of the European Communities** (CEC). Directives are legally binding for all Member States (MSs) but only as to the result to be achieved – it leaves to the national authorities the choice of which form of enactment will be used to achieve it. In other words, Directives are legally binding as to the result to be achieved upon each **Member State** (MS), whereas **Regulations** are binding *per se*. Regulations are passed through the European Parliament and applied to all MSs while Directives leave the means of achieving the desired results up to the individual MS. Directives do not have uniformity as their objective, but instead

the **approximation** of national laws. The text of the Directives themselves usually sets a time limit upon their implementation. Even so, the MSs may not always comply promptly with the agreed timetable for implementation. Like Regulations, Directives have to be based on the powers in the **Treaty of Rome**. If national laws are inconsistent with the Directives, it is usually assumed that the Directive has the overriding effect. Most of the pharmaceutical sector legislations have been Directives originating from the Council of Ministers. Some of the more recent Directives (e.g. 89/341/EEC, 89/342/EEC, 89/343/EEC) have, however, been created by the Committee for Technical Adaptation. The technical Directives are likely to be CEC Directives.

In some countries, like the UK, there are, however, a number of national guidelines for areas not yet covered by the EC guidance (see **Medicines Advice Leaflet** (MAL)).

See also **Communications, Decisions, Opinions, Recommendations, Regulations**.

Directive 65/65/EEC

The first of the European pharmaceutical Directives that was drawn up and adopted by the Council of Ministers on 26 January 1966. The Directive is 'On the approximation of the provisions laid down by law, regulation or administrative action relating to **medicinal products**'. It has the following principal features:
- The definition of a **proprietary medicinal product** (Article 1)
- The requirement for the **Member States** to issue authorizations for medicinal products (Article 3)
- The need for documents and particulars to accompany an application for a **marketing authorization** (MA) (Article 4)
- The obligation on the authorities to refuse an application for a product if it is 'harmful in its normal conditions of use' or lacking in therapeutic **efficacy**; if efficacy is not sufficiently shown; or if its qualitative or quantitative composition is not declared (Article 5)
- The time allowed for the authorities to process applications is within 120 days of submitting the application, with an extension of 90 days in exceptional cases (Article 7)
- The conditions where a MA may be suspended or revoked (Articles 11–12)
- Container and outer package **labelling** requirements (Articles 13–20). These Articles were later repealed by **Directive 92/27/EEC**.

This Directive was amended by **Directive 83/570/EEC**, 81/21/EEC, **89/341/EEC, 89/342/EEC, 89/343/EEC** and **89/381/EEC**.

See also **Proprietary Medicinal Product**.

Directive 75/318/EEC

A **European Union** (EU) Council Directive, adopted on 20 May 1975 and implemented within 18 months. It deals with the approximation of laws of **Member States** relating to analytical, pharmacological and clinical standards and protocols in respect of the testing of **medicinal products** (as amended by **83/570/EEC** and **91/507/EEC**). It has a definition for the term 'documents and particulars to accompany an application for a **marketing authorization**' which was in article 4.8 of **Directive 65/65/EEC**.

Directive 75/319/EEC

A **European Union** (EU) Council Directive, adopted on 20 May 1975, to set the legal and administrative framework for the authorities in the **Member States**. It relates to the following issues:
- The submission and processing of **marketing authorization** (MA) applications
- The establishment of a new European Committee (the **Committee for Proprietary**

Medicinal Products (CPMP)) to consider questions referred to it concerning approval, refusal, suspension, or revocation of MAs
- The requirements for the inspection of manufacturers, issue of manufacturing authorizations, and the need for a '**Qualified Person** (QP)' who is responsible for ensuring that the manufacture is in accord with the MA
- The need for the national authorities to inspect manufacturing and contract test laboratories to ensure that the testing is carried out as laid down in the MA
- An exemption from the Directives for immunologicals, **radiopharmaceuticals**, **homeopathics** and blood products.

Council Directive 75/319/EEC as amended (Chapter Va), together with Council Regulation (EEC) No 2309/93 (title II, Chapter 3), describe the respective obligations of the MA holder and of the competent authorities to set up a system for **pharmacovigilance** in order to collect, collate and evaluate information about suspected adverse reactions.

Directive 75/320/EEC

A **European Union** (EU) Council Directive, adopted on 20 May 1975 to create a new body, the pharmaceutical committee, which consists of Director of Pharmacy (or their equivalents) in each of the **Member States**. The committee considers any proposals relating to new Directives (or amends existing Directives) from the **Commission of the European Communities**. It also considers the broad policy issues in relation to the control of medicinal products.

Directive 78/25/EEC

A **European Union** (EU) Council Directive adopted on 12 December 1977. It created a list of colouring matters which may be used in medicinal products.

Directive 81/464/EEC

A **European Union** (EU) Council Directive amending **Directive 78/25/EEC**.

Directive 83/570/EEC

A **European Union** (EU) Council Directive, adopted on 26 October 1983 and implemented by all **Member States** on 1 November 1985, to amend the first three Directives. This Directive established the obligation for the applicant to produce a draft **Summary of Product Characteristics** (SPC) as an element of the documentation to be submitted with the **marketing authorization** application. It also modified the **Committee for Proprietary Medicininal Products** procedures and made provision for the **multi-state procedure**.

Directive 83/189/EEC

A **European Union** (EU) Council Directive, issued on 28 March 1983, that deals with the provision of information in the field of technical standards and regulations. It was amended by Directive 88/189/EEC.

Directive 83/571/EEC

A **European Union** (EU) Council Directive defining pre-clinical and **clinical guidelines** as an annex to **Directive 75/318/EEC**.

Directive 86/609/EEC

A **European Union** (EU) Council Directive, issued on 24 November 1986, that deals with the provisions of **Member States** regarding the protection of animals used for experimental and other scientific purposes.

Directive 87/18/EEC
A **European Union** (EU) Council Directive applying **good laboratory practice** to animal safety work on chemical substances with reference to the Organization of Economic Cooperation and Development.

Directive 87/19/EEC
A **European Union** (EU) Council Directive adopted on 22 December 1986 and implemented on 1 July 1987. It introduced the requirement for data on developmental pharmaceuticals and on process validation and also rapid procedure for adapting the technical requirements in the 'norm and **protocols**' **Directive (75/318/EEC)** for the dossier to be submitted with a **marketing authorization**.

Directive 87/21/EEC
A **European Union** (EU) Council Directive adopted on 22 December 1986 and implemented on 1 July 1987. It deals with abridged applications for 'copy products' and protection of innovation (particularly biotechnology products) and guarantees greater harmonization of all the requirements for 'copy products'.

Directive 87/22/EEC
A **European Union** (EU) Council Directive adopted on 22 December 1986 and implemented on 1 July 1987. The Directive introduced the concertation procedure (i.e. a procedure to obtain a mutual agreement on the authorization) for high technology/biotechnology products. That is a procedure by which the competent authorities in the **Member States** are obliged to consult each other before deciding to authorize, refuse, or withdraw a medicinal biotechnology product. The directive contains two lists of products: List A, the biotechnology products, and List B, the high technology products.

Directive 87/176/EEC
A **European Union** (EU) Council **Recommendation** defining further pre-clinical and **clinical guidelines** as an annex to **Directive 75/319/EEC**.

Directive 88/320/EEC
A **European Union** (EU) Council Directive relating to the inspection and verification of **good laboratory practice** by establishing a harmonized system for study audits and inspections.

Directive 89/105/EEC
Adopted on 21 December 1988. This Council Directive deals with the transparency of measures regulating pricing of medicines and their inclusion in the national health insurance systems.

Directive 89/341/EEC
A **European Union** (EU) Council Directive, adopted on 3 May 1989, which has the main objective of improving the information given to consumers of medicines by requiring more systematic provision of patient leaflets. It was this Directive that made the insertion of a package insert in all medicinal products obligatory after 1 January 1992. This was the consequence of the request that the European Council of Health Ministers had from the European Parliament. It was in Article 1 of this Directive that the term '**proprietary medicinal product**' was replaced with '**medicinal product**.'

Directive 89/342/EEC
A **European Union** (EU) Council Directive, adopted on 3 May 1989, extending the scope of **Directives 65/65/EEC** and **75/319/EEC** and laying down additional provisions for immunological medicinal products consisting of vaccines, toxins, sera and allergens.

Directive 89/343/EEC

A **European Union** (EU) Council Directive, adopted on 3 May 1989, extending the scope of **Directives 65/65/EEC** and **75/319/EEC** and laying down additional provisions for radiopharmaceuticals. It requires labels to be in accordance with the requirements of the Regulations for Safe Transport of Radioactive Materials laid down by the International Atomic Energy Agency.

Directive 89/381/EEC

A **European Union** (EU) Council Directive, adopted on 14 June 1989, extending the scope of **Directives 65/65/EEC** and **75/319/EEC** to cover medicines derived from human blood or plasma (blood products).

Directive 90/18/EEC

A **European Union** (EU) Council extension/modification Directive to amend the annex to **Directive 88/320/EEC** and providing the text of the OECD.

Directive 90/219/EEC

A **European Union** (EU) Council Directive issued on 23 April 1990 on the deliberate release into the environment of genetically modified organisms. This directive was modified by the Commission Directive 94/15/EC of April 1994 which introduced the issue of releasing genetically modified higher plants.

Directive 90/220/EEC

A **European Union** (EU) Council Directive issued on 23 April 1990 on the contained use of genetically modified micro-organisms.

Directive 90/356/EEC

A **European Union** (EU) Council Directive defining **good manufacturing practice** principles.

Directive 90/385/EEC

A **European Union** (EU) Council Directive, established on 20 June 1990, which focuses on the contents of the **active implantable medical devices**.

Directive 91/356/EEC

A **European Union** (EU) Commission Directive, which came into force on 13 June 1991, and provides the principles and guidelines of **good manufacturing practice** for medicinal products for human use.

Directive 91/412/EEC

A **European Union** (EU) Council Directive, which came into force on 13 June 1991, that provides the principles and guidelines of **good manufacturing practice** for veterinary medicinal products.

Directive 91/507/EEC

A **European Union** (EU) Council Directive to modify the annex of **Directive 75/318/EEC**. It focuses on the format of the **marketing authorization** application and details the obligatory basis for the implementation of **good laboratory practice** and **good clinical practice**.

Directive 92/25/EEC

A **European Union** (EU) Council Directive on wholesale distribution of medicines for human use.

Directive 92/26/EEC
A **European Union** (EU) Council Directive on the legal classification of medicines intended for human use.

Directive 92/27/EEC
A **European Union** (EU) Council Directive, which came into force on 1 January 1994. This Directive deals with the **labelling** of medicinal products for human use and for the format and content of **patient information leaflets** (PILs) to be supplied with each medicine when dispensed in the EU. It also established the requirement for use of the recommended **International Non-proprietary Name** (rINN) for medicinal substances.

Directive 92/28/EEC
A **European Union** (EU) Council Directive, which came into force on 31 March 1992, that provides guidance on advertising medicinal products intended for human use.

Directive 92/73/EEC
A **European Union** (EU) Council extension Directive on homeopathic medicines.

Directive 93/42/EEC
A **European Union** (EU) Council Directive, published on 12 July 1993 in the Official Journal (L169), concerning the Classification of **medical devices**. This Directive covers a vast range of products from first-aid bandages and walking frames to CT scanners and non-active implants. Medical devices, covered by this Directive, are grouped into four classes:
1. Class I   generally regarded as low risk
2. Class II   generally regarded as medium risk
3. Class IIb   generally regarded as medium risk
4. Class III   generally regarded as high risk.

Directorate General (of the European Commission)
The departments of the **Commission of the European Communities** (CEC) which cover all aspects of the Community's work. The **European Medicines Evaluation Agency** participates in meetings of some of the DGs, namely:

DG III   Internal Market and Industry – Pharmaceutical Committee
DG VI   Agriculture
DG XII   Science and Research
DG XXIV   Consumer Policy and Consumer Health Protection.

Directory of Physician Groups & Networks
Online directory of **Individual Practice Associations** (IPAs), medical group practices, **Provider Health Plans**, practice management companies and management service organizations. It is the official directory of the IPA Association of America. It is published by Dorland Health Care Information.

Direct Payment to Contractors (DPC) (UK)
A system used to pay the reimbursement and remuneration costs, calculated by the pricing systems. Each month the DPC system pays monies owed direct to the bank accounts of the following contractors only:
- pharmacy contractors
- appliance contractors
- oxygen concentrators suppliers.

The system reimburses:

- pharmacy and appliance contractors for the supply of drugs, chemical reagents and appliances
- oxygen concentrator suppliers for the provision and maintenance of oxygen concentrator equipment
- pharmacy contractors for locally authorized payments (e.g. rota, high cost drug advances, payment under the Essential Small Pharmacy Scheme).

A schedule of payment is also sent to the contractor 5 working days before monies are transferred. In addition, the DPC system produces Financial Information Systems Reports for the **National Health Service** (NHS) Executive.

See also **Prescription Pricing Authority**.

Direzione Generale Del Servizo Farmaceutico, Ministero Della Santia (Italy) see Ministry of Health, Directorate-General of the Pharmaceutical Division.

disallowance (US)
When a payer declines to pay for all or part of a claim submitted for payment.

discharge planning (US)
Required by **Medicare** and the **Joint Commission of Accreditation of Healthcare Organizations** for all hospital patients. A procedure where aftercare services are determined after discharge from the inpatient facility.

disclosure procedure (Clinical Trials)
A procedure designed to identify, in the event of an emergency, the nature of treatment given to a subject.

discontinued subject see subject withdrawal.

disease management
Refers to the concept considering all health needs of a patient with a particular disease and then managing the whole process of their delivery in an efficient manner with an emphasis on **cost-effectiveness**, rather than treating individual components of a disease in isolation. For example, a cancer patient may be given **chemotherapy** for a particular malignancy, without regard to the costs of **side-effects** such as serious nausea and vomiting, which often require medical treatment. A disease state management approach would be to determine which therapeutic combination would result in the highest overall cost-effectiveness (taking into account all foreseeable side-effects) and treating the patient accordingly during the entire course of the disease.

In the US, the term is also used to describe a type of product or service now being offered by many large pharmaceutical companies to get them into broader health care services. Grouping the use of prescription drugs with physician and allied professionals, linked to large databases created by the pharmaceutical companies, to treat people with specific diseases. The claim is that this type of service provides higher quality of care at more reasonable price than alternative, presumably more fragmented, care.

From a **managed care** perspective, disease management involves aspects of case and outcomes management, but the approach focuses on specific diseases, looking at what creates the costs, what treatment plan works, educating patients and **providers**, and coordinating care at all levels: hospital, pharmacy, physician, etc.

disease state management see disease management.

disinfection
The destruction of micro-organisms, but not usually bacterial spores; it does not necessarily

kill all micro-organisms but reduces them to a level which is harmful neither to health nor to the quality of perishable goods. The term is applicable to the treatment of inanimate objects and materials and may also be applied to the treatment of the skin and other body membranes and cavities.

disintegrant
An agent used in the pharmaceutical preparation of **tablets**, which causes them to disintegrate and release their medicinal content on contact with gastric and/or intestinal fluids.

dispense as written (DAW)
When physicians write a prescription, they may designate on the form that the prescription must be dispensed as written. This means substitutions (usually generic drugs) may not be used. This is called a physician DAW. Under certain circumstances the pharmacy or the card holder may also request that the prescription be dispensed as written, but that type of DAW may involve an additional payment.

Compare **generic substitution**.

dispensing contractors (UK)
Community pharmacies, dispensing general practitioners and appliance contractors under contract to the local Health Authorities. These are collectively known as dispensing contractors.

Dispensing Doctor Analysis see Prescription Cost Analysis.

dispersant
Chemical agent with the property of separating concentrations of organic material, e.g. detergent on oil.

disposition see drug disposition.

Dispute Resolution Meeting (US)
During the new product development process of a medical product, disputes may surface between the **Food and Drug Administration** (FDA) and the **manufacturer**. If these cannot be resolved amicably, the manufacturer may request a Dispute Resolution Meeting with the FDA. The FDA is obliged to grant such a meeting, subject to the conditions described in the **Code of Federal Regulations**.

distomer
The enantiomer of a chiral compound that is the less potent for a particular action. This definition does not exclude the possibility of another effect or **side-effect** of the distomer.

See also **eutomer**.

distribution
The reversible transfer of drug from one location to another within the body. Once a drug has entered the vascular system it becomes distributed throughout the various tissues and body fluids in a pattern that reflects the physiochemical nature of the drug and the ease with which it penetrates different membranes. The one compartment model assumes rapid distribution but it does not preclude extensive distribution into various tissues.

Distribution can be thought of as following one of four types of patterns:
1. The drug may remain largely within the vascular system. Plasma substitutes are an example of this type, but drugs which are strongly bound to plasma protein may also approach this pattern.

2. Some low molecular weight water soluble compounds such as ethanol and a few sulfonamides become uniformly distributed throughout the body water.
3. A few drugs are concentrated specifically in one or more tissues that may or may not be the site of action. Iodine is concentrated by the thyroid gland. The antimalarial drug chloroquine may be present in the liver at concentrations 1000 times those present in plasma. Tetracycline is almost irreversibly bound to bone and developing teeth. Consequently tetracyclines should only be given to young children or infants in extreme conditions as it can cause discoloration and mottling of the developing second set of teeth. Another type of specific concentration may occur with highly lipid soluble compounds which distribute into fat tissue.
4. Most drugs exhibit a non-uniform distribution in the body with variations that are largely determined by the ability to pass through membranes and their lipid/water solubility. The highest concentrations are often present in the kidney, liver, and intestine usually reflecting the amount of drug being excreted.

Pattern 4 is the most common being a combination of patterns 1, 2 and 3.

The rate of distribution depends on: membrane permeability, and blood perfusion while the extent of distribution depends on: lipid solubility, pH–pKa, plasma protein binding, and intracellular binding.

See also **pharmacokinetics**, **volume of distribution**.

District Health Authorities (DHA) (UK)

The bodies responsible for purchasing hospital and community health services for their residents and managing the services provided in directly-managed units. DHAs also have a number of traditional public health responsibilities. There are around 190 DHAs in England. The DHA works as a corporate body and used to be accountable to the **Regional Health Authority** (RHA). As part of the Health Authorities Act, regional health authorities were abolished with effect from April 1996 and replaced by eight regional offices of the **National Health Service** (NHS) Executive. Each DHA has a chairman appointed by the Secretary of State, five non-executive members who were appointed by the RHA and up to five executive members. Two of the executives, the General Manager and the Chief Finance Officer are *ex-officio* members. The remainder are appointed by the chairman and non-executive members together with the general manager. DHAs perform a number of functions in the NHS.

See also **Family Health Services Authorities**, **National Health Service**, **Regional Health Authority**, **Special Health Authorities**.

diuretic

A drug that increases the amount of water in the urine, removing excess water from the body; used in treating high blood pressure and fluid retention.

DLT see **dose-limiting toxicity**.

DMF see **Drug Master File**.

DMOS (France)

Diverses Mesures d'Ordre Social. French law Act controlling payment from pharmaceutical industry to physicians.

DMR see **Device Master Record**.

DMRC see **Defective Medicines Report Centre**.

DN

District Nurse.

DoB
    Date of birth.

docking studies
    Molecular modelling studies aimed at finding a proper fit between a ligand and its binding site.

Doctors' and Dentists' Exemption Scheme (DDX) (Clinical Trials) (UK)
    A British scheme for those trials where the pharmaceutical company is not the originator of the trial. There should be a clinician-initiated request for materials to be made available so that they may carry out the trial. In such cases, the clinician should obtain **Ethics Committee** approval and should, in the case of a new ingredient or new dosage form (or for a **placebo** to be used with marketed products), apply for a DDX from the **Medicines Control Agency (MCA)**. Provided that the MCA is not aware of any problems associated with the material or the proposed trial, the trialist may continue, but under their own responsibility.
    See also **Clinical Trial Certificate, Clinical Trial Exemption**.

documentation (Clinical Trials)
    All records in any form (including written documents, magnetic, optical records and scans, X-rays and electrocardiograms) describing methods and conduct of the trial, factors affecting the trial and the action taken. These include **protocol**, copies of **investigator**(s)' *curriculum vitae*, **consent forms**, **monitor** reports, **audit certificates**, relevant letters, reference ranges, **raw data**, completed **case record form** and the **Final Report**.

DoH see **Department of Health**.

DOP
    Data Operating Procedures.

dosage form
    The physical state in which a drug is dispensed for use. The most frequent dosage form of aspirin, for example, is a **tablet**.

dosage regimen
    (a) The number of doses per given time period; (b) the time that elapses between doses (for example, every 6 hours) or the time that the doses are to be given (for example, at 08:00 and 16:00 daily); or (c) The quantity of a drug that is given at each specific time intervals.

dose
    The quantity of drug prescribed (normally) by a doctor to be given to a patient at any one time. Dose may be described as an absolute dose (the total amount administered to a subject) or as a relative dose (relative to some property of the subject such as body weight or surface area, mg/kg, or mg/m^2).
    Compare **dosage, multiple dose regimens**.

dose-comparison concurrent control study
    A **clinical trial** when at least two **doses** or treatment dose regimens of the **investigational product** are compared. A dose-comparison study may include additional treatment groups, such as **placebo** or active controls. It can be considered as 'adequate and well-controlled **clinical trial**' when at least three doses or treatment regimens of the study drug are evaluated.

dose-escalation study (Clinical Trials)
    A type of **clinical trial** (usually conducted during phase I) in which different groups of study

patients are given progressively higher doses of the study agent to determine the **maximum tolerated dose** for future trials.

dose-limiting toxicity
Side-effects that are severe enough to prevent giving more of the treatment.
See **phase I trial**.

dose proportionality
The situation where certain bioavailability parameters (C_{max} and **area under the curve**) are linear over a certain dose range.

dose-ranging clinical trials
Trials designed to identify the **maximum tolerated dose**, minimum effective dose, and effective dose range for maintenance therapy and starting dose to initiate treatment.

dose–response
The relationship between the dose administered and the pharmacodynamic effect with time.

dosimeter
Instrument for measuring dose or exposure to radiation.

double-blind clinical trial (Clinical Trials)
A clinical study of an **investigational product** or a marketed **drug**(s) where neither the **investigator**s (**outcome** assessors) nor the participants know which subjects will be treated with the active principle/intervention and which ones will receive a **placebo**. The purpose of blinding the participants (recipients and providers of care) is to prevent performance **bias**. The purpose of blinding the investigators (outcome assessors, who might also be the care providers) is to protect against **detection bias**.

See also **blinding/masking, blinding system, detection bias, single-blind clinical trial, triple-blind clinical trial**.

double-blind study see double-blind clinical trial.

double dummy (Clinical Trials)
A procedure for achieving blindness when comparing two different drugs wherein, for example, an active injection and **placebo** tablets are given to one group and the matching placebo injection and active tablet are given to the other group.

double-masked design see double-blind clinical trial.

double prodrug
A biologically inactive molecule which is transformed *in vivo* in two steps (enzymatically and/or chemically) to the active species.
Also called pro-prodrug.

DPC see Direct Payment to Contractors.

DPC-PTR see Drug Price Competition and Patent Term Restoration Act.

DPLM
Direction de la Pharmacie et du Médicament.

DPR (UK)
Data Protection Registrar.

D

DRA
Drug Regulatory Authority.

DRG
1. See **diagnosis-related group**.
2. (US) Division of Research Grants.

DRL see **WHO-DRL**.

DRLS (US)
Drug Registration and Listing System.

DSI (US)
Division of Scientific Investigations (**Food and Drug Administration**).

DSM
Diagnostic and Statistical Manual.

DSM-IV see **Diagnostic and Statistical Manual of Mental Disorders, Fourth Edition**.

drug
A substance or a chemical compound used in the diagnosis, treatment, or prevention of disease in human beings or in animals or for restoring, correcting, or modifying physiological functions (e.g. the contraceptive pill). Drugs may occur naturally in animals (e.g. insulin) or plants (e.g. morphine); it may be semi-synthetic (e.g. aspirin) or wholly synthetic (e.g. phenobarbital).

As defined in the **Food, Drug and Cosmetic Act**, drugs are '(a) articles recognized in the official **United States Pharmacopoeia**, Official Homeopathic Pharmacopoeia of the US, or Official National Formulary, or any supplement to any of them, and (b) articles intended for use in the diagnosis, cure, mitigation, treatment, or prevention of disease in man or other animals, and (c) articles (other than food) intended to affect the structure or any function of the body of man or other animals, and (d) articles intended for use as a component of any articles specified in clause (a), (b), or (c), but does not include devices or their components, parts or accessories.'

drug abuse
Persistent or sporadic, intentional excessive use of drugs inconsistent with or unrelated to the recommendations of the **Summary of Product Characteristics** or acceptable medical practice. It also describes use of a drug to an extent, considered 'more harmful than helpful for both the individual or society.'

Compare **addiction**, **dependence**, **habituation**, **Harrison Act**.

Drug Analysis see **Prescription Cost Analysis**.

Drug Analysis Print (DAP) (UK)
A report provided by the UK authority, the **Medicines Control Agency** (MCA), upon request. DAPs can also be downloaded by the **marketing authorization** (MA) holder if they have subscribed for access to the **ADROIT Electronically Generated Information Service (AEGIS)**. The report print is a complete historical record of all suspected adverse reactions reported in association with the named drug substance since the introduction of the Register of Adverse Reactions in 1964. The inclusion of a particular reaction on the print, however, does not necessarily mean that it has been caused by the drug. Causality evaluation factors have to be taken into consideration in assessing causal relationship. A DAP provides a:

- List of all the reactions reported to have occurred in association with the named suspect drug substance
- List of all reactions included on the original report. This means that because some reports contain more than one reaction, the total number of reactions usually exceeds the number of reports received for the drug. The number of reports is shown at the end of the print. Each report relates to one patient
- List of reactions reported for a particular drug substance irrespective of whether the reporter provided the approved drug substance name or a brand name of the substance. Brand names are shown on the print if they have been associated with at least one reported adverse reaction to one patient
- Data for reports where:
    1. The approved drug substance was given as a single constituent
    2. The approved drug substance was used in combination (multi-constituent) products. It may not be possible to decide which (if any) of the drug substances in the combination products was responsible for a particular reaction.
- List of reactions grouped within broad categories, System Organ Classes (SOC), (e.g. gastrointestinal disorders). Reactions are grouped also under High Level Terms (HLT) within a SOC (e.g. the reaction diarrhoea is listed under the HLT 'Gastro-intestinal system, symptoms and signs' in the gastro-intestinal SOC. The ADROIT listing of classified reactions (preferred terms) is comprehensive and classification hierarchy permits a preferred term to be represented in more than one SOC. However, in order to prevent multiple counting of a term, a Preferred Term appears only under its designated 'Primary SOC' on the print
- List of the number of deaths associated with each reaction when the reaction is thought to have contributed to death
- The date on which the information was extracted from the computer, the date of the earliest reported reaction, the total number of reactions and the total number of reports for the drug substance.

The print groups adverse reaction terms in a hierarchical structure. The 'preferred term' (e.g. ventricular fibrillation) is grouped under the broader heading the 'high level term, HLT' (e.g. ventricular arrhythmias). HLTs are contained within the SOC.

See also **causality, causality assessment of suspected adverse reactions**.

drug candidate

The compound qualified for further research after methods of detection, such as **high throughput screening**, have been employed.

drug dependence see **dependence**.

drug disposition

All processes involved in the **absorption**, **distribution**, **metabolism** and excretion of **drugs** in a living organism.

drug–drug interaction

The situation where there is an influence of one drug on the **bioavailability**, pharmacokinetic parameters, **adverse events**' profile or pharmacological **outcome**s of another drug given concomitantly or recently. Drug interactions can be:
- Pharmacokinetic interactions: Where the interaction is based on a change in one of the pharmacokinetic aspects of the drugs. Also known as **ADME** interactions.

- **Metabolism**: the metabolism of one drug can be increased or decreased by the enzyme-inducing effects of another drug resulting in increased toxicity or reduction in efficacy respectively (e.g. cimitidine and warfarin)
- **Distribution** (e.g. tricyclic antidepressants and debrisoquine)
- **Elimination** (e.g. sodium bicarbonate effect on salicylate excretion)
- **Absorption** (e.g. tetracyclines and antacids)
- Pharmaceutical; occurring outside the body when mixing different drugs (e.g. precipitation or inactivation).
- Pharmacodynamic interactions; These are sometimes sub-classified as:
  - Direct
    - Antagonistic (e.g. opiates and naloxone)
    - Augmented or potentiated (antiarrhythmic drugs)
    - Non-specific (e.g. alcohol and some antihistamines)
  - Indirect. Affecting normal physiological processes (e.g. sulphonylureas and corticosteroids, diuretics and digoxin, or NSAIDs and anticoagulants.

See also **food–drug interaction, P-450**, and **enzyme-inducing drugs**.

drug–food interaction see **food–drug interaction**.

Drug Formulary (US)

Varying list of prescription drugs approved by a given health plan for distribution to a covered (by insurance) person through specific pharmacies.

See also **formulary**.

Drug Information Association, The (DIA)

Founded in 1964 as a non-profit, scientific, member-driven association whose professionals are from academia and the pharmaceutical industry. The organization had over 20 000 members in 1999. The DIA provides a neutral global forum for the exchange and dissemination of information on the discovery, development, evaluation, and utilization of medicines and related health care technologies. Through these activities, the DIA provides development opportunities for its members.

The DIA does not exert editorial control over materials that are posted by third parties onto its internet site or materials that are emailed by third parties to any other persons. DIA early publications included the *Drug Information Bulletin* that became the quarterly *Drug Information Journal*. The publishing activities increased with a quarterly DIA Newsletter and an annual **PCSO** Register.

The DIA has a European office in Basel. There is also a DIA office in Sydney and Tokyo. As of January 1999 the number of DIA meetings, training courses and symposia, held around the world, exceed 100 per year.

drug intolerance

A type of **adverse drug reactions** in which the expected pharmacological effects of the drug occur with an unusually small dose.

drug latentiation

The chemical modification of a biologically active compound to form a new compound, which *in vivo* will liberate the parent compound. Drug latentiation is synonymous with **prodrug** design.

Drug Master File (DMF) (US)

DMFs provide a way for companies other than drug product manufacturers, such as chemical manufacturers or contract manufacturing facilities, to submit information to the **Food and Drug Administration** (FDA) which can then be referenced by a drug manufacturer in an **Investigational New Drug** or **New Drug Application** submission. This eliminates the same information being submitted to the FDA several times if the chemical manufacturer or contract laboratory works with several different **drug product** manufacturers. In the UK and the US (unlike the EC), DMFs are not normally assessed until an application is made which cross-refers to them, and it is the product and not the DMF that is subject to approval.

In the UK, a DMF is a set of documents submitted voluntarily to the **Medicines Control Agency** by the manufacturer of the **active ingredient, excipient**, or container component or by the manufacturer's agent. The information is submitted on a commercially confidential basis and access to it is authorized by the person or the company originally supplying the information.

DMFs may be submitted at any time but are not assessed until **marketing authorization** or a **Clinical Trial Certificate** application is submitted which cross refers to it, and for which a letter of authorization of access has been received from the DMF provider. Reference to a DMF is not usually permitted in connection with a **Clinical Trial Certificate Exemption** application, and 'approval' in such cases would in any case be of limited value in the light of the negative vetting procedure applied to this type of application.

DMFs are accepted in Denmark, France, Greece, Ireland, and The Netherlands. European DMFs are usually equivalent to FDA DMFs for drug substances, excipients, and occasionally containers. The German authorities do not accept DMFs.

See also **European Drug Master File**.

drug misuse see drug abuse.

drug overdose

Administration or taking a drug dose in excess of the recommended dose in the **Summary of Product Characteristics** which can lead to serious **adverse drug reactions**.

Drug Price Competition and Patent Term Act, 1984 (DPC-PTR) (US)

An extension of the **Abbreviated New Drug Application**. The aim of this Act was to include drugs approved for marketing after 1962. This was meant to make it easier for **generic drugs** to gain **Food and Drug Administration** (FDA) **approval (marketing authorization)**, and by way of reparation for the research industry, to make provision for their patents to be extended in view of the time lost while the **New Drug Application** was being reviewed by the FDA.

drug product

Generally, it is a finished dosage form, for example: ointments, **suspensions, solutions, capsules creams**, etc., that contains an **active ingredient** generally, but not necessarily, in association with **inactive ingredients**. The **European Union** (EU) definition is 'finished dosage form (e.g. **tablet, capsule, solution**, etc.) that may contain an active drug ingredient with an inactive ingredient' According to the US **Food, Drug and Cosmetic Act** definition, they are 'articles intended for use in the diagnosis, cure, mitigation, treatment, or prevention of disease in man or other animals and articles, other than food, intended to affect the structure or any function of the body of man or other animals and any article intended for use as a component of any articles specified above.' Drug products are further defined in 21 **CFR (Code of Federal Regulations)** 210.3 (4) as a 'finished dosage form, for example, tablet, capsule, solution, etc., that contains an active drug ingredient generally, but not necessarily, in association with inactive ingredients.' The term also includes finished dosage forms that do not contain active ingredients, but are intended to be used as **placebo**.

Compare **active ingredient**.

drug redistribution
This applies to certain drugs whose action can be terminated not by **elimination** or **biotransformation** but by redistribution from their sites of action to other *in vivo* areas. For this to happen, the drug must be delivered to its site of action much more rapidly than to its site of redistribution and this depends on its physiochemical properties, blood flow and route of administration.

Drug Safety Unit (DSU)
Usually the name given to the **Pharmacovigilance** Department in a pharmaceutical company.

drug substance see **active ingredient**.

Drug Surveillance Unit see **Prescription Event Monitoring**.

drug targeting
A strategy aiming at the delivery of a compound to a particular tissue of the body.

drug tariff (UK)
A monthly publication, compiled by the **Prescription Pricing Authority** on behalf of the **Department of Health**, setting out details of payments to be made in respect to the supply of pharmaceuticals, appliances, and chemical reagents.

Drug Utilization Review (DUR)
Continuing analysis of an insured population's drug use and cost from which patterns of prescribing, dispensing, and use can be determined. The aim of DUR is to determine how to reduce the cost of utilization and to detect inappropriate prescribing and drug use. Reviews often result in recommendations to practitioners, including generic substitutions, use of formularies, use of co-payments for prescriptions and education. In some cases, practitioners are now penalized or rewarded depending on their drug prescription-related costs and utilization. Some speculate that these incentives can adversely affect doctor decisions.

Drugs Action Team-Inter-Agency-Group (DAT) (UK)
A Local Authority, Health Authority, Prison Service, or a Probation, which consults and works with the community to establish and implement a strategy on drugs.

Drugs and Therapeutics Bulletin **(DTB)** (UK)
A regular publication listing all drugs and their indications. It is distributed to all prescribers.

Drugs and Therapeutics Committee (DTC) (UK)
A hospital-based committee which sets policy on medicines management issues within a hospital.

DSD
Drug Safety Department.

DSM III
Diagnostic and Statistical Manual, third edition.

DSMB see **Data and Safety Monitoring Board**.

DSNP
Development of Standardized Nomenclature Project.

DSRU
Drug Safety Research Unit.

DSS
Department of Social Security.

DSU see **Drug Safety Unit.**

DTB see *Drugs and Therapeutics Bulletin.*

DTI (UK)
: Department of Trade and Industry.

dual action drug
: A compound which combines two desired different pharmacological actions at a similarly efficacious **dose**.

duplicate products
: Products with the same **active ingredient**(s), route of administration, **labelling**, **dosage** form, **strength**, or condition of use that may be made by different **manufacturers**. In the US, it is allowed for duplicates of **drug products** which were first approved before 10 October 1962 and for certain other drugs which are described in the CFR to submit an application for approval (**marketing authorization**) consisting of an abbreviated version of the **New Drug Application** (i.e. ANDA). An ANDA is reserved for drug products that duplicate products previously approved (e.g. generics) under a full NDA.
  See also **Abbreviated New Drug Application, Bioequivalence.**

duplication of benefits (US)
: When a person is covered under two or more health plans with the same or similar coverage.

DUR see **Drug Utilization Review.**

Durham–Humphrey Amendment (US)
: An amendment issued in 1951 to the Federal **Food, Drug and Cosmetic Act** of 1938. It laid down the list of drugs to be labelled as **prescription only medicines**. It also stipulated that such products bear the **Rx** legend.
  See also **Food, Drug and Cosmetic (FDC) Act, prescription only medicine.**

E102
Tartrazine; a synthetic organic food or drug additive colourant.

E104
Quinoline yellow; food or drug additive colourant.

E110
Sunset yellow FCF; food or drug additive.

E123
Amaranth; a red acid azo dye used to colour food or drugs.

E124
Ponceau 4R; an azo dye which gives a red colour and used in food, biological stains or drug colourant.

E127
Erythrosine; a synthetic organic food or drug additive colourant.

E132
Indigo carmine; food or drug additive colourant.

E142
Green S; food or drug additive.

E171
Titanium dioxide; an inorganic food or drug additive colourant.

E172
Iron oxides, iron dioxides; an inorganic food or drug additive colourant.

E211
Sodium benzoate; food or drug additive.

E322
Lecithins; food or drug additive.

E420
Sorbitol; a faintly sweet alcohol that occurs in fruits of the mountain ash. It is made synthetically and is used specially as a softener, sweetener, in making ascorbic acid in food and drug formulations.

E421
Mannitol; a slightly sweet crystalline alcohol found in many plants and used as a food or drug additive.

E422
Glycerol; a sweet syrupy hygroscopic trihydroxy alcohol used in foods and drugs as a solvent, plasticizer, moisturizing agent, emollient, lubricant and emulsifying agent.

E1 guidance document
An **International Conference on Harmonization** (ICH) guidance document entitled 'The extent of population exposure to access clinical safety'.

E2A guidance document
An **International Conference on Harmonization** (ICH) guidance document entitled

'Clinical Safety Data Management: Definitions and Standards for Expedited Reporting'. It was written to provide for the harmonization of the ways to gather, and if necessary, to take action on the importance of clinical **safety** information arising in clinical development. However, because clinical **drug** development does not take place at the same pace in all countries or regions, the guidance recognizes that drugs may be marketed in some areas of the world while still in clinical development in others. Thus, the definitions and procedures were harmonized for all drugs being tested or used in humans. Therefore, both pre- and post-marketing phases are covered. It should be recognized that the post-marketing phase is of particular importance to the area of **pharmacoepidemiology** due to the limited sample size in the pre-marketing **controlled clinical trials** and the non-representative nature of the population included in these trials. The guidance makes provisions for **expedited reporting** of **adverse drug reactions** (ADRs) that are both serious and unexpected. Specific criteria for being classified as a 'serious **adverse event** (SAE)' are that it results in death, is **life-threatening**, requires or prolongs hospitalization, results in disability, is a congenital anomaly, jeopardizes the patient according to medical judgment, or requires intervention to prevent one of the other outcomes. In order for the reaction to be subject to expedited reporting rules, it would also need to be 'unexpected', i.e. not be described in the information provided to the researchers or practitioners, and have a reasonable possibility of being related to the drug (i.e. the distinction between an AE and an ADR). By definition, all spontaneous reports are considered to fulfil this last criterion. ADRs that qualify for expedited reporting must be provided to regulatory authorities within 15 calendar days, and if the ADR is either life-threatening or fatal a preliminary communication must be made within 7 days.

See also **CIOMS I, E2B guidance document, E2C guidance document, International Conference on Harmonization, Serious Adverse Event (SAE)/ Serious Adverse Drug Reaction.**

E2B guidance document

An **International Conference on Harmonization** (ICH) guidance document entitled 'Data Elements for Transmission of Individual Case Safety Reports'. This guidance serves as the basis for electronic data interchange. It is to facilitate the transmission of information from one database to another allowing for a more efficient process by eliminating duplicate data entry. The standards for electronic data interchange required some structuring of the clinical history and **adverse event** (AE) information as well as the mechanism to ensure accuracy of the data transmission process. The subtopics are handled by the M1 and M2 expert working groups. Medical terminology (M1) is a terminology designed to support the classification, retrieval, presentation and communication of medical information, especially as it relates to pharmaceuticals. It includes terminology from **ICD-9**, the **WHO-ART**, and the **Food and Drug Administration** (FDA) **COSTART** developed for their AE database. In addition, it includes nomenclature for standard laboratory tests and terms for social history.

The M2 expert working group for 'Electronic Standards for the Transfer of Regulatory Information and Data' has developed the procedures needed to ensure data integrity and security when transmitted electronically. In addition, they have developed the file format needed to accommodate the information provided in the single E2B case transmission.

See also **CIOMS 1A, E2A guidance document, E2C guidance document, International Conference on Harmonization.**

E2C guidance document

An **International Conference on Harmonization** (ICH) guidance document entitled '**Periodic Safety Updates Reports** (PSUR)' which provides guidance on the content, format, and frequency of reports to regulators which summarizes the safety experience with pharmaceuticals. The objective of E2C is to avoid duplication of effort and to ensure that important data are submitted with consistency to regulatory authorities.

See also **CIOMS II, E2A guidance document, E2B guidance document, International Conference on Harmonization, Periodic Safety Update Report**.

E3 guidance document
An **International Conference on Harmonization** (ICH) guidance document entitled 'Study Reports'.

E4 guidance document
An **International Conference on Harmonization** (ICH) guidance document entitled 'Dose–Response Information to Support Drug Registration'.

E5 guidance document
An **International Conference on Harmonization** (ICH) guidance document entitled 'Ethnic Factors in the Acceptability of Foreign Clinical Data'.

E6 guidance document
An **International Conference on Harmonization** (ICH) guidance document entitled 'Good Clinical Practice: Consolidated Guidelines'.

E7 guidance document
An **International Conference on Harmonization** (ICH) guidance document on 'Special Populations' entitled 'Studies in Support of Special Populations: Geriatrics'.

E8 guidance document
An **International Conference on Harmonization** (ICH) guidance document on 'Clinical Trial Design' entitled 'General Considerations for Clinical Trials'.

E9 guidance document
An **International Conference on Harmonization** (ICH) guidance document on 'Statistical Considerations' entitled 'Statistical Principles for Clinical Trials'.

EAACI
European Academy of Allerology and Clinical Immunology.

EAB
Ethical Advisory Board (term used in some countries).

EAG
Expert Advisory Group.

EAN
European Article Number.

Early and Periodic Screening, Diagnosis, and Treatment (EPSDT)
Covers screening and diagnostic services to determine physical or mental defects in recipients under age 21, as well as health care and other measures to correct or ameliorate any defects and chronic conditions discovered.

EASR
European Age Standardized Rate. A measure of the **incidence** of disease.

EASSI
European Association of Surgical Sutures Industry.

Eastern Cooperative Oncology Group scale (ECOG)

A scale for measuring performance status, in clinical trials, on a scale from 0 to 4. Most trials require ECOG 0 or 1, but it is not unusual to find trials that admit patients with ECOG status 2. Only very few trials admit patients with ECOG status 3. It can be hard to objectively rate your own performance status.

See also **Karnofsky status**.

ECOG Performance Status Scale and Comparison to Karnofsky Status

ECOG status	Meaning	Karnofsky status
0	No Symptoms, fully active, able to work	100
1	Symptomatic, but not spending extra time in bed. Able to do light work	80 or 90
2	In bed less than 50% of the day, unable to work, but can take care of self	60 or 70
3	In bed more than 50% of the day, but not bedridden, limited self care	40 or 50
4	Completely bedridden	20 or 30

EBD see **EU birth date**.

EBHC see **evidence-based health care**.

eBNF

Electronic version of the **British National Formulary** on a CD-ROM.

EBP

Evidence-based practice.

EBSA

European Biosafety Association.

e-c

Enteric-coated.

EC

1. see **Ethics Committee**.
2. see **European Community/European Commission**.

ECACC

European Collection of Animal Cell Cultures.

Ecbolic

Oxytocic.

ECF see **Extended Care Facility**.

ECJ see **European Court of Justice**.

ECOG scale see **Eastern Cooperative Oncology Group scale**.

ecological epidemiology

A branch of epidemiology which views disease as a result of the ecological interactions between populations of hosts and parasites.

Compare **classical epidemiology**.

ecological survey (Epidemiology)
Based on aggregated data for some **populations** as it exists at some point or points in time; to investigate the relationship of an exposure to a known or presumed **risk factor** for a specified **outcome**.

economic analysis
Comparison of the **costs** and **outcomes** of alternative health care interventions.
Also called **economic evaluation**.
See **cost–benefit analysis, cost-effectiveness analysis, cost-utility analysis**.

economic credentialing (US)
The use of economic criteria, unrelated to quality of care or professional competency, in determining an individual's qualifications for initial or continuing hospital medical staff membership or privileges. Economic credentialing has become a controversial topic involving much concern about ethics, yet, it remains the most powerful form of controlling the behaviour of doctors. Other forms of control include utilization review, certification, exclusive provider panels and more.
See also **credentialing**.

economic efficiency
In a health care context, economic efficiency is a measure of how well resources are distributed to achieve the most favourable outcomes at the lowest cost. In the current environment, many believe that the marginal cost of care exceeds the marginal benefits, i.e., that the current system is economically inefficient.

economic evaluation see **economic analysis**.

ECPHIN
European Community Pharmaceutical Information Network.

ECR see **extra contractual referral**.

ECS (UK)
The Export Certificate System at the **Medicines Control Agency**.

ECT
Enteric-coated tablet.

EC Text see **Rules Governing Medicinal Products in the EC**.

ED see **enumeration district**.

ED$_{50}$ see **median effective dose**.

EDL
Essential Drug List.

EDM see **Essential Drugs and Medicines Policy**.

EDMA
European Diagnostic Manufacturers Association.

EEA see **European Economic Area**.

EEC
European Economic Community, see **European Union**.

EER
　　Experimental event rate, see **event rate**.

EERC
　　European Ethical Review Committee.

effectiveness
　　The extent to which a medical intervention achieves its intended benefit in an ideal situation. It is a measure of the drug's or the intervention's desired influence on a disease condition when used under ordinary circumstances. Effectiveness must be proven by substantial evidence consisting of adequate and well controlled investigations. The investigations must include human studies by qualified experts that prove the drug will have the effect claimed in its **labelling**. **Clinical trials** that assess effectiveness are sometimes called **management trials**.
　　See also **intention-to-treat**.

effect size
　　1. A generic term for the estimate of effect in a study.
　　2. A dimensionless measure of effect that is typically used for continuous **data** when different scales (e.g. for measuring pain) are used to measure an **outcome** and is usually defined as the difference in means between the intervention and **control** groups divided by the **standard deviation** of the control or both groups.

efficacy
　　It is the property that enables drugs (or any medical intervention) to produce beneficial responses under ideal conditions. The properties of drugs are differentiated into two groups, those which cause them to associate with the **receptors** (**affinity**) and those that produce stimulus (efficacy). It is often used to characterize the level of maximal responses induced by **agonists**. Not all agonists of a receptor are capable of inducing identical levels of maximal responses as maximal response depends on the efficiency of receptor coupling, i.e. from the cascade of events, in which, the binding of the drug to the receptor leads to the observed biological effect. Efficacy is not synonymous with **intrinsic activity**. Clinical trials that assess efficacy are sometimes called **explanatory trials** and are restricted to participants who fully cooperate.
　　See also **affinity**, **effectiveness**, **intrinsic activity**.

EFGCP
　　European Forum on Good Clinical Practice.

EFL see external finance limit.

EFPIA see European Federation of Pharmaceutical Industries Association.

EFTA see European Free Trade Association.

EGA
　　European Generic Manufacturers Association.

EHMA
　　European Health care Management Association.

EHR
　　Electronic Health Record.

EINECS
　　The European Inventory of Existing Chemical Substances.

EIR (US)
Establishment Inspection Report (**Food and Drug Administration**).

ELA see **Establishment License Application**.

electrolyte
A substance (e.g. acid, base, salt) that dissociates into ions when in aqueous solution and that provides ionic conductivity. Electrolytes are lost from the body through perspiration as salts, causing impairment of central nervous system functions if not adequately replaced.

Electronic Data Interchange (EDI)
The automated exchange of data and documents in a standardized format. In health care, some common uses of this technology include claims submission and payment, eligibility and hospital referral authorization.

electronic medical record (EMR)
A system whose objective is to facilitate meeting the needs of provider for real-time data access and evaluation in medical care. Together with clinical workstations and clinical data repository technologies, the EMR provides the mechanism for longitudinal data storage and access. A motivation for health care entities to implement this technology derives from the need for medical outcome studies, more efficient care, speedier communication among providers and management of health plans.

Electronic Prescribing Analysis and Cost (ePACT) (UK)
ePACT is designed to give authorized users early access to their prescribing data from the PPA database, as opposed to waiting until a quarterly PACT Standard report is issued.

ePACT for Health Authorities (HAs)
HAs can use this system to view prescribing data at the following levels:
- Practice
- **Primary care group** (PCG)
- HA.

Regional Offices and the Prescribing Support Unit (on behalf of the **National Health Service Executive**) also have access to this system.

Each month a user requests data from the **Prescription Pricing Authority** (PPA), which is then downloaded to a PC ready for analysis. The 'Request Generator' allows the user to formulate requests based on one or more reporting periods, prescribing organizations and **British National Formulary** (BNF) classification. A 'tagging' facility is included to permit a user to create specific prescribing requests (e.g. inner city practices or new drugs). Generated requests are maintained using the 'Request Explorer', which allows a user to download, merge or cancel a request.

The 'Analysis Tool' allows the user to interpret the downloaded data and display it in user defined graphs and tabular reports. These can be viewed on screen, saved to disk or printed.

ePACT for PCGs:
This is the internet version of ePACT available at the PPA Website address (www.ppa.nhs.uk). It differs from ePACT for HAs in that it allows users real time on-line access to their prescribing data held on the database. Like ePACT for HAs, data can be selected according to reporting period, prescribing organization, and BNF classification. A 'tagging' facility for specific requests is also available. Information is presented in graph format or tabular reports and can be viewed on screen or printed.

ePACT for Community Units:
Like ePACT for PCGs, this is an on-line system available at the PPA website. This system is used by CUs to monitor community nurse prescribing at the following levels:
- Nurse prescriber
- Community Unit.

User-defined graphs and tabular reports can be produced according to reporting period, prescribing organization and BNF classification.

Electronic Standards for the Transfer of Information (ESTRI)
An expert working group (EWG) established by **International Conference on Harmonization** (ICH) to harmonize the standards of the transfer of electronic information to promote communication between industry and the regulators as well as between the regulators.

eligible patients (Clinical Trials)
Patients who meet the **inclusion** and **exclusion criteria** indicated in the **protocol**.

elimination
The process achieving the reduction of the concentration of a **xenobiotic** including its **metabolism**.
See also **biliary excretion, biotransformation, metabolism**.

elimination half-life
The time it takes for the body to eliminate or break down half of a dose of a pharmacological agent.

ELISA see enzyme-linked immunosorbent assay.

elixir
A clear sweetened, usually hydroalcoholic liquid containing flavouring substances, and sometimes active medicinal agents, used orally as a vehicle or for the effect of the medicinal agent contained.

EMACOLEX
A group of European lawyers from health departments and regulatory agencies.

emancipated minor (Clinical Trials) (US)
A legal status conferred upon persons who have not yet attained the age of legal competency as defined by State law (for such purposes as consenting to medical care), but who are entitled to treatment as if they had by virtue of assuming adult responsibilities such as being self-supporting and not living at home.
See also **mature minor**.

EMBASE see Excerpta Medica database.

embrocation
A liniment; a preparation designed to be applied to the intact skin.

embryo
Early stages of a developing organism, broadly used to refer to stages immediately following fertilization of an egg through implantation and very early pregnancy (i.e. from conception to the eighth week of **pregnancy**).
See also **fetus**.

embryotoxin
A material harmful to a developing **embryo** at a concentration that has no adverse effect on the pregnant female.

EMEA see **European Medicines Evaluation Agency**.

emergency drug release programme (Clinical Trials) (Canada)
An **investigator** can ask the Bureau of Human Prescription Drugs of Health and Welfare Canada for the release, on emergency basis, of an experimental drug if the drug **manufacturer** has authorized its release. The programme applies to new drugs not yet marketable and drugs currently used in **clinical trials**.

emetic see **emetogenic**.

emetogenic
A substance that causes vomiting; used to treat some cases of poisoning and **drug overdose**.

emmenagogue
An agent that induces menstruation.

emollient
An agent that softens or soothes the skin.

empirical
Results based on experience (or observation) rather than on reasoning alone.

emulsion
A preparation of one liquid distributed in small globules throughout a second liquid.

EN
Harmonized Standard; a European Norm (EN) that has been accepted by all **Member States** and published in the Official Journal of the European Community.

endemic
A term used to describe a disease that is always present in a certain **population** of people or where the levels of infection do not exhibit wide fluctuations through time in a defined place. For microparasites like measles, the term is used slightly differently to indicate an infection which can persist in a population in the long-term without needing to be reintroduced from outside.
See also **endemic fadeout**, **stable endemicity**.

endemic fadeout
Parasite extinction occurring because **endemic** levels are so low that it is possible for small **stochastic** fluctuations to remove all parasites.
See also **epidemic fadeout**.

End-of-Phase II Meeting (US)
The **Food and Drug Administration** allows for meetings with **sponsors** after the completion of their **Phase II clinical trials**. These are known as end-of-phase II meetings and are intended to provide a forum for discussion of phase II results and plans for upcoming phase III clinical trials.

end point (Clinical Trials)
An indicator measured in a **subject/patient** or biological sample to assess the **safety**,

efficacy, or other objective or goal of a **clinical trial**. It is scientifically very important that the goals for clinical trials be selected and clearly defined in advance and documented in the **protocol**. Typical end points include measurements of **toxicity**, response rate and survival.
See also **surrogate marker**.

Engineering and Analytical Center (US)
A centre for testing **medical devices**, radiation-emitting products and **radioactive drugs**. It is based at Winchester, Massachusetts and operated by the **Food and Drug Administration**.

enrolled subject (Clinical Trials)
Any **subject/patient** signing an **informed consent** or any subject/patient having a **legally acceptable representative** signing an informed consent to permit participation in a **clinical trial**.
Compare **entered subject**.

ENS see European Nervous System.

ENT
Ear, nose and throat.

entered subject (Clinical Trials)
Any **subject** who has signed the **informed consent** form, met all the **inclusion** and **exclusion criteria** set out in the **protocol**, and has been administered or exposed to the **investigational product**.
Compare **enrolled subject**.

enteric coating (ec, or ECT)
Coating given to a tablet or pill to prevent the disintegration in the stomach and ensure that the ingredients pass unchanged through the stomach into the intestines.

enumeration district (ED)
The smallest unit for census data – about 200 homes.

enzyme-inducing drugs
Drugs that induce a proliferation of smooth endoplasmic reticulum in hepatocytes and hence lead to an increase in **P450** enzymes. This can lead to **tolerance** that develops with certain drugs. The extent of this induction depends on the nature of the drugs in question as well as their dose. Examples include phenytoin, rifampicin, the barbiturates, carbamazepine and ethanol.
See also **P450**.

enzyme induction
The process whereby an (inducible) enzyme is synthesized in response to a specific inducer molecule. The inducer molecule (often a substrate that needs the catalytic activity of the inducible enzyme for its **metabolism**) combines with a repressor and thereby prevents the blocking of an operator by the repressor leading to the translation of the gene for the enzyme.

enzyme-linked immunosorbent assay (ELISA)
A technique using the antigen binding properties of antibodies to detect specific antigens or antibodies. Visualization is typically made possible by enzyme induced colour formation.

enzyme repression
The mode by which the synthesis of an enzyme is prevented by repressor molecules. In many cases, the end product of a synthesis chain (e.g. an amino acid) acts as a feedback co-repressor

by combining with an intracellular aporepressor protein, so that this complex is able to block the function of an operator. As a result, the whole operation is prevented from being transcribed into mRNA, and the expression of all enzymes necessary for the synthesis of the end product enzyme is abolished.

EOF see **Greek National Drug Service.**

EOQ
European Organization for Quality.

EORTC
European Organization for Research and Treatment of Cancer.

EP
European Parliament.

ePACT see **Electronic Prescribing Analysis and Cost.**

EPAR see **European Public Assessment Report.**

EPC
European Patent Convention.

EPhMRA
European Pharmaceutical Market Research Association.

EPID
Extended (also Expanded) Public Information Document. It is provided by the pharmaceutical industry to the public, and contains information about their products.

epidemic
A rapid increase in the levels of an infection. It is distinctive of the microparasitic infections (with long-term immunity and short generation times) that an epidemic is typically heralded by an exponential rise in the number of cases in time and a consequent decline as prone numbers are exhausted. Epidemics may begin from the introduction of a novel pathogen (or strain) to a previously unexposed (naïve) population or as a consequence of the regrowth of susceptible numbers some time after an earlier epidemic due to the identical infectious agent.
Compare **endemic**, **pandemic**.

epidemic fadeout
Parasite extinction occurring because numbers are so low immediately following an **epidemic** that it is possible for small **stochastic** fluctuations to remove all parasites.
Compare **endemic fadeout**.

epidemiology
('*Epi*' – upon, '*demos*' – the people, 'logos' – study of.) The logical and systematic study of the distribution and determinants of health-related states or events in specified populations to understand the complexities of disease and the application of this study to the control of health problems (Center for Disease Control).

Epidemiology includes (1) the methods for measuring the health of groups and for determining the attributes and exposures that influence health; (2) the study of the occurrence of disease in its natural habitat rather than the controlled environment of the laboratory; and (3) the methods for the quantitative study of the distribution, variation, and determinants of health-related outcomes in specific groups (populations) of individuals, and the application of

this study to the diagnosis, treatment, and prevention of these states or events (Last, 1995). This broad science includes the following disciplines:
1. Descriptive (Observational) Epidemiology: The most basic form of epidemiology, which is the description of the patterns of occurrence of health-related states or events in groups. Descriptive epidemiology is usually one of the first things done at the scene of any disease outbreak.
2. Analytical Epidemiology: The design, execution and analysis of studies in groups to evaluate potential associations between risk factors and health outcomes.
3. Clinical Epidemiology: The application of the logical and quantitative concepts and methods of epidemiology to problems (diagnostic, prognostic, therapeutic, and preventive) encountered in the clinical delivery of care to individual patients. The population aspect of epidemiology is present because these individual patients are members of conceptual populations.
4. Infectious Disease Epidemiology: Classica epidemiology; the study of epidemics; the study of the dynamic factors involved in the transmission of infectious agents in populations. Some include the products of the application of the methods of this discipline, the natural history of disease (information about how each disease spreads through groups and how a case of that disease develops in an individual).

EPIF (Finland)
The Finnish Pharmaceutical Industry Association.

episode of care (US)
A term used to describe and measure the various health care services and encounters rendered in connection with identified injury or period of illness.

epispastic (vesicant)
A blistering drug or agent.

EPO
1. See **Exclusive Provider Organization**.
2. European Patent Office.

EPRG
European Pharmacovigilance Research Group.

equilibrium (Epidemiology)
A state in which a system is not changing. A population size might be at a static equilibrium at which nothing is happening (there are no births or deaths) or a dynamic equilibrium at which different processes are balanced (there are the same numbers of births and deaths). More generally, the state to which a system eventually evolves, for example sustained periodic oscillations, might be called an equilibrium.

equipoise (Clinical Trials)
A concept in medical ethics that entails the requirement to believe that, in initiating a controlled study, there is no reason to suppose that one therapy is necessarily superior to another. Ethically, without this belief, patients must receive the perceived superior treatment.

equitable (Clinical Trials)
Fair or just; used in the context of selection of subjects to indicate that the benefits and burdens of research are fairly distributed.

equivalence
In simple terms, drugs that share the same **bioavailability**, or chemical structure, or therapeutic response are called 'equivalent'. In the US, the federal Task Force on Prescription Drugs recommended, in 1969, that the words 'generic equivalents' no longer be used in describing and comparing drug preparations.
Compare **bioavailability, generic drugs**.

ER
1. See **essential requirements**.
2. Extended release **medicinal product** formulation, see **sustained release**.

ergonomics
The study of human characteristics for appropriate design of living and work environments.

escape medication (Clinical Trials)
The additional medication provided to a patient to treat any pain occurring during a study and which is not being controlled despite the use of the study medication. Such additional therapy is necessary when the pain killing activity of a new drug has not been established yet in man. Escape medication may also be necessary if the study design involves periods of only **placebo** medication. The additional pain killing therapy is then taken by the patient as needed. It would be unethical to conduct such a study without providing escape medication to alleviate pain.
See also **rescue medication**.

ESCP
European Society of Clinical Pharmacy.

ESOP
European Society Of Pharmacovigilance.

Essential Community Providers (US)
Providers such as community health centres that have traditionally served low-income populations.

essential documents (Clinical Trials)
Documents which individually and collectively permit evaluation of the conduct of a study and the quality of the data produced.

Essential Drugs and Medicines Policy (EDM)
All activities related to medicines are carried out by the **World Health Organization** Department of EDM. The department is responsible for the development, harmonization and promotion of international standards of modern and traditional medicines, and for the exchange of pharmaceutical information with the private and public sector. EDM aims to provide governments and pharmaceutical **manufacturers** with the means to establish and maintain mechanisms which ensure the **quality, safety, efficacy** and rational use of pharmaceutical products, supports drug **regulatory authorities** and prevention of counterfeit drugs. EDM also collaborates with the United Nations (UN) on substance abuse related to the UN Conventions on Narcotic Drugs (1961) and Psychotropic Substances (1971). Activities in this area are carried out by the EDM Quality assurance and Safety of Medicines (QSM) team, and Traditional Medicines (TRM) team with support from the other teams.

essential requirements (ER)
The requirements, laid down in Annex I of the **Medical Device Directives**, which any device

must fulfil before a **CE** marking may be affixed. Compliance with most ERs is presumed when the company is deemed in compliance with certain harmonized standards.

ESRA see **European Society of Regulatory Affairs**.

ESTRI see **Electronic Standards for the Transfer of Information**.

Establishment License Application (ELA) (US)

An application to the **Center for Biologics Evaluation and Review** group at the **Food and Drug Administration** requesting **approval** for a facility to be used in the manufacture of a **biological product**.

estimate of effect

In studies of the effects of health care, the observed relationship between an intervention and an **outcome** expressed as, for example, a **number needed to treat**, **odds ratio**, risk difference, **relative risk**, standardized mean difference, or weighted mean difference.

Also called treatment effect.

ethical drug see **prescription only medicine**.

Ethics Committee (EC)

An independent body (a review board, a committee, institutional, regional, national, or supranational) that consists of medical/scientific professionals and non-medical/non-scientific members. The responsibility of an EC is to ensure the protection of the rights, **safety** and well-being of human subjects involved in a trial and thereby provide public assurance of their protection. They achieve this by reviewing and approving/providing favourable opinion on: the trial **protocol**, the suitability of the **investigator**(s), the eligibility of trial subject groups, facilities, adequacy of **confidentiality** safeguards and the methods and material to be used in obtaining and documenting **informed consent** of the trial subjects.

The Committee reviews all of these trial's aspects on behalf of investigators who may be located in different institutions or practices within or across national boundaries. The legal status, composition, function, operations and regulatory requirements pertaining to independent EC may differ among countries, but should allow the Independent EC to act in agreement with **good clinical practice**. A list of the EC members, their positions and a description of its working procedures including response times should be publicly available. The EC Review Committee and the Quorn Research Review Committee are examples of central ECs.

See also **Institutional Review Board, Research Ethics Board**.

Ethics Committee decision (Clinical Trials)

The decision of the Ethics Committee whereby it is documented by the following outcomes:
1. approvable/favourable opinion
2. modification(s) required prior to **approval**/favourable opinion
3. disapproval/negative opinion, and
4. suspension of any prior approval/favourable opinion.

ethnographic research

Ethnography is the study of people and their culture. Ethnographic research, also called fieldwork, involves observation of and interaction with the persons or group being studied in the group's own environment, often for long periods of time.

See also **fieldwork**.

etiology see **aetiology**.

EU see **European Union**.

EU birth date (EBD)
The date for the first **marketing authorization** (MA) for a **medicinal product** in the European Union (EU) to the MA holder:
* For medicinal products authorized through the **centralized procedure**, the EBD is the date of the MA granted by the **European Commission** (Commission Decision Date)
* For medicinal products authorized through the **mutual recognition procedure**, the EBD is the date of the MA granted by the **Reference Member State**
* For products authorized nationally, the MA holder may propose an EBD which can be applied to reporting requirements across the **Member States**.

EUCOMED
European Confederation of Medicinal Suppliers Association.

eudismic ratio
The **potency** of the **eutomer** relative to that of the **distomer**.

EUDRA
European Union Drug Regulatory Authorities.

EUDRANET see **European Union Drug Regulatory Authorities Network**.

EUDRATRACK
Tracking system for procedures for **marketing authorization** of **medicinal products** carried out by **Member States** through the **mutual recognition procedure**.

EudraWatch
A **pharmacovigilance** database installed at the **European Medicines Evaluation Agency** to manage and to transmit individual case safety reports of **adverse drug reactions** (ADRs) suspected to have been provoked by medicines for human use. It was established in parallel with the **EUDRANET** to meet the pharmacovigilance and information exchange requirements of the **marketing authorizations** system. It comprises two similar applications – one for veterinary and one for human products. The content and format specifications of EudraWatch pharmacovigilance reports follow the **International Conference on Harmonization** (ICH) guidelines. **Member States** send suspected ADR reports electronically to the EMEA using the ICH E2b guidelines.

EURATOM
European Atomic Energy Community.

EuroDMF see **European Drug Master File**.

EuroDirect Service (UK)
A **Medicines Control Agency** (MCA) publication service set up in October 1993 for two reasons: to enable companies to obtain texts of draft and finalized **Committee for Proprietary Medicinal Products** (CPMP) guidelines including those developed under the auspices of the **International Conference on Harmonization** (ICH); and secondly the **European Commission** had asked **Member States** if they would distribute these guidelines for them since they did not have resources to do so. Eurodirect provides unpublished draft and finalized texts (CPMP, ICH, and selected European Commission documents), as well as selected CPMP position papers covering the major technical and operational areas of **quality**, biotechnology, clinical (general), clinical (therapeutic class), herbal medicinal products, pharmacological-

toxicological, pharmacovigilance, core **Summary of Product Characteristics** for groups of products and information for applicants for **marketing authorizations**.

Eurom VI
European Federation of Precision Mechanical and Optical Industries.

Euromcontact
European Federation of National Associations of Contact Lens Manufacturers.

Euro-SPC
The concept/plan to harmonize the **Summary of Product Characteristics** (SPCs) for high technology (**centralized procedure**) and **mutual recognition procedure** within the **Committee for Proprietary Medicinal Products** where there is a common SPC throughout the **European Union**.

Eur Ph see European Pharmacopoeia.

EuropaBio
European Association for BioIndustries.

European Clearing House on Health Systems Reforms (ECHHSR)
Aims to set up a Europe-wide network of researchers and policy analysts, provide a forum for exchanging information on health systems reform, promote cross-national policy research and facilitate rapid feedback into practice, and encourage multi-centre comparative research. In support of these activities the Network is developing a database of published and 'grey' literature on European health systems reform, together with details of ongoing research projects. The database contains information on major changes in the structure and financing of health services in **European Union (EU) Member States** and other European countries. Topics covered include:
- **Managed care**
- Competition
- The shift from secondary to **primary care**
- Health insurance
- Decentralizaton
- **Purchaser/Provider** split.

European Commission see Commission of the European Communities.

European Community (EC)
The legal foundation of the **European Union** (EU) comprising UK, Germany, Netherlands, Greece, Spain, Portugal, Sweden, Finland, Austria, Ireland, Italy, France, Belgium, Luxembourg and Denmark. It used to be called the EEC. It is often used to refer to the EU but the two are not synonymous. It is a single institutional structure managing the three Treaties: European Coal & Steel Community, European Atomic Energy Community, and European Economic Community. The five Institutions of the EC are:
- The **European Commission** (EC)
- The **Council of Ministers**
- The **European Parliament** (EP)
- The **European Court of Justice** (ECJ)
- The Court of Auditors.

European Court of Justice (ECJ)
The ECJ exists to safeguard European Community Law. It also rules on whether actions by the

Commission, the Council of Ministers, and Members of Governments are compatible with Treaties. Judgment is achieved by a majority vote between the ECJ's judges. The ECJ is a final court of appeal against decisions in **Member States**.

European Drug Master File (EuroDMF)
A file procedure that the **Committee for Proprietary Medicinal Products** (CPMP) is introducing for **active ingredients** (AIs) in association with the **EC Pharmaceutical Directives** to rationalize current arrangement. The document is to be available to any **active ingredient** manufacturer (AIM) who is not the applicant for **marketing authorization** (MA) as an alternative option to the inclusion of all data within the MA application. The EuroDMF documentation should include sufficient information to establish the quality of the AI and to show that the material is adequately controlled by the specification proposed by the MA applicant.

See also **Drug Master File**.

European Economic Area (EEA)
Includes all the **Member States** of the **European Community** together with Iceland, Liechtenstein and Norway.

European Electrotechnical Standards Coordinating Committee (CENELEC) *(Comité Européen de Coordination des Normes Electrotechniques)* (European Union)
The recognized source of published standards for technical requirements in the **Directives**. This body, like **CEN**, start with the available standards from the International Electrotechnical Commission (IEC) and, if deemed suitable, are taken and adopted unchanged. CEN standards are not obligatory but compliance by the manufacturer is considered to be confirmatory evidence for compliance with relevant essential requirements.

European Federation of Pharmaceutical Industries Association (EFPIA)
The representative voice of the pharmaceutical industry in Europe. It was founded in 1978 and is currently based in Brussels. Through its membership (national pharmaceutical industry associations and major companies), EFPIA represents the common views and interests of over 2000 pharmaceutical companies undertaking research, development and manufacturing of medical products for human use in Europe. The aim of EFPIA is to promote pharmaceutical research and development in order to bring new medicines onto the market in the interest of patients and human health world-wide. The objectives of EFPIA are:
- Provides a link between the research-driven pharmaceutical industry and policy-makers at European and international level
- Maintains close links with **European Union** (EU) institutions (Parliament, Commission, Council, Economic & Social Committee), regulatory authorities (**European Medicines Evaluation Agency**), health care professionals and patient and consumer associations
- Is consulted and informs its members on European initiatives and developments affecting the pharmaceutical industry
- Organizes conferences, 'info days', visits to pharmaceutical companies, etc. to keep its target audiences informed of the contribution of the pharmaceutical industry to society, its needs and recent developments
- Produces and distributes economic surveys, publications and position papers on a wide range of priority issues such as:
  - Single market and industrial policy
  - Research and innovation
  - EU enlargement

- National pricing and reimbursement policies
- **Regulatory affairs**
- Product liability
- **Clinical trials**
- Orphan medicinal products
- **Intellectual property** rights (patents, trade marks, etc.)
- Biotechnological inventions
- Environmental legislation
- Marketing and electronic commerce, etc.

European Free Trade Association (EFTA)

Founded by the Stockholm Convention as a response to the **EEC** in 1960, with the objectives of removing import duties, quotas and other obstacles and of upholding liberal, non-discriminatory practice in world trade. It consisted of: Austria, Switzerland, Sweden, Ireland, Denmark, UK, Portugal and Norway. Finland became an associate member in 1961 (full member in 1986) and Iceland joined the EFTA in 1970 while Liechtenstein became a member in 1991. Three countries then left to join the EC: Denmark and the UK in 1972 and Portugal in 1985. In 1979, the registration authorities in these countries agreed on a 'Scheme for the Mutual Recognition of Pharmaceutical Evaluation Reports (see **PIC**). Under this scheme, a participating authority may be requested, either by the manufacturer, or by another participating authority, to draw up an evaluation report on any registered pharmaceutical product (including products developed outside the EFTA countries) which may be used by the other member countries for guidance in considering an application for **marketing authorization**. In May 1992, EFTA and EC Ministers signed the agreement establishing the EEC.

European Medicines Evaluation Agency (EMEA) (European Union)

A **European Union** (EU) body whose task it is to authorize **medicinal products** and provide scientific advice of high quality to the Community institutions and **Member States** in relation to authorization and supervision of medicinal products. The Council of the EU adopted, in June 1993, three **Directives** and a **Regulation**, which together form the legal basis of the EMEA system.

The EMEA was established by Council **Regulation (EEC) No 2309/93** of 22 July 1993 (OJ EC L 214 of 24/8/1993) and London was chosen as its seat by decision of the Heads of State and Governments on 29 October 1993. The EMEA mission is to contribute to the protection and promotion of public and animal health by:

- Mobilizing scientific resources from throughout the EU to provide high quality evaluation of medicinal products, to advise on research and development programmes and to provide useful and clear information to users and health professionals
- Developing efficient and transparent procedures to allow timely access by users to innovative medicines through a single European **marketing authorization** (MA)
- Controlling the safety of medicines for human and animals, in particular through a **pharmacovigilance** network and the establishment of safe limits for residues in food-producing animals.

Main tasks of the EMEA

- Provide the **Member States** (MSs) and the Community institutions with the best possible scientific advice on questions concerning quality, safety and efficacy of medicinal products for human and veterinary use.
- Establish a multinational scientific expertise through the mobilizaton of existing national resources in order to achieve a single evaluation via a centralized or decentralized MA system.

- Organize speedy, transparent and efficient procedures for the authorization, surveillance and, where appropriate, withdrawal of products in the EU.
- Advise companies on the conduct of pharmaceutical research.
- Reinforce the supervision of existing medicinal products in coordinating national pharmacovigilance and inspection activities.
- Create the necessary databases and telecommunication facilities to promote a more rational drug use.

Procedures for authorizing medicinal products in the EU
Since 1995, two new registration procedures for human and veterinary **medicinal products** have become available throughout the EU: The **centralized procedure** and the **mutual recognition procedure** (de-centralized procedure).

Structure of the EMEA
- An Executive Director who is the legal representative of the Agency
- A Management Board which comprises two representatives from each MS, of the **European Parliament** and of the EC. The Board meets four times a year.
- Two scientific committees responsible for formulating the Agency's opinion on any question relating to the evaluation of medicines for human use (the **Committee for Proprietary Medicinal Products** (CPMP)) and veterinary use (the **CVMP**). Both committees meet every month and have two members per Member State, appointed to give independent scientific advice to the EMEA.
- A technical and administrative Secretariat under the supervision of the Executive Director.

See also **centralized procedure, Committee for Proprietary Medicinal Products, Committee for Veterinary Medicinal Products, mutual recognition procedure**.

European Nervous System (ENS)

It is an EC **pharmacovigilance** telematics pilot joint project between the pharmacovigilance centres in Spain, France and the UK (Post Licensing Division of the **Medicines Control Agency**).

European Parliament (EP)

A parliament representing all **Member States** (MSs) of the **European Union**. The members (MEPs) are elected by the people of the MS as in any other parliamentary election for a term of 5 years. Its powers are somewhat different to those of the national parliaments (such as the UK Parliament) in that it can only suggest new legislation, and then react to what is brought to it by the Commission.

European Pharmaceutical Wholesaler Association (GIRP) *(Groupement International de la Répartition Pharmaceutique Européenne)*

The international umbrella organization of pharmaceutical wholesalers' associations in Europe. Founded in 1960, GIRP has 20 national member associations and represents more than 450 pharmaceutical full-line wholesalers serving 18 European countries, including every member state of the **European Union** (EU). Employing around 70 000 staff, these companies distribute medicines valued annually at more than 65 billion EURO from their **manufacturers** to community and hospital pharmacies and dispensing doctors.

GIRP facilitates the exchange of views between its member organizations, and co-ordinates opinions and actions needed to safeguard this essential aspect of health care provision. GIRP examines proposed legislation where there may be an adverse impact on the distribution of medicines, possibly resulting in a reduced level of service to the community, or higher costs to national authorities and in turn, the taxpayer. GIRP full members are the national associations of pharmaceutical wholesalers in each country. There are two other classes of membership – the Associate Professional Members are full-line pharmaceutical wholesalers that are members of their national association, which also have direct representation, and the Associate External Members who may be companies or organizations whose business interests are related to the pharmaceutical industry and its distribution. These latter members do not need to be based in Europe.

European Pharmacopoeia (Eur Ph)

A convention signed in 1964 by **six Member States** of the Council of Europe and currently by 19 European countries (EC and non-EC). It focuses on pharmaceutical controls, standardization of quality specifications for **active ingredients, excipients,** and **finished products**. The European Pharmacopoeia publication (Eur Ph) is published under the direction of the Council of Europe in accordance with the convention on the Elaboration of a European Pharmacopoeia (1964).

European Public Assessment Report (EPAR)

A report by the **Committee for Proprietary Medicinal Products** of the reasons for its opinion in favour of granting authorization of a **medicinal product**. The report is made available by the **European Medicines Evaluation Agency** upon request from any interested person after deletion of all commercially confidential information in accordance with Article 12 of Council **Regulation EEC No. 2309/93**.

European Society of Regulatory Affairs (ESRA)

The association for individual **regulatory affairs** professionals with members drawn from over 30 countries worldwide. Although largely focused on Europe, its interests are international, noting that drug development and registration have in most cases to be global in application and that many professionals will therefore be operating in a global environment.

The society, managed by professionals, is dedicated to enabling its members to further their professional standing and capability through the sharing of their experience and knowledge. ESRA has a well-developed meetings programme, including an introductory Course on European Regulatory Affairs, update seminars run in collaboration with the **Committee for Proprietary Medicinal Products** (CPMP) Working Parties, and an annual meeting with representatives of the **European Medicines Central Agency**, CPMP, national agencies and the EC. Its journal, '*ESRA Rapporteur*', published 6 times a year, provides articles on drug development, practical aspects of regulatory affairs and related topics, and other information of interest, as well as summaries and discussion of current and proposed European legislation and guidelines. Its website also provides a members' forum for information and discussion of current regulatory issues.

European Standardization Committee (*Comité Européen de Normalization* (CEN))

The recognized source of published standards for technical requirements in the **Directives**. This body, like **CENELEC**, starts with the available standards from the ISO and, if deemed suitable, are taken and adopted unchanged. CEN standards are not obligatory but compliance by the **manufacturer** is considered to be confirmatory evidence for compliance with relevant **essential requirements**.

European Union (EU)

A group of countries in Europe established by the **Treaty of Rome** in 1957. The members of the EU, united by treaty to establish a unified market, are gradually bringing the economic and monitory affairs closer together. In 1957, the EU consisted of six **Member States** – France, the Federal Republic of Germany, Italy, Belgium, The Netherlands and Luxembourg. Denmark,

UK, and the Republic of Ireland joined the EU in 1973 and completed a transition period to full membership in 1977. Greece joined the EU in 1981 while Portugal and Spain in 1989 and Austria, Finland, and Sweeden in 1995. The founding Treaties have been revised three times: in 1987 (the Single Act), in 1992 (the Treaty on European Union) and in 1997 (Treaty of Amsterdam).

'The EU is the **Competent Authority**, and responsible for the adoption of Decisions on the basis of **Committee for Proprietary Medicinal Products** (CPMP). **Opinions** relating to centrally authorized products and those products subject to the procedure of Articles 13 and 14 Council **Directive 75/319/EEC** as amended' (CPMP/PhVWP/108/99 corr.).

European Union Drug Regulatory Authorities Network (EUDRANET)

An electronic communications system that allows **Member State** authorities to exchange information rapidly with the **European Medicines Evaluation Agency** and the **European Community**. It enables a rapid and reliable communication, as well as mutual trust among all parties involved for the efficient operation of the pharmaceutical authorization system and pharmacovigilance.

Eurosurveillance

A bilingual bulletin, in French and English, which features news of recent **epidemics**, reports of national outbreaks and public health policies of interest to other countries, current trends in **communicable diseases** in **Member States** of the **European Union** (EU), reports of European concerted actions, and collates material of international interest from the national bulletins. It was produced as part of a feasibility study for the development of a European bulletin on communicable diseases as a direct response to the **European Parliament's** call on the **European Community** 'to develop the exchange of information between national health systems'. The study was coordinated by the European Centre for the Epidemiological Monitoring of AIDS of the *Institut de Médecine et d'Épidémiologique Africaines* in Paris, in collaboration with the **Communicable Disease Surveillance Centre** of the **Public Health Laboratory Service** in London, and was funded by Directorate General V of the EC. A permanent French and English editorial team was established which works in liaison with the editorial board composed of the editors of national surveillance bulletins and representatives of countries without such bulletins of the Member States of the EU.

In 1996 the Directorate General V of the **European Commission** agreed to fund the first year of *Eurosurveillance*. In July, *Eurosurveillance* became a monthly publication. It is also available electronically on the world wide web as full text articles in English, French, Portuguese and Spanish at the home page of the European Centre for the Epidemiological Monitoring of AIDS in France.

eutomer

The enantiomer of a chiral compound that is the more potent for a particular action.

See also **distomer**.

event rate (ER) (Clinical Trials)

The proportion of participants in a group in whom an event is observed. Thus, if out of 100 patients the event (e.g. a myocardial infarction) is observed in 19, the event rate is 0.19. **Control event rate** (CER) and **experimental event rate** (EER) are used to refer to this in control and experimental groups of patients respectively.

evidence-based health care (EBHC)

A concept that extends the application of the principles of **evidence-based medicine** to all professions associated with health care, including purchasing and management.

evidence-based medicine (EBM)

'The conscientious, explicit and judicious use of current best evidence in making decisions about the care of individual patients' (Sackett DL *et al.* BMJ 1996; 312: 71–2). 'It is also a way of ensuring that clinical practice is based on the best available evidence through the use of strategies derived from clinical **epidemiology** and **medical informatics**.' (Geddes J *et al.* Br J Psych 1997; 171: 220–225). The practice of EBM means integrating 'individual clinical expertise' with the best available 'external clinical evidence' from systematic research. Despite its very old origins, EBM remains a relatively young field.

'Individual clinical expertise' means the proficiency and judgement that individual clinicians acquire through clinical experience and clinical practice. External clinical evidence both invalidates previously accepted diagnostic tests and treatments and replaces them with new ones that are more powerful, more accurate, more efficacious, and safer. Good doctors use both types of clinical expertise.

EBM is not cost-cutting medicine for the benefit of purchasers and managers to cut the costs of health care. EBM practice aims to identify and apply the most efficient interventions to exploit the **quality** and quantity of life for individual patients; this may raise rather than lower the cost of their care. Evidence-based medicine is not restricted to randomized trials and meta-analyses and their reviews. It involves tracking down the best external evidence with which to answer clinical questions.

Evidence-Based On Call (UK)

This web-based service by the evidence-based medicine organization in the UK aims to provide accurate, up-to-date and evidence-based information created by and for clinicians. The site is planned to feature:
1. detailed description of evidence-based guidelines for key areas, so that a doctor can be in touch with the latest thinking
2. a database of critically appraised topics: one-page summaries of the literature, slanted towards solving clinical problems
3. texts which explore issues around these topics, enabling doctors to develop their background knowledge and pursue areas of interest.

Excerpta Medica database (EMBASE)

A European-based electronic database, produced by Elsevier Science, of pharmacological and biomedical literature covering 3500 journals from 110 countries whilst concentrating in particular on European and Asian sources. It provides current information on drugs and **pharmacology**, and all other aspects of human medicine and related disciplines. Articles are indexed within 15 days of receipt and are online very soon after that. Additional areas of coverage are human medicine and biological sciences, health affairs (occupational and environmental health, **health economics**, policy and management), drug and alcohol **dependence**, psychiatry, forensic science, and pollution control. It contains over 6.5 million documents from 1974 to date, with 375 000 records added annually. Information on veterinary medicine, nursing and dentistry is covered selectively. The database provides the full author abstract for 85% of recent articles.

excipient

Any inert substance added to a **formulation** in order to confer a suitable consistency or form to a drug.

exclusion criteria (Clinical Trials)

A list of criteria, any one of which would exclude a patient from participating in a clinical study.

They are the medical or social reasons why a person may not be allowed to enter a certain trial. For example, most trials do not allow pregnant women to enter, others do not allow people taking certain drugs, while others exclude people with certain illnesses.
See also **inclusion criteria**.

Exclusive Provider Organization (EPO) (US)

A plan which limits coverage of non-emergency care to contracted health care providers. People who belong to an EPO must receive their care from affiliated providers as services rendered by unaffiliated providers will not receive reimbursement. EPO operates similarly to a **Health Management Organization** (HMO) plan but is usually offered as an insured or self-funded product. Sometimes it acts as a **Managed Care Organization** (MCO) that is organized similarly to a **Preferred Provider Organization** in that physicians do not receive capitated payments, but the plan only allows patients to choose medical care from network providers. If a patient elects to seek care outside of the network, then he or she will usually not be reimbursed for the cost of the treatment. It uses a small network of providers and has **primary care** physicians serving as care coordinators (or **gatekeepers**). Typically, an EPO has financial incentives for physicians to practice cost-effective medicine by using either a prepaid **per-capita rate** or a discounted fee schedule, plus a bonus if cost targets are met. Most EPOs are forms of POS plans because they pay for some out-of-network care.

excretion

Ridding the body of waste. The major routes included are renal, biliary, pulmonary and salivary.

expanded access (Clinical Trials)

A general term for the policy and procedure/programme that permits individuals who have serious or **life-threatening** diseases for which there are no alternative therapies, who
- do not qualify for **clinical trials**, or
- live too far from a trial site, or
- do not want to participate for any other reason

to have access to **investigational products** and devices that may be beneficial to them. Examples of expanded availability mechanisms include **treatment INDs**, **Parallel Track Mechanism**, **compassionate use** and **open study protocols**.

Expansion of Quality of Care Measures (Q-SPAN)

A scheme initiated by the **Agency for Health Care Policy and Research** designed to strengthen the science base of quality measurement while expanding the scope and availability of validated, ready-to-use measures. Q-SPAN builds on past work in **quality** measurement by public and private organizations through eight cooperative agreements to develop and test additional clinical performance measures for specific conditions, patient populations and health care settings.

expectedness/unexpectedness of AEs/ADRs

An unexpected **adverse drug reaction** (ADR) is one, the nature or severity of which is not consistent with information in the relevant source document(s). For reporting requirements, all such ADRs should be reported by expedited routes. When the source document for a product not yet approved for marketing in a country does not exist the company's **Investigator's Brochure** will serve as the source document in that country. Reports which add significant information on specificity or severity of a known, already documented serious ADR constitute unexpected events. The term should also include class-related ADRs which are mentioned in the **Summary of Product Characteristics** but which are not specifically described as occurring with this product.

See also **adverse drug reaction, adverse event, expedited reporting**.

expectorant medicine
A **medicinal product** having the property of promoting the ejection of phlegm or other fluid from the respiratory tract.

expedited reporting
The accelerated reporting of **adverse events** (AEs). The purpose of expedited reporting is to make regulators, **investigators** and other appropriate people aware of new, important information on serious **adverse drug reactions** (ADRs). Such reporting will generally involve events previously unobserved or undocumented. In the EU, companies are required to report only serious **unexpected ADRs** using the definitions and standards for expedited reporting in the **Committee for Proprietary Medicinal Products** (CPMP) note for guidance **E2C guidance document** 'Clinical Safety Data Management – Definitions and Standards for Expedited Reporting' (ICH-III.3375/93 Final). All expedited reports should be reported immediately and in no case later than 15 calendar days from receipt. The criteria for when the clock for expedited reporting starts is defined in the Notice to Marketing Authorization Holders Pharmacovigilance Guidelines (CPMP/PhVWP/108/99 corr.).

See also **E2C guidance document**.

expedited review (Clinical Trials) (US)
Review of proposed research by the **Investigational Review Board** (IRB) chair or a designated voting member or group of voting members rather than by the entire IRB. Federal rules permit expedited review for certain kinds of research involving no more than minimal risk and for minor changes in approved research.

experimental group (Clinical Trials)
The arm of a **randomized trial** which gets the new or 'experimental' treatment. In some randomized trials, both of the treatments are standard treatments, or both equally well known new treatments, and in such cases there is no experimental group.

See also **control group**.

experimental study
A true experimental study is one in which subjects are randomly assigned to groups that experience carefully controlled interventions manipulated by the experimenter according to a strict logic allowing causal inference about the effects of the interventions under investigation.

See also **quasi-experimental study**.

expert patients (UK)
Part of the Healthy Citizens Programme announced in 'Saving Lives: Our Healthier Nation'. It is designed to help people with chronic conditions take control over the management of their condition.

expert reports
Reports required by the **regulatory authorities** regarding some aspect of a drug (e.g. **toxicology**, chemistry and **pharmacy**, clinical). The author of such a report must be an expert in that particular field, or may be a company employee, or an external person. Three reports are required in the case of applications for products containing new chemical **active ingredients**. These are chemical, pharmaceutical and biological documentations; on the

toxicological and pharmacological documentation, each is to be written by a specialist in the field respectively.

expiry date
As applied to a **medicinal product**, the term refers to the date after which the product should not be used (administered to a human or animal).

explanatory trial
Trials that are designed to explain how a treatment works, in which patients are typically analysed by treatment received and not as assigned.

exploratory studies (Clinical Trials)
These are the series of studies on which, always, rests the rationale and design of **confirmatory studies**. Like all **clinical trials**, these exploratory studies should have clear and precise objectives. However, in contrast to confirmatory studies, their objectives may not always lead to simple tests of predefined hypotheses. In addition, exploratory studies may sometimes require a more flexible approach to design so that changes can be made in response to accumulating results. Their analysis may entail data exploration; tests of **hypothesis** may be carried out, but the choice of hypothesis may be data-dependent. Such studies cannot be the basis of the formal proof of **efficacy**, although they may contribute to the total body of relevant evidence.

Any individual study may have both confirmatory and exploratory aspects. For example, in most confirmatory studies the data are also subjected to exploratory analyses which serve as a basis for explaining or supporting their findings and for suggesting further hypotheses for later research. The **protocol** should make a clear distinction between the aspects of a study which will be used for confirmatory proof and the aspects which will provide data for exploratory analysis.

See also **confirmatory studies**.

(CPMP/PhVWP/108/99 corr.), The author wishes to thank the European Medicines Evaluation Agency for their contribution.

exponential decay (Epidemiology)
A decline in which the rate of decay is always proportional to the amount of material remaining; the constant of proportionality is the rate constant.

exponential growth (Epidemiology)
An increase in which the rate of growth is always proportional to the amount of material remaining; the constant of proportionality is the rate constant.

exposure odds ratio see **odds ratio**.

extemporaneous preparation
(*Extempore* = spoken or done without preparation, *Ex tempore* Latin for 'on the spur of the moment). It refers to medicinal preparations formulated by pharmacists on their premises. It is recommended that such preparations are freshly prepared no longer than 24 hours before they are dispensed for use as they are prone to rapid deterioration.

external assessment
The part of a **SWOT** analysis where a company's **external environment** is examined.
See also **internal assessment**.

external validity see **applicability**.

extra-amniotic
Injection between chorion and amnion.
Compare **intra-amniotic**.

extradural anaesthesia
Injection of anaesthetic into the space outside the dura mater, the fibrous membrane that envelops the spinal cord.

extravascular administration
Refers to all routes of drug administration except those where a drug is directly introduced into the bloodstream.

eyewash
Sterile solution used to bathe the eye or dilute and flush out irritating foreign matter.

F

F see **availability**.

facility registration (US)
A process dictated by **Food and Drug Administration** regulations requiring the submission of a short form, on an annual basis, which identifies **drug product manufacturers** and their facilities.

FACP (US)
Fellow of the American College of Physicians. A title often used by physicians following their MDs that denotes meeting challenging professional standards in internal medicine, indicating a high level of expertise.

FACS (US)
Fellow of the American College of Surgeons. An honorary degree awarded to surgeons for professional excellence and having met requirements of full surgical training, certification and taking a special examination.

factorial treatment structure
A treatment structure in which one **investigational product** is used in combination with at least one other study treatment in a trial, or where multiples of a defined dose of a specified treatment are used in the same trial.

false negative
The situation that arises in a **clinical trial** whereby an effective treatment is considered ineffective. The term is often used in reference to a diagnostic test when a diseased individual is deemed not to have the disease.
Also known as **beta error, producer's risk, type II error**.

false positive
The situation that arises in a **clinical trial** whereby an ineffective treatment is considered to be effective. The term is often used in reference to a diagnostic test when a non-diseased individual is deemed to have the disease.
Also known as **alpha error, consumer risk, type I error**.

familial
A term describing a disorder or characteristic (such as male pattern baldness) that occurs within a family more often than would be expected.

Family Health Services (FHS) (UK)
Services provided by general practitioners, general dental practitioners, optometrists and pharmacists etc.

Family Health Services Authorities (FHSA) (UK)
Authorities that manage the services provided by general practitioners (GPs), general dental practitioners, retail pharmacists and opticians. These family practitioners are independent contractors and are not employees of the **National Health Service** (NHS). The FHSA works as a corporate body and is accountable to the **Regional Health Authority** (RHA). The terms and conditions under which family practitioners work in the NHS is negotiated nationally. FHSAs are responsible for implementing the national contracts in their areas. There are 90 FHSAs in England. Each conforms to a major local authority area and generally follows the geographical boundaries of each **District Health Authority** (DHA). Each FHSA has a chairman appointed by the Secretary of State, five lay non-executive members and four professional non-executives appointed by the RHA. The FHSA also has a General Manager appointed by the chairman and

non-executive members. FHSAs perform a number of functions. These include managing the contracts of family practitioners, paying practitioners in accordance with contracts, providing information to the public and dealing with complaints made by patients. They also set up and monitor indicative prescribing amounts and work with RHAs on the introduction of GP fundholding.

See also **District Health Authorities, GP Fundholder, National Health Service, Regional Health Authority, Special Health Authorities.**

Family Practice Associates (FPA) (US)
A company that has acquired the practices of many **primary care** physicians and specialists, beginning in San Diego, but now in 28 States, and has gone public, is rapidly growing, and has been emphasizing managed care products.

FAO
United Nations Food and Agricultural Organization.

FAPA
Federation of Asian Pharmaceutical Associations.

FÄPI (Germany)
Fachgesellschaft der Ärzte In der Pharmazeutischen Industrie. German society of physicians in the pharmaceutical industry.

Farmacopoeia Ufficiale della Repubblica Italiana (Italy)
The Italian Pharmacopoeia.

FBC (UK)
1. See **full business case**.
2. Full blood count.

f-c
Film-coated drug product.

FCE see **finished consultant episode**.

FDA see **Food and Drug Administration**.

FDA Advisory Committee (US)
Standing Committees of the **Food and Drug Administration** (FDA) that are called upon, on a regular basis, to provide advice regarding the approvability of new drugs, biologicals and **medical devices**. The opinions rendered at Advisory Committee meetings are non-binding on the FDA. They are, however, generally followed by the Agency.

FDA Advisory Councils
Groups of experts that provide advice and recommendations to the **Food and Drug Administration**.

FDA Approval (US)
A permission granted by **Food and Drug Administration** to market a **drug product**, biological, or **medical device**. It is given only after review of the appropriate market application.

FDA Center for Devices and Radiological Health (US)
The **Food and Drug Administration's** (FDA's) section responsible for ensuring the **safety**

and **effectiveness** of **medical devices** and eliminating unnecessary human exposure to manmade radiation from medical, occupational and consumer products. There are thousands of types of medical devices, from heart pacemakers to contact lenses. Radiation-emitting products regulated by FDA include microwave ovens, video display terminals, medical ultrasound and X-ray machines. The Center accomplishes its mission by:
- reviewing requests to research or market medical devices
- collecting, analysing, and acting on information about injuries and other experiences in the use of medical devices and radiation-emitting electronic products
- setting and enforcing good manufacturing practice regulations and performance standards for radiation-emitting electronic products and medical devices
- monitoring **compliance** and surveillance programmes for medical devices and radiation-emitting electronic products
- providing technical and other non-financial assistance to small **manufacturers** of medical devices.

FDA Code of Federal Regulations see Code of Federal Regulations.

FDA Form 356h (Clinical Trials) (US)
The form that has to be completed when filing for a **New Drug Application**.

FDA Form 483 (Clinical Trials) (US)
The form that has to be completed when filing for inspectional observation.

FDA Form 484 (Clinical Trials) (US)
The form that has to be completed when confirming receipt of samples.

FDA Form 1571 (Clinical Trials) (US)
This is the form that has to be completed when an **investigational new drug** submission is made to the **Food and Drug Administration**.

FDA Form 1572 (Clinical Trials) (US)
Also referred to as a 'Statement of **Investigator**'; it is a requirement of Section 505(I) of the **Food, Drug and Cosmetic Act** and 312.1 of Title 21 **Code of Federal Regulations,** that an investigator complete, sign and date this form as a condition for receiving and conducting clinical studies involving investigational drug(s) in the US for a **sponsor** under an **investigational new drug** application. It includes details of the investigator's training and experience and provides for legal certifications. All principal and **co-investigators** performing a **clinical trial** must sign this form.

FDA Form 1639 (Clinical Trials) (US)
The form on which **adverse events** are reported to the **Food and Drug Administration**.

FDA Guideline (US)
A document published by the **Food and Drug Administration** (FDA) to clarify **regulations**. Although they do not have the force of law, the FDA usually enforces them as though they do.
Compare **Communications, Decisions, Opinions, Recommendations, Regulations**.

FDAMA (US)
Food and Drug Administration Modernization Act of 1997.

FDLI (US)
Food and Drug Law Institute.

febrifuge
A drug or medicine that relieves or reduces fever. **Antipyretic** is the more commonly used term.

Federal FDC Act (US) see **Food, Drug and Cosmetic FDC Act** (US).

Federal Institute for Drugs and Medical Devices *(Bundesinstitute für Arzneimittel und Medizinprodukte)* **(BfArM)** (Germany)
BfArM is an independent higher federal authority under the responsibility of the Federal Ministry of Health of Germany. It was established on 1 July 1994 under the Act on the Reform of the Central Institutions of the Public Health System (*Gesetz zur Neuordnung zentraler Einrichtungen des Gesundheitswesens* [GNG]). BfArM is the successor to the Institute for Drugs (Institut für Arzneimittel) founded on 1 July 1975 as part of the now dissolved Federal Health Office – known as the **BGA**.

BfArM is responsible for:
1. Authorization of finished medicinal products
   Medicines Act (AMG), enforced in 1978 of **efficacy**, **safety** and adequate pharmaceutical quality is reviewed in the process of product authorization. Provided all legal requirements for authorization are fulfilled, the pharmaceutical company is granted the authorization it has applied for. Product authorization is limited to 5 years; renewal of authorization must be applied for and is granted if the documentation has passed new review. Changes to products on the market need to be notified to BfArM as well. The institute checks whether the changes are acceptable according to current scientific knowledge and in agreement with the provisions of the AMG. Authorization is also needed for the great number of so-called 'old products', i.e. products that had already been on the market before the AMG was in force. This process, which is still ongoing, is referred to as post-marketing authorization, or, shorter, post-approval.
2. Registration of homeopathic products
3. Recording and assessment of risks
   At BfArM, the reports of **adverse drug reactions** in Germany are centrally recorded and assessed; it takes measures under the graduated plan (Stufenplan) where necessary. When drug-associated risks become known benefits and risks are evaluated, followed by a decision on whether a product authorization is to be restricted or even to be revoked to protect consumers from dangers.
4. Control of legal marketing of narcotic drugs and starting materials
   The Federal Opium Agency, a department of BfArM, is responsible for controlling the manufacture and legal trade in narcotic drugs, psychotropic substances and precursors. Issuing general licences and granting import and export authorizations are parts of the duties as well as (on-site) inspections of the licence holders.
5. Activities in connection with medical and technical safety, suitability and performance of medical devices according to national and European regulations. When the Medical Devices Act (**MPG**) came into force on 1 January 1995, BfArM was assigned the medical devices matters, such as central recording and assessment of observed and reported risks associated with medical devices as well as coordination of measures where necessary.

Federal Opium Agency (*Germany*) see **Federal Institute for Drugs and Medical Devices** (*Bundesinstitutes für Arzneimittel und Medizinprodukte*) **(BfArM)**

Federal Policy (The) (US)
Provides regulations for the involvement of human subjects in research. The Policy applies to

all research involving human subjects conducted, supported, or otherwise subject to regulation by any federal department or agency that takes appropriate administrative action to make the Policy applicable to such research. Currently, 16 federal agencies have adopted the Federal Policy.

Also known as the Common Rule.

Federal Register (FR) (US)

A register where all public official matters, rules, proposed rules and notices of federal agencies and organizations such as **Health Care Finance Administration** and **Food and Drug Administration** are published in a daily bulletin. It also encompasses Executive Orders and other Presidential Documents. This publication, which can be several hundred pages long, contains information about proposed **Regulations**, final regulations, **advisory committee** meetings, and other regulatory issues that are of critical importance to the health care industry.

Recent FR Notices pertaining to medical devices may be found on the CDRH website. To obtain a Federal Register published after 1994 one can search the FR Online via GPO Access.

feedback inhibition

Mechanism that maintains constant secretion of a compound, hormone, or enzyme by exerting inhibitory control.

fetal material

The placenta, amniotic fluid, fetal membranes and umbilical cord.

fetus

The product of conception from the time of implantation until delivery. If the delivered or expelled fetus is viable, it is designated an infant. The term 'fetus' generally refers to later phases of development; the term 'embryo' is usually used for earlier phases of development.

See also **embryo**.

FFPM (UK)

Fellow of the Faculty of Pharmaceutical Medicine.

FFS (US)

Fee-for-service basis patients. See **Individual (Independent) Practice Association (IPA) or Organization (IPO)**.

FHS (UK) see **Family Health Services**.

FHSA (UK) see **Family Health Services Authorities**.

FIDE

Federation of European Dental Industry.

fiduciary

A legal term relating to, or founded upon, a trust or confidence. A fiduciary relationship exists where an individual or organization has an explicit or implicit obligation to act on behalf of another person's or organization's interests in matters which affect the other person or organization. This fiduciary is also obligated to act in the other person's best interest with total disregard for any interests of the fiduciary. Traditionally, it was generally believed that a physician had a fiduciary relationship with patients. This is being questioned in the era of **managed care** as the public becomes aware of the other influences which are effecting physician decisions. Doctors are provided incentives by **managed care** companies to provide less care, by pharmaceutical companies to order certain drugs and by hospitals to refer to their hospitals.

With the pervasive monetary incentives influencing doctor decisions, consumer advocates are concerned because the patient no longer has an unencumbered fiduciary.

fieldwork
Behavioural, social, or anthropological research involving the study of persons or groups in their own environment and without manipulation for research purposes (distinguished from laboratory or controlled settings).
See also **ethnographic research**.

Final Report (Clinical Trials) see **Clinical Trial/Study Report**.

Financial Agreement Letter (Clinical Trials)
A written, dated and signed agreement between the **sponsor** and an **investigator** or an institution. It sets out any arrangements in financial matters.

financial PR
A type of **public relations** (PR) that can be used to improve the relationship between the financial community and the company by affecting share price but also, increasingly in the pharmaceutical industry, to help facilitate mergers and acquisitions.

financial target (UK)
The return on assets that a **National Health Service (NHS) Trust** must pay. It is a pre-interest payment and is currently set at 6% of the average opening and closing assets in the Trust's financial accounts.

finished consultant episode (FCE)
An episode where the patient has completed a period of care under one consultant within one hospital **provider** and is either transferred to another consultant or discharged or has died.

finished product
A **medicinal product** which has undergone all stages of production, including packaging and is in its final container.
Compare **bulk product**.

FIP
International Pharmaceutical Federation.

first-dollar coverage (US)
Insurance coverage with no front-end deductible where coverage begins with the first dollar of expense incurred by the insured for any covered benefit.

first-in-humans study see **phase I clinical trial**.

first-in-man study see **phase I clinical trial**.

first-order kinetics
Because drug concentrations are usually too low to saturate the processes involved in drug pharmacokinetics, it follows that their rate is governed by the law of mass action and is proportional to drug concentration. Thus for most drugs the rates of accumulation and elimination follow first-order (exponential) kinetics. These drugs' half-lives are independent of dosage (compare drugs that follow zero-order kinetics).
Compare **half-life**, **zero-order kinetics**.

first pass effect see **first pass metabolism**.

first pass metabolism

Refers to **metabolism** of a drug that occurs en route from the gut lumen to the systemic circulation. For the majority of drugs administered orally, absorption occurs across the portion of the gastrointestinal epithelium that is drained by veins forming part of the hepatoportal system. Before reaching the systemic circulation such drugs must pass through the liver and are, therefore, exposed to enzymes in the liver that metabolize them. First pass metabolism depends on:
1. Hepatic function
2. Portosystemic shunting.

First pass metabolism is a major reason for apparent differences in drug absorption between individuals. Consequently, in patients with severe liver disease a far greater proportion of drugs are absorbed unchanged.

Also called first pass effect and pre-systemic metabolism.

See also **bioavailability**.

flare

A period of time in which disease symptoms reappear or become worse.

flat fee-per-case (US)

Flat fee paid for a client's treatment based on their diagnosis and/or presented case. For this fee, the **provider** covers all of the services the client requires for a specific period of time. It often characterizes 'second generation' **managed care** systems. After the **Managed Care Organizations** press out costs by discounting fees, they often adopt this method.

FOI

Freedom of information.

See also **Freedom of Information (FOI) Act**.

FOIA see **Freedom of Information (FOI) Act**.

Food

As defined by the US **Food, Drug and Cosmetic Act** is-'1. Articles used for food or drink for man or other animals, 2. chewing gum, and 3. articles used for components of any such article.'

Food and Drug Administration (FDA) (US)

An agency, headed by a Commissioner, that operates within the **Public Health Service**, which in turn is a part of the **Department of Health and Human Services**. The FDA is one of the US's oldest consumer protection agencies. Its approximately 9000 employees monitor the manufacture, import, transport, storage and sale of products with the aim of protecting American consumers by enforcing the **Food, Drug and Cosmetic Act** and several related public health laws.

The FDA has some 1100 investigators and inspectors who cover the country's almost 95 000 FDA-regulated businesses. These employees are located in district and local offices in 157 cities across the country.

These investigators and inspectors visit more than 15 000 facilities a year, ensuring proper manufacture and **labelling** is carried out. As part of their inspections, they collect about 80 000 domestic and imported product samples for examination by FDA scientists or for label checks.

If a company is found violating any of the laws that the FDA enforces, the FDA can encourage the firm to voluntarily correct the problem or to recall a faulty product from the market. When a company cannot or will not correct a public health problem with one of its products voluntarily, the FDA has legal sanctions it can use. The agency can go to court to force a company to stop selling a product and to have items already produced seized and destroyed. When warranted, criminal penalties – including prison sentences – are sought against manufacturers and distributors.

About 3000 products a year are found to be unfit for consumers and are withdrawn from the marketplace, either by voluntary **recall** or by court-ordered seizure. In addition, about 30 000 import shipments a year are detained at the port of entry because the goods appear to be unacceptable.

The scientific evidence needed to back up the FDA's legal cases is prepared by the agency's 2100 scientists, including 900 chemists and 300 microbiologists, who work in 40 laboratories in the Washington area and around the country. Some of these scientists analyse samples to see, for example, if products are contaminated with illegal substances. Other scientists review test results submitted by companies seeking agency approval for drugs, vaccines, food additives, colouring agents and **medical devices**.

The FDA also operates the National Center for Toxicological Research at Jefferson, Arkansas, which investigates the biological effects of widely used chemicals. The agency also runs the Engineering and Analytical Center at Winchester, Massachusetts, which tests **medical devices**, radiation-emitting products and **radioactive drugs**.

In deciding whether to approve new drugs, the FDA does not itself do research, but rather examines the results of studies done by the manufacturer. The agency must determine that the new drug produces the benefits it's supposed to without causing side-effects that would outweigh those benefits.

Other major FDA functions include ensuring the safety and wholesomeness of food, blood supply, **biologics**, **cosmetics**, medical devices and monitor unexpected adverse reactions.

Contact:
> United States of America Bureau of Drugs, FDA
> DHHS
> 5600 Fishers Lane, Rockville, MD 20857, USA
> Tel: + 1 301 443 3380

See also **Food, Drug and Cosmetic Act**.

Food, Drug and Cosmetic (FDC) Act (US)

The law governing the manufacture, storage, distribution, licensing, sale, and use of foods, drugs and **cosmetics** in the US. Originally passed in 1938, it has since been amended and supplemented by other laws and regulations to include **medical devices** and **biologics**. The FDC Act requires that the **safety** and **efficacy** of drugs, devices, and biologics be proven before they can be distributed.

Food–drug interaction

The *in vivo* influence of food on **bioavailability**, pharmacokinetic parameters, **adverse events**' profile, or pharmacological outcomes of a drug.

force of infection

The per capita rate at which susceptibles are infected.

formulary

An approved list of prescription drugs, selected pharmaceuticals and their appropriate dosages felt to be the most useful and cost-effective for patient care. In the US, organizations often develop a formulary under the auspices of a pharmacy and therapeutics committee. In the US, **Health**

Maintenance Organizations, physicians are often required to prescribe from the formulary. The US formulary is a list of **medicinal products** that most hospitals, **Managed Care Organizations** and State **Medicaid** programmes maintain. This list can be used to describe any of the following:
1. Drugs which are routinely kept in inventory
2. Drugs which they permit their personnel to prescribe
3. Drugs which they will provide payment/reimbursement for.

Many organizations limit the numbers and/or types of products on their formulary to contain costs.

See also **British National Formulary, drug formulary**.

formulation
The combination and concentrations of ingredients of a **drug product**. With any drug, it is possible to alter its **bioavailability** considerably by modifying the formulation. With some drugs, an even larger variation between a good formulation and a bad formulation can be observed. Since a drug must be in solution to be absorbed from the gastrointestinal tract, the **bioavailability** of a drug decreases in the order solution > suspension > capsule > tablet > coated tablet. This order may not always be followed but it is a useful guide. One example is pentobarbital where the order is aqueous solution > aqueous suspension = capsule > tablet of free acid form.

See also **capsule, solutions, suspensions, tablet**.

FP10 (UK)
The prescription form used by general practitioners.

FP10 (HP) (UK)
The prescription form used by hospital doctors but dispensed by community pharmacists.

FPA (UK)
Family Planning Association.

FPC (UK)
1. Family Practitioner Committee.
2. Family Planning Clinic.

FPI (Clinical Trials)
First patient in.

FPIF
Finnish Pharmaceutical Industry Federation.

FPLA (US)
Fair Packaging and Labeling Act.

FPO (Clinical Trials)
First patient out.

FPS
Family Planning Services.

fraud
An intentional deception committed to secure an unjust gain. The term 'research fraud' or 'scientific fraud' is also used to mean an intentional deception about scientific results, a type of research misconduct.

FRCOG (UK)
: Fellow of the Royal College of Gynaecology.

FRCP (UK)
: Fellow of the Royal College of Physicians.

FRCPath (UK)
: Fellow of the Royal College of Pathologists.

FRCS (UK)
: Fellow of the Royal College of Surgeons.

freedom of choice
: A principle of **Medicaid** which allows a recipient the freedom to choose among participating Medicaid providers.

Freedom of Information (FOI) Act (FOIA) (US)
: The FOI Act states that certain government-held information is public and must be made available upon request. In the context of **medical products**, certain parts of license applications become public after **Food and Drug Administration** approval is granted.

free radical see **oxygen free radical.**

FTC (US)
: Federal Trade Commission.

full agonist
: An agonist that can elicit a **maximum agonist effect** in a tissue by occupying only a fraction of the **receptors**.

Full Board/Committee Review (US)
: Review of proposed research at a convened meeting at which a majority of the membership of the **Investigational Review Board** are present, including at least one member whose primary concerns are in non-scientific areas. For the research to be approved, it must receive the approval of a majority of those members present at the meeting.

full business case (FBC) (UK)
: A business plan submitted to the **National Health Service** Executive for approval when a potential choice for development has been made and the costs are known.

full protective clothing
: Fully protective gear that prevents skin contact, inhalation, ingestion of gases, vapour, liquids, and solids (dusts, etc.). Includes SCBA (self-contained breathing apparatus).
  See also **chemical-protective clothing.**

functional genomics
: The study of the roles genes play in directing different biological processes, including how they contribute to or cause disease.

FVAR
: Final Variation Assessment Report.

gag clause
A provision of a contract between a **Managed Care Organization** and a health care **provider** that restricts the amount of information a provider may share with a **beneficiary** or that limits the circumstances under which a provider may recommend a specific treatment option.

'Gaiyo'
The Japanese name for the 'Summary of Findings' document.

galenical
A preparation, in a form suitable for therapeutic use, derived from natural non-synthetic source (animal or vegetable).

gargle
A solution used for rinsing or medicating the mouth and throat.

gastric lavage
Washing out of the stomach with water, often to treat poisoning; commonly called 'stomach pumping'.

gatekeeper (US)
A **primary care** physician (PCP) or **managed care** entity responsible for determining when and what services a patient can access and receive reimbursement for. It applies to a PCP who is involved in overseeing and coordinating all aspects of a patient's medical care. In order for a patient to receive a specialty care referral or hospital admission, the PCP must pre-authorize the visit, unless there is an emergency. The term gatekeeper is also used in health care business to describe anyone (EAP, employer-based case-manager, underwriting entity, etc.) that makes the decision of where a patient will receive services.

GATT (US)
General Agreement on Tariffs and Trade (**Food and Drug Administration**).

Gaussian distribution see **normal distribution**.

GCP see **good clinical practice**.

GCRP (UK)
Good Clinical Research Practice. Term sometimes used in the UK to describe **good clinical practice**.
See also **good clinical practice**.

GCTP
Good Clinical Trial Practice, see **good clinical practice**.

GDC
General Dental Council.

GDP
1. Good distribution practice.
2. General Dental Practitioner.

gel
A semi-solid formulation which, although containing a great deal of liquid, is firm in consistency; a colloid in a gelatinous form.

general controls (US)
Certain **Food and Drug Administration** statutory provisions designed to control the safety of marketed drugs and devices. The general controls include provisions on adulteration, misbranding, banned devices, **good manufacturing practice**, notification and record keeping, and other sections of the Medical Device Amendments to the **Food, Drug and Cosmetic Act**.

generalizability see **applicability**.

General Medical Council (GMC) (UK)
The competent authority for the purposes of recognition and registration of specialist medical qualifications in the UK.

General Professional Training (GPT)
The two-year post taken, following the professional medical registration, that is spent in one of a number of approved hospitals.

General Sales List (GSL) medicine (UK)
A medicine that is widely available and can be sold at any shop without the supervision of a pharmacist or a doctor.
See also **controlled drug**, **pharmacy drug**, **prescription only medicine**.

generic drug
A **drug product** that has the same **active ingredients** but different **formulation** to an already licensed drug product which is no longer covered by a patent. The term is the opposite of 'proprietary medicinal product'.
In the US, federal regulations allow for generic drugs to be licensed using a much simpler process than other drugs, which results in lower costs. Most payers now provide patients with financial incentives to use generic drugs, which save the payers money.
See also **bioavailability**, **biopharmaceutics**, **equivalence**, **United States Pharmacopoeia**.

generic name
The established, non-proprietary or common name of the **active ingredient** in a **drug product**.

generic substitution
The dispensing, by a pharmacist, of a **generic drug** in place of the brand-name entity prescribed. The generic drug, however, is not the generic version of the brand-name pharmaceutical but may be a generic version of another product that is in the same class as the brand name prescribed. In the US, every State permits generic substitution under certain circumstances. Regulations vary considerably, however, from State to State.

gene therapy
The treatment of genetic disease accomplished by altering the genetic structure of either somatic (non-reproductive) or germline (reproductive) cells.

genetic engineering
The alteration of genetic information to change an organism; mainly used to produce vaccines and drugs such as insulin.

genetic screening
Tests to identify persons who have an inherited predisposition to a certain phenotype or who are at risk of producing offspring with inherited diseases or disorders.

German Medicines Act (*Arzneimittelgesetz*) (AMG)
The AMG, enforced in 1978, stipulates that finished **medicinal products** need to be authorized before they are allowed to be placed on the market, i.e. before they are made available to patients. Proof of **efficacy**, **safety** and adequate pharmaceutical **quality** is reviewed in the process of product authorization. Provided all legal requirements for authorization are fulfilled, the pharmaceutical company is granted the authorization it has applied for. Product authorization is limited to 5 years, renewal of authorization must be applied for and is granted if the documentation has passed the new review. Changes to products on the market need to be notified to **BfArM**.

germicide
A chemical agent that kills micro-organisms.

Gesetz zur Neuordnung zentraler Einrichtungen des Gesundheitswesens (GNG) (Germany)
Act on the Reform of the Central Institutions of the Public Health System in Germany.
See also **Federal Institute for Drugs and Medical Devices**.

GHIA (US)
Group Health Insurance Association. Trade association of **Health Maintenance Organizations**.

GHTF see **Global Harmonization Task Force**.

Global Harmonization Task Force (GHTF)
The GHTF was conceived in 1992 in an effort to respond to the growing need for international harmonization in the regulation of **medical devices**. The Chairmanship of the GHTF is rotated amongst the regulatory representatives of the five founding members.

Global Health Network (US)
An alliance of experts in health and telecommunications who are actively developing the architecture for a health information structure for the prevention of disease in the 21st century.

global introspection
An unstructured mental process whereby the facts concerning a patient and their disease are integrated to form a diagnosis.

GLP see **good laboratory practice**.

gluten
A protein found in wheat, rye, barley and oats. Many **medicinal products** contain gluten as part of their inert ingredients.
See also **celiac disease**.

gluten intolerance see **celiac disease**.

GMC see **General Medical Council**.

GMO
Genetically modified organism.

GMP
1. See **good manufacturing practice**.
2. General Medical Practitioner (same as GP)

GMS
General Medical Services.

GMSC (UK)
General Medical Services Committee (London).

GNG see *Gesetz zur Neuordnung zentraler Einrichtungen des Gesundheitswesens*.

good clinical practice (GCP)
The **International Conference on Harmonization** Note for Guidance on GCP (CPMP/ICH/135/95) defines GCP as 'a standard for the design, conduct, performance, monitoring, auditing, recording, analyses and reporting of clinical trials that provides assurance that the data and reported results are credible and accurate, and that the rights, integrity, and confidentiality of trial subjects are protected.'
Also known as good clinical research practice.

good clinical research practice see **good clinical practice**.

good laboratory practice (GLP)
GLP is a regulation governing the conduct of *in vitro* 'bench top' and *in vivo* animal studies for collecting data.

good manufacturing practice (GMP)
GMP is a regulation governing the manufacturing and distribution of approved **drug products**. It is a quality system incorporating the elements of the international quality standard **ISO** 9000 but with additional requirements and recommendations pertinent to the manufacture of medicines. It is the part of the pharmaceutical **quality assurance** which ensures that products are consistently produced and controlled to the quality standards appropriate for their intended use and as required by the product specification.

Any reference to GMP, in the **European Union**, should be understood as reference to the current EEC GMP (cf. Vol. IV of the **Rules Governing Medicinal Products in the European Community**). In the UK, GMP is described in the 'Rules and Guidance for Pharmaceutical Manufacturers and Distributors 1997' which is published by and available from the Stationary Office.

GP
1. General practitioner.
2. Gas permeable (contact lenses).

GPCC
General Practitioner Commissioning Consultant.

GP Fundholder
A general practitioner practice which has elected to hold its own funds for negotiating **contracts** and purchasing a range of health care for their patients.

GPFC (UK)
General Practice Finance Corporation.

GPRA
Government Performance and Results Act of 1993.

GPT see **General Professional Training**.

grade
1. A numeric scale, usually I through to IV, representing the microscopic extent of the abnormality and aggressiveness of cancer cells.
2. (Clinical Trials) A numeric scale to rate the severity of **toxicity** from a treatment. Each specific **side-effect** such as 'nausea and vomiting' is rated on a scale from 0 to 4. Grade 0 toxicity always means the side-effect is not present, grade 1 means it is present but relatively minor, grade 2 means it is moderate, grade 3 means it is severe, and grade 4 means it is potentially **life-threatening**. The exact definition of each number in the scale depends on the particular side-effect. Treatments are often stopped or temporarily delayed for grade 3 or 4 toxicity. Sometimes treatments are resumed at a lower dose.

grandfather drug
Drug brought to market before 1938. These products are allowed to be sold without providing safety or effectiveness data, because they are generally recognized as safe and effective – provided no evidence to the contrary develops.

grant (US)
Financial support provided for research study designed and proposed by the principal investigator(s). The granting agency exercises no direct control over the conduct of approved research supported by a grant.
Compare **contract**.

GRAS (US)
Generally Recognized As Safe (**Food and Drug Administration**).

GRIP
International group for pharmaceutical distribution in the EC.

group comparison (Clinical Trials)
A trial design in which patients are randomly allocated to one of two or more treatment groups and the responses of each group are compared.

Group Model HMO (US)
Health care plan involving contracts with physicians organized as a partnership, professional corporation, or other legal association. It can also refer to a **Health Maintenance Organization** (HMO) model in which the HMO contracts with one or more medical groups to provide services to members. In either case, the payer or health plan pays the medical group, which is, in turn, responsible for compensating physicians. The medical group may also be responsible for paying or contracting with hospitals and other providers.

group practice
A group of persons licensed to practise medicine as a group responsibility, engage in the coordinated practice of their profession primarily in one or more group practice facilities, and who in their connection share common overhead expenses. Group practices in the US use the acronyms **PA**, **IPA**, **MSO** and others. The American Group Practice Association, the **American Medical Association** and the Medical Group Management Association define medical group practice as 'provision of health care services by a group of at least three licensed physicians engaged in a formally organized and legally recognized entity sharing equipment, facilities, common records and personnel involved in both patient care and business management.' Group practices are far more common now than a decade ago because physicians seek to lower costs, increase contracting power and share payer contracts.

GSL see **General Sales List medicine**.

GTAC (UK)
Gene Therapy Advisory Committee.

guar
A naturally occurring carbohydrate gum used as a thickening agent in foods and in weight-loss preparations.

guardian
An individual who is authorized under applicable State or local law to give permission on behalf of a child to general medical care or participation in a **clinical trial**.

guidelines
Instructions that are proposed for applicants for **marketing authorizations** (MAs) for **medicinal products**. They are intended to clarify obscurities and avoid national differences in the understanding of the comprehensive technical requirements for **safety**, **quality**, and **efficacy** in EU **Directives** by giving national explanation; and to facilitate the applications for MA which will be accepted by all of the **EEC Member States**. Guidelines set out the main points to be dealt with in the dossiers and **Expert Reports**; the minimum requirements (such as the number of batches of a medicinal product in its intended pack which will need to be subjected to stability test), and the methods in general terms (but taking care to maintain flexibility, so as not to restrict the freedom to use legitimate alternative test methods). Guidelines are not mandatory but are complementary to the legal requirements of directives and expected to be observed when assessing applications for MAs.

See also **Decisions, Directives, Recommendations, Regulations**.

HA
Health Authority.

habituation
A condition resulting from the repeated consumption of a drug. It is characterized by a psychological desire (but not compulsion) to continue taking the drug for the sense of improved well-being. There is normally little or no tendency to increase the dose and there is absence of physical dependence.
Compare **addiction, dependence, drug dependence, narcotic, tolerance**.

HACCP (US)
Hazard Analysis Critical Control Point (inspection technique) (**Food and Drug Administration**).

HAD see Health Development Agency.

haematinic
An agent that tends to increase the concentration of haemoglobin, but more broadly may refer to any substance having anti-anaemic properties.

haematology
1. The study of blood, its physiology and pathology.
2. Laboratory investigations of patients using a wide range of biological, chemical, and physical techniques.

haematopoietic
A drug that stimulates the production of blood cells, especially by furnishing deficient vitamins or other essential substance.

haemodialysis
'Artificial kidney' therapy used in renal failure to remove toxic waste material, otherwise, normally removed by the kidneys, from the patient's blood. In the procedure, blood is diverted externally and allowed to flow across a semi-permeable membrane that is bathed with an aqueous isotonic solution. Nitrogenous waste products and some drugs will diffuse from the blood, thus these compounds will be eliminated. Therefore in patients with kidney failure, haemodialysis will be an important route of drug elimination.
This technique is particularly important with drugs which:
1. have good water solubility;
2. are not tightly bound to plasma proteins;
3. have smaller (less than 500) molecular weight; and
4. have a small apparent **volume of distribution**.

Conversely drugs which are tightly bound or extensively stored or distributed into tissues are only poorly removed by this route, or process.

haemostatic
An agent that stops bleeding.

Hahnemann, Samuel see homeopathic medicine.

half-life ($t_{1/2}$)
The time taken for the plasma concentration of a drug to fall to half its original value. It depends on drug **clearance** and **volume of distribution** and if the processes involved **first-order kinetics**. A drug obeying first-order elimination kinetics has a constant half-life and its

elimination time will be a multiple of this value. This is to say that a 50% drop in plasma concentration will occur in one half-life. For most drugs, the plasma half-life is independent of dosage since they obey first-order kinetics. However, for the few drugs which obey **zero-order kinetics**, the plasma half-life increases with increasing plasma concentration. Plasma half-life can either be estimated by noting the time taken for any concentration to fall by half, or it can be obtained by measuring the slope of the linear plot and calculating the rate constant for elimination (k_{el}) and the ($t_{1/2}$).

Compare **biotransformation, elimination, first-order kinetics, pharmacokinetics, volume of distribution**.

hallucinogen
A drug, such as LSD, that induces hallucination.

HAM-A
Hamilton Anxiety Scale.

HAM-D
Hamilton Depression Scale.

Hansch analysis
The investigation of the quantitative relationship between the biological activity of a series of compounds and their physicochemical substitutes or global parameters representing hydrophobic, electronic, steric and other effects using multiple regression correlation methodology.

hard drug
A non-metabolizable compound, characterized either by high lipid solubility and accumulation in adipose tissues and organelles, or by high water solubility. In the lay press the term 'hard drug' refers to a powerful **drug** of abuse such as cocaine or heroin for which the proper name is **controlled drug**.

Compare **soft drug**.

hard end point
Any **outcome** measure that is not subject to serious errors of interpretation or measurement. Usually death, infection or some other explicit clinical event.

See also **end point, surrogate marker**.

harmonization
The term used to describe the efforts among countries to make food and drug regulatory requirements more uniform.

See also **International Conference on Harmonization**.

HASSASSA (UK)
Health and Social Services and Social Security Adjudication Act.

Hawthorne effect
Named after a study performed in the 1930s in Hawthorne, Illinois in which it was discovered that the act of merely studying individual behaviour can influence it. The Hawthorne effect in **clinical trials** is sometimes associated with the **placebo effect** and can best be dealt with by having both a treatment and **control group**.

Also known as the experimenter effect.

HAZ see Health Action Zone.

hazard
All chemicals, given in sufficient doses, are capable of producing harm. Three categories of information are needed to define a hazard: specific descriptions of the harms it can produce, specific identification of the species or kinds of subjects that can be harmed, and specification of the kinds of exposure to the chemical (including dose) which can result in the respective harms.
Compare **safety, risk, therapeutic index**.

hazardous chemical, material.
In a broad sense, any substance or mixture of substances having properties capable of producing adverse effects on the health or safety of a human. Included are substances that are carcinogens, toxic, irritants, corrosives, sanitizers and agents which damage the lungs, skin, eyes, mucous membranes, etc.

HCA see **Home Care Assistant**.

HCFA see **Health Care Finance Administration**.

HCFA 1500 see **Health Care Finance Administration 1500**.

HCFA Common Procedure Coding System (HCPCS) (US)
The HCPCS (pronounced 'hick picks') is a system of codes and descriptive terminology used for reporting the provision of supplies, materials, injections and certain services and procedures to **Medicare**. It is a three level coding system, consisting of **current procedural terminology**, National and Local Codes used primarily to report services to Medicare fiscal intermediaries and carriers.

HD
Harmonization document.

HEA see **Health Education Agency**.

health
'Health is a state of complete physical, mental and social well-being and not merely the absence of disease or infirmity' (**World Health Organization**). It is recognized, however, that health has many dimensions (anatomical, physiological and mental) and is largely culturally defined. The relative importance of various disabilities will differ depending upon the cultural milieu and the role of the affected individual in that culture. Most attempts at measurement have been assessed in terms of **morbidity** and **mortality**.

Health Action Zone (HAZ) (UK)
An initiative, covering parts of the UK, which aims to bring together organizations within and beyond the **National Health Service** to develop and implement a locally agreed strategy for improving the health of local people.

Health Canada Online
In partnership with provincial and territorial governments, Health Canada provides national leadership to develop health policy, enforce health regulations, promote disease prevention and enhance healthy living for all Canadians.

Health Care Finance Administration (HCFA) (US)
The federal government agency within the Department of **Health and Human Services** which directs and oversees a State's administrations of **Medicare** while directly administering

Medicaid programmes (Titles XVIII and XIX of the Social Security Act), overseeing Child Health Insurance Programs and conducting research to support those programmes.
Website: http://www.hcfa.gov.

Health Care Finance Administration 1500 (HCFA 1500) (US)
The HCFA's standard form for submitting provider service claims to third party companies or insurance carriers. It is the form accepted by the majority of payers (payers = payors in the US).

Health Care Information Service (HCIS) (UK)
A division within the British Library that deals with all health care information. Facilities include: advice on accessing and searching **MEDLINE** and other **NLM** Databases; production of the Allied and Alternative Medicine (AMED) database; Current Awareness Topics Searches (CATS); training and consultancy; document delivery.

health care professional
For the purpose of the regulations regarding reporting **adverse drug reactions** and clinical research, a health care professional includes medically-qualified doctors, coroners, dentists, pharmacists and nurses.

health care reform (US)
The movement that resulted as a reaction to the health care crisis in the US. This movement has resulted in action in both the public and private sectors. The main impact the reform movement is having on private payers is an increased reliance on **managed care** to deliver health care services. In the public sector, **Medicare** and other public payers are working toward better **cost-containment**. In addition, Congress has drafted over 30 bills to reform health care delivery and payment systems, while in 1994 the White House issued daily statements calling for universal coverage. Although pressure for legislative action at the Federal level has greatly decreased since the 1994 election, state legislatures have been quite successful in passing incremental healthcare reform bills, and will continue to do so throughout.

health care system participants
The people and organizations that rely in some way on the health care system. This group includes **patients**, **providers**, health care **manufacturers**, payers and others.

Health Development Agency (HAD) (UK)
An organization which supersedes the **Health Education Agency**. It was introduced to map and disseminate the evidence base for public health and set standards for public health and public health practice.

Health Economic Evaluations Database (HEED) (UK)
A database, designed by health economists for use by health economists, that was developed as a joint initiative between the **Office of Health Economics** and the **International Federation of Pharmaceutical Manufacturers Association** and contains information on studies of **cost-effectiveness** and other forms of economic evaluation of medicines, other treatments and medical interventions. HEED also includes, in bibliographic detail, entries from the Wellcome and Battelle databases of economic evaluation literature.

HEED, as of January 2000, contains approximately 18 500 references. There are two types of reference in HEED, bibliographic references and references which have been reviewed by a health economist according to a standard report format. The latter constitute nearly half of the references. HEED includes relevant literature covered by other published registries and bibliographies of health economic studies as well as additional material.

HEED can be searched using a combination of the 54 available search fields, in addition to keyword and free text searching. HEED can be interrogated by tailoring the search criteria to pick up only the relevant data, which is then presented in easy-to-read formats. The search criteria are grouped into a number of subject groupings, with each subject group containing criteria that can be specified in any number of combinations to search the database. Boolean operator and wild card functions can also be used to increase the power of the search capabilities. The search criteria can be modified and refined to produce information in manageable amounts, and each search strategy can be saved and used at a later date. The quality and quantity of information available on HEED can only be appreciated by carrying out specific searches using defined search parameters. HEED can also be searched using two different types of searching technique, namely, compound and expert search modes.

The process of selecting suitable articles for review is complex and to arrive at the monthly target of 150 to 200 fully reviewed as well as additional bibliographic articles, a precise screening and selection process is implemented.

Contact:
Project Manager
OHE-IFPMA Database Ltd
12 Whitehall, London SW1A 2DY, UK
Tel: +44 171 930 3477, Ext. 1474
Fax: +44 171 747 1419

See also **International Federation of Pharmaceutical Manufacturers Associations**, **Office of Health Economics**.

health economics

The science concerned with the measurement of the total value of particular courses of therapy. It is based on the principle that every clinical intervention produces a change in the health status of a patient, which has an intrinsic, measurable value impacting the patient's future use of the health care system and productive output to society. Sometimes referred to as '**health outcomes research**' or, when referring strictly to pharmaceuticals, '**pharmacoeconomics**'.

Health Economics Research Centre (HERC) (UK)

A specialist unit within the University of Oxford, Division of Public Health and Primary Health Care. It undertakes independent research in **health economics**, and supports other academic and **National Health Service** (NHS) research activities through teaching, research and dissemination. It is a collaborative venture between the University and the NHS Executive. Members of the Centre undertake applied and methodological research in health economics. They also teach at undergraduate and postgraduate level, and supervise research students pursuing the MSc, MPhil and DPhil degrees of the University. HERC runs short courses in health economics methodology for professionals in the field, and a seminar series.

Contact:
The Administrator
Health Economics Research Centre
University of Oxford
Institute of Health Sciences
Headington, Oxford OX3 7LF, UK
Tel: (+44) (0)(1865) 226679
Fax: (+44) (0)(1865) 226842
Email: herc@ihs.ox.ac.uk
Website: http://www.ihs.ox.ac.uk/herc/

Health Education Agency (HEA) (UK)
Now superseded by the **Health Development Agency**.

health gain
The improvement in the health of a given population. Sometimes described as adding years to life and life to years. The concept encompasses such other concepts as quality and related measures e.g. **QUALY**s.

Health Impact Assessment (HIA) (UK)
An assessment used in central government and its agencies and in local government to consider the consequences for health of all major policies.

Health Improvement Programme (HImp) (UK)
A 3-year rolling strategy, led by the health authority, to improve health and health care locally. It involves **National Health Service (NHS) Trusts**, **primary care groups**, and other **primary care** professionals working in partnership with the local authority and engaging other local interests.

Health Level Seven (HL7) (US)
A data interchange protocol for health care computer applications that simplifies the ability of different vendor-supplied IS systems to interconnect. Although not a software program in itself, HL7 requires that each health care software vendor program HL7 interfaces for its products.

Health Maintenance Organization (HMO) (US)
A Nixon-administration name that has remained in use to describe a capitated prepaid health plan. They are a type of **Managed Care Organization** that may be group models organization, hospital-based models, or individual physicians contracting. They offer prepaid, comprehensive health coverage for both hospital and physician services that presents an organized, coordinated system of healthcare within a specific geographic area. The HMO is paid monthly premiums or capitated rates by the payers, which include employers, insurance companies, government agencies, and other groups representing covered lives. The HMO must meet the specifications of the federal HMO act as well as meeting many rules and regulations required at the state level. There are four basic models: group model, individual practice association, network model and staff model. The system provides a comprehensive set of basic and supplemental health services, including doctors, specialists, inpatient facilities, outpatient facilities and, often, prescription drugs. An HMO contracts with health care providers. The members of an HMO are required to use participating or approved providers for all health services and generally all services will need to meet further approval by the HMO through its utilization programme. Subscribers are enrolled for a specified period of time and prepay a fixed amount of money at regular intervals. HMOs may turn around and sub-capitate to other groups. For example, it may carve-out certain benefit categories, such as mental health, and subcapitate these to a mental health HMO. Alternatively the HMO may subcapitate to a provider, provider group or provider network. HMOs are the most restrictive form of managed care benefit plans because they restrict the procedures, providers and benefits.

health needs assessment
A technique of measuring the health status of a given population. It is often undertaken on a disease specific basis and the subject of some contention. It may also be described in terms of the ability to benefit from a range or specific type of intervention.

health outcome see outcome.

health outcomes research
The discipline concerned with the measurement of the total worth of particular options of therapy. It encompasses research on measures of changes in patient **outcomes**, that is, patient health status and satisfaction, resulting from specific medical and health interventions. It is based on the theory that every clinical intervention produces an alteration in the health status of a patient, which has an intrinsic, measurable value impacting the patient's future use of the health care system and productive output to society. Attributing changes in outcomes to medical care requires distinguishing the effects of care from the effects of the many other factors that influence patients' health and satisfaction. With the exclusion of the physician's **fiduciary** responsibility to the patient, outcomes **data** is gaining increasing importance for patient advocacy and consumer protection. Outcomes research will also be used in the future by payers to identify potential partners on the basis of good outcomes. Sometimes referred to as '**health economics**' or, when referring strictly to pharmaceuticals, '**pharmacoeconomics**'.

See also **pharmacoeconomics**.

health plan organization
An organization that acts as insurer for an enrolled population.

See **managed care**.

health promotion
The science and art of helping people change their lifestyle to move toward a state of optimal health. Optimal health is defined as a balance of physical, emotional, social, spiritual and intellectual health.

Health Reimbursement Services Agency (HRSA) (US)
The branch of the federal government with primary responsibility for paying for health care. HRSA runs **Medicaid** and **Medicare**.

Health-Related Quality of Life (HRQoL) indicators as a pharmaceutical outcome
In pharmacotherapy, there are several criteria for determining whether HR-QoL measures are appropriate **end points** for **pharmacoeconomic** analysis. When the primary purpose of a drug is palliative rather than curative, as is often the case in chronic disease, HR-QoL endpoints can help weigh the beneficial and **adverse effects** of a drug.

When a drug is somewhat effective but is also associated with significant toxicity, HR-QoL endpoints can help answer whether the benefits of therapy outweigh **side-effects** (e.g., cancer **chemotherapy**). When lifelong therapy is administered to prevent complications of a relatively asymptomatic disease, HR-QoL instruments can help determine whether patient **quality of life** (QoL) impairment is worth the abstract reduction in risk associated with the original condition (e.g. reduction in the risk of stroke by **antihypertensive** treatment).

When there are several equally effective therapies for a specific condition, but their adverse effect profiles differ, HR-QoL instruments can be used to decide the relative value of **QoL** differences and incremental differences in cost associated with the several therapies (e.g. antibiotics for upper respiratory tract infection).

Health Resources and Services Administration (HRSA) (US)
A component of the US **DHHS**. Included in HRSA responsibilities, is the administration of the Ryan White Care funds with a budget of about $1 billion/year to support a continuum of care services for persons with HIV infection.

Health Security Act (US)
The health care reform bill introduced to Congress by the Clinton administration. This bill was

known as S1757 in the Senate and HR3600 in the House of Representatives. The original Act, which was heavily marked up and amended in both houses of Congress, was the subject of vigorous debate, and had the following key provisions:
1. Universal coverage for all Americans
2. Health care alliances for purchasing **insurance** in bulk
3. A National Health Board for controlling health care costs
4. Employer mandates for covering most of the cost of the programme
5. A modern claims processing system to reduce paperwork
6. A tobacco tax to help fund the programme.

This bill did not pass during the 103rd session of Congress.

Health Service Circular (HSC) (UK)
A series of management letters from the **Department of Health**, replacing Executive Letters, Health Service Guidance, Finance Directorate Letters and other circulars.

Health Service Price Index (UK)
An index which takes a **National Health Service** shopping basket of goods and services (excluding pay) and weighs them according to use. It is used to measure price movements on a monthly basis and sometimes it is used to influence budget and financial allocations.

Health Service Agreement (HSA) (US)
Detailed explanation of procedures and benefits provided to an employer by a health plan.

Health Services Act of 1993 (US)
A Washington State law enacted in May 1993 that sets forth early implementation measures and a process for overall reform of the health services system. The intent is to stabilize health services costs, assure access to essential services for all residents, actively address the health care needs of persons of colour, improve the public's health, and reduce unwarranted health services costs.

health status
A measure of the overall state of health of a specified defined individual, group, or **population**. It may be measured by obtaining alternatives such as people's subjective assessments of their health; by one or more indicators of **mortality** and **morbidity** in the population, such as longevity or maternal and infant mortality; or by using the incidence or **prevalence** of major diseases (communicable, chronic, or nutritional). Conceptually, health status is the proper **outcome** measure for the **effectiveness** of a specific population's medical care system, although attempts to relate effects of available medical care to variations in health status have proved difficult.

Health Technology Assessment (HTA)
Systematic critical appraisal of the available research evidence to provide practitioners and policy makers with recommendations on the best way forward.

healthy, normal volunteer (Clinical Trials)
Someone without disease or other known health problems who volunteers to participate in a **clinical trial** for reasons other than medical and receives compensation (normally) but no direct health benefit from participating. It is the type of subject frequently used in **phase I clinical trial** studies to assess the **safety** of a new medical intervention. 'Normal' may not mean normal in all respects. For example, patients with broken legs (if not on medication that will affect the results) may serve as **normal volunteers** in studies of **metabolism**, cognitive development and the like. Similarly, patients with heart disease but without diabetes may be the 'normals' in a study of diabetes complicated by heart disease.

healthy volunteer see **healthy, normal volunteer**.

HEED see **Health Economic Evaluation Database**.

Helsinki Declaration see **Declaration of Helsinki**.

hepatotoxicity
How much injury/harm a medicine or other substance does to the liver.

herbal product
Medicinal product containing, as **active ingredients**, exclusively plant material and/or vegetable **drug** preparations.

HERC see **Health Economics Research Centre**.

HES
Hospital Episode Statistics.

heteroreceptor
A **receptor** regulating the synthesis and/or the release of mediators other than its own ligand. See also **autoreceptor**.

HEW (US)
The predecessor of The Department of Health and Human Services.
See also **Department of Health and Human Services**.

HFEA
Human Fertilization and Embryology Authority.

HFMA (UK)
Healthcare Financial Management Association.

HHS see **Department of Health and Human Services**.

HIA see **health impact assessment**.

HIBCC (UK)
Health Index Bar Code Council.

high level performance indicator (HLPI) (UK)
Part of the **National Health Service** performance management system. It is used in conjunction with the **clinical indicator**.

high throughput screening (HTS)
Rapid *in vitro* screening of large numbers of compounds (libraries); generally tens to thousands of compounds, using robotic screening assays.

HIMA
Health Industry Manufacturers Association.

HImP see **Health Improvement Programme**.

HIP see **Health Improvement Programme**.

HIPC
Health Insurance Purchasing Cooperative.

Hippocratic oath
The pledge taken by doctors that binds them to observe the code of their conduct and practice.

It originates from the Greek physician Hippocrates (470–370 BC) whose famous statement is 'It is the duty of the physician not only to do that which immediately belongs to him, but likewise to secure the cooperation of the sick, of those in attendance, and of all external agents.'

histogram
A way of graphically showing the characteristics of the distribution of items in a given **population** or **sample**. In a histogram, each measure is represented by a single block that is placed over the midpoint of the class interval into which the measure falls.

historical controls (Clinical Trials)
A group of patients (may be loosely or explicitly defined) considered to have the same disease or condition as the study group, but who were diagnosed and treated in a period of time prior to that of the study group and who received the conventional form of therapy for that time. They represent control subjects (followed at some time in the past or for whom data are available through records) who are used for comparison with subjects being treated concurrently. The study is considered historically controlled when the present condition of subjects is compared with their own condition on a prior regimen or treatment. Historical control groups are generally only useful for evaluations of treatments involving rare diseases with highly predictable outcomes and where it is considered impractical or unethical to carry out a controlled **clinical trial**.

historical control studies (Clinical Trials)
Trials where the results of the **investigational product** are compared with experience historically derived from adequately documented natural history of the disease or condition, or from the results of active treatment, in comparable subjects or populations and is described and documented in the **protocol**.

HIV ADR Reporting Scheme (UK)
An extension (launched end of October 1997) of the **Yellow Card Scheme** that involves reporting suspected **adverse drug reactions**, occurring in HIV patients undergoing treatment, which are analysed and regularly fed back to reporters. The Scheme is a collaboration between: the **Medicines Control Agency (MCA)**, the Medical Research Council (MRC) – HIV Clinical Trials Centre and the **Committee on Safety of Medicines**. Cases are analysed individually and as case series by scientists, pharmacists and doctors at the MCA and MRC. Data are used to assess the causal relationship between the drugs and reported reactions and to identify possible **risk factors** contributing to the occurrence of reactions, for example, age, dose, pre-existing liver disease etc. Assessment includes analysis of relevant data from other sources, for example, case reports in the literature, pre- and post-marketing clinical studies, epidemiological studies, **record linkage** databases, and data from drug regulatory authorities such as the US **Food and Drug Administration**. The risk of a newly identified hazard is considered in the context of the overall safety profile for the drug in comparison with relevant therapeutic alternatives, and its benefits in terms of effectiveness and therapeutic indication.

HLPI see High Level Performance Indicator.
HMO see Health Maintenance Organization.
HMR
Hospital medical record.

HMR1 (UK)
This is usually the front sheet of hospital medical record forms. It is used to record personal

and medical details in summary form. It is used in all hospital records except maternity and mental illness.

HMSO (UK)
Her Majesty's Stationery Office.

HNA
Health needs assessment.

HO
House Officer (junior hospital doctor)

hold harmless clause (US)
A clause frequently found in **managed care** contracts whereby the **Health Maintenance Organization** and the physician hold each other not liable for malpractice or corporate malfeasance if either of the parties is found to be liable. Many **insurance** carriers exclude this type of liability from coverage. It may also refer to language that prohibits the provider from billing patients if their managed care company becomes insolvent. State and federal regulations may require this language.

Home Care Assistant (HCA)
A social care worker who provides domiciliary care. Formerly known as 'home helps'.

homeopathic medicine
A system of therapeutics founded by Samuel **Hahnemann** (1755–1843) in which diseases are treated by drugs (administered in minute doses) which are capable, in larger quantities, of producing, in healthy persons, symptoms like those of the disease to be treated.

homologue
A compound belonging to a series of compounds differing from each other by a repeating unit, such as a methylene group, a peptide residue, etc.

horizontal integration
Merging of two or more firms at the same level of production in some formal, legal relationship. In hospital networks, this may refer to the grouping of several hospitals, the grouping of outpatient clinics with the hospital or a geographic network of various health care services. Integrated systems seek to integrate both vertically with some organizations and horizontally with others.

horizontal study
A study that involves the observation of a defined **population** (a community), perhaps stratified by age, sex, ethnicity etc., at one point in time or time interval. Most clinical studies are of this type. Exposure and **outcome** are determined simultaneously. Although a snapshot, horizontal studies of prevalence and intensity within different age classes of a community can nevertheless provide valuable information on the rate at which hosts acquire infection through time, provided that the host and parasite populations have remained approximately stable for a period of time (i.e. **stable endemicity**). These studies tend to be cheap and simple to design and run and well accepted by ethical committees. They, however, tend to incur recall and Neyman's biases, have unequal group sizes and at most establish 'association' not 'causality'.
   Also called cross-sectional study.

horizontal survey see **horizontal study**.

hospital days (per 1000) (US)
A measurement of the number of days of hospital care **Health Maintenance Organization** members use in a year. It is calculated as follows: total number of days spent in a hospital by members divided by total members. This information is available through **HHS**, **OHMO** and a variety of sources.
Compare **hospital stay**.

hospital stay
The number of days a patient stays in one hospital during a period of treatment. It also refers to the length of stay and may be affected by the **finished consultant episode** concept.

hotel costs
The costs of heating, lighting, catering, domestic and other non-clinical services.

HPB (Canada)
Health Protection Board.

HPLC
High performance liquid chromatography.

HPRU see **Human Psychopharmacology Research Unit**.

HRSA see **Health Resources and Services Administration**.

HSAC
Health Service Advisory Committee.

HSC (UK)
1. Health and Safety Commission.
2. see **Health Service Circular**.
3. Health Service Commissioner.

HSE
Health and Safety Executive

HSPI
Health Service Price Index.

HTA see **health technology assessment**.

HTS see **high throughput screening**.

Human Genome Project
A multi-billion dollar project to sequence the entire human genome by identifying the, approximately, 100 000 human genes.

Human Psychopharmacology Research Unit (HPRU) (UK)
A part of the University of Surrey and a centre with a high research rating. It has a multidisciplinary team combining the experience of clinicians, nurses, pharmacologists, electrophysiologists, psychologists and statisticians.

Over the years, HPRU has built a psychopharmacological database with profiles of over 200 psychoactive agents, including analgesics, anaesthetics, anxiolytics, antidepressants, anti-dementia agents, neuroleptics, cognitive enhancers, antihistamines and hypnotics. HPRU has a 12-bedded ward with full clinical service support and handles data from various kinds of clinical studies and for many purposes:

- **bioavailabilty**, including first dose in man
- **safety** and **tolerance**
- **drug–drug interaction** (especially alcohol)
- **bioequivalence** and dose-ranging effects
- in **volunteers** (healthy, atypical and elderly)
- in **patients** (hospital, general practice, long-term follow-up)
- **post-marketing surveillance**.

human subject (Clinical Trials)
An individual who is or becomes a participant in a **clinical trial**, either as a recipient of the **investigational product** or **comparator** or as a control and/or by signing an **informed consent** to participate in a clinical trial where his/her physiologic or behavioural characteristics and responses become the object of study in a research project.

In the US, under the federal regulations, human subjects are defined as: living individual(s) about whom an investigator conducting research obtains: (1) data through intervention or interaction with the individual; or (2) identifiable private information. A human subject, defined in 21 **Code of Federal Regulations** 50.3, is an 'individual who is or becomes a participant in research, either as a recipient of the test article or as a control. A subject may be either a healthy human or a patient'. Synonym: subject/trial subject.

See also **healthy volunteer**.

Humphrey–Durham Act See **Durham-Humphrey Amendment**

Huriet Law (France)
France's regulations on the initiation and conduct of clinical trials.

HV
Health Visitor.

hyperglycaemic
A drug that elevates blood glucose level, especially for the treatment of hypoglycaemic states.

hypersensitivity
An excessive response of the body's immune system to a foreign protein; the state is dependent on the administration of a haptene or allergen to a susceptible individual, and the development of antibodies and immune mechanisms capable of being activated by a subsequent administration of the haptene.
Compare **allergic response**, **idiosyncratic response**.

hypersensitivity reaction
Reactions in certain individuals which occur at therapeutic or lower doses of a drug. Examples include the reaction of some asthmatics to aspirin or anaphylaxis to penicillin.

hypoallergenic
A product from which most known allergens have been removed to minimize chance of **allergic response**.

hypodermic needle
A thin, hollow needle attached to a syringe; used to inject a medication under the skin, into a vein, or into a muscle.

hypoendemic (Epidemiology)
An area with little transmission.

hypothesis
A statement that is believed to be true or one that is used as a basis for argument that has not yet been proven. It is a statement of the goal of any scientific research.

A scientific hypothesis is a provisional or temporary assumption about something's function or status that is based on limited or no preliminary evidence and that evidence from further investigation will either support or refute. In this sense, a list of differential diagnoses represents a set of hypotheses for which more evidence must be obtained in the diagnostic process before a level of certainty is reached that is sufficient for action.

Research hypothesis is the conclusion a study sets out to support (or disprove); for example, 'blood pressure will be lowered (by specific **end point**) in **subjects** who receive the **investigational product**'. In **clinical trials** there are typically two hypotheses: the '**null hypothesis**', which is a statement of no difference between treatment and **control** (see **equipoise**) and the '**alternative hypothesis**', which is a statement that the treatment has an effect over and above the control. The goal of most clinical studies is to reject the null hypothesis in favour of the alternative.

A logical problem is that although the facts derived from the test of a hypothesis are correct, the broader underlying theory from which the hypothesis was derived can still be wrong. Proponents of any hypothesis can defend it against contrary evidence by *ad hoc* modifications of the underlying theory. Science often progresses by researchers noting discrepant observations and pursuing their explanation with investigations based on further hypotheses. Note that in non-scientific contexts what most people call a 'theory' is actually a hypothesis or speculation.

See also **null hypothesis**.

IAPM
International Association of Medical Prosthetics Manufacturers.

IARC see **International Agency for Research on Cancer.**

IASBM
International Association of Surgical Blade Manufacturers.

iatrogenic
A term used to describe a disease, disorder, or medical condition that is a direct result of medical treatment produced by physicians; usually applied to disorders directly attributable to medical or surgical procedures.
See also **idiosyncratic reaction/response**.

IB see **Investigator's Brochure.**

IBD see **International Birth Date.**

ICD-9-CM see **International Classification of Diseases, Ninth Revision, Clinical Modification.**

ICD-9-CM I
International Classification of Diseases – Ninth Revision – Clinical Modification part I.

ICD-10
International Classification of Diseases, 10th edition (1992).

ICD-O
International Classification of Diseases. It is the **World Health Organization** International Classification of Diseases for Oncology.

ICDRA
International Conference on Drug Regulatory Authorities.

ICE
International Chemical Extension.

ICEC
Institute for Clinical Evaluative Sciences.

ICH see **International Conference on Harmonization.**

ICHS
International Committee for Standardization in Haematology.

ICIDH
International Classification of Impairments, Disabilities, and Handicaps.

ICMJE
International Committee of Medical Journal Editors.

ICP see **integrated care pathway.**

ICPC
International Classification of Primary Care.

ICSU
International Council for Science.

IDE see **Investigational Device Exemption.**

identification code see **subject identification code.**

idiosyncratic reaction/response
(Greek; *Idios* = personal/individual, *Syn* = together, and *krasis* = mix) An abnormal, most probably non-allergic, reaction of a person to a drug. The reaction is uniquely individualistic in nature and not seen in the general population.
Compare **adverse drug reaction, adverse event, allergic response, hypersensitivity reaction, iatrogenic.**

IDMC see **Independent Data Monitoring Committee.**

IDR
Idiosyncratic drug reaction, see **idiosyncratic reaction/response.**

IDRAC
A division of IMS HEALTH that was formed in 1993 to help pharmaceutical companies register products more quickly. To accelerate the time-consuming process of developing a drug in accordance with stringent regulations, IDRAC developed a regulatory affairs (RA) database for the pharmaceutical industry. The IDRAC first release covered the **European Union** (EU) and its **Member States**. The US were added in 1995, Central and Eastern Europe in 1997 and Japan in 1998. The objective of IDRAC is to provide RA departments with an intelligent tool in order:
- to construct dossiers more efficiently
- to simplify global registration
- to optimize in-house resources and free them for more value creating tasks.

The Database consists primarily of regulatory and legal texts issued by the EU, **European Free Trade Association**, Central and Eastern Europe member states, the US **Food and Drug Administration** and Japan, technical and scientific texts issued by a wide range of organizations, and practical information such as organizational structures, presentation and explanation of Community and National procedures and specific technical requirements for compiling registration dossiers.

The database is continuously updated. IDRAC On-line (updated every week) gives direct access to the database, IDRAC on CD-ROM is updated 6 times per year and can be completed with the synchronization option for weekly updates.

The sources of information used to build and maintain the IDRAC Database consist of:
- Official explanatory texts and guidelines from different supervisory organizations (e.g. **Committee for Proprietary Medicinal Products, International Conference on Harmonization**)
- National procedures and guidelines from the Medicines Agencies
- Legislative and regulatory texts from official journals
- Information on national regulatory happenings from external consultants
- Information on latest publications issued or modified from periodicals, reviews and publications
- Information regarding upcoming changes, new publications, new procedures and regulatory strategy from attendance at congresses, seminars and fairs
- Feedback and interaction with current and potential IDRAC customers through meetings and presentations of IDRAC at seminars, congresses and trade shows.

IEC
1. International Electrotechnical Commission.

2. (Clinical Trials) Independent Ethics Committee, see **Ethics Committee**.

IEC decision (Clinical Trials)
Independent Ethics Committee decision, see **Ethics Committee decision**.

IFAPP see **International Federation of Associations of Pharmaceutical Physicians**.

IFCC
International Federation of Clinical Chemistry.

IFDES
International Federation for Drug Efficacy and Safety.

IFPMA
International Federation of Pharmaceutical Manufacturers Association.

IFPP
International Federation of Pharmaceutical Physicians.

IHRIM (UK)
Institute of Health Record Information and Management.

IHSM see **Institute of Health Service Managers**.

IIS see **Institute of Information Scientists**.

IKS (Germany)
Interkantonale Kontrollstelle Für Heilmittel.

IMMP see **Intensive Medicines Monitoring Programme**.

immunizing agent, active
An antigenic preparation (**toxoid** or vaccine) used to induce formation of specific antibodies against a pathogenic micro-organism, which provides delayed but permanent protection against the associated disease.

immunizing agent, passive
A biological preparation (antitoxin, antivenin or immune serum) containing specific antibodies, against a pathogenic micro-organism, which provides immediate but temporary protection against the associated disease.

immunogenicity
The ability of a vaccine to stimulate the immune system, as measured by the proportion of individuals who produce specific antibody or T cells, or the amount of antibody produced. Not the same as **efficacy**.

immunopathology
A branch of medicine that deals with immune responses associated with disease.

immunosuppression
A pathological or medically-induced reduction in the capability of the immune system. It is caused by infection (e.g. HIV), drug treatment (to reduce rejection of a transplanted organ/tissue), pregnancy and malnutrition among others. Immunosuppressed individuals are commonly referred to as immunocompromised.

immunotherapy
A medical treatment or prophylaxis of disease using agents that may modify the

immune response. It is a largely experimental approach, studied most widely in the treatment of cancer.

impartial witness (Clinical Trials)
A person, who is independent of the trial, who cannot be influenced by people involved with the trial, who attends the **informed consent** process if the subject or the subject's **legally acceptable representative** cannot read, and who reads the informed consent form and any other written information supplied to the subject.
See also **informed consent, legally acceptable representative**.

implant
An organ, tissue, or device surgically inserted and left in the body.

imprint code (US)
Any single letter or number or any combination of letter(s) and numbers assigned by a US drug firm to a specific **drug product**.

imputability see **causality**.

IMS Health Global Services
IMS HEALTH is one of the world's leading providers of pharmaceutical information operating in over 90 countries with over 40 years' experience. Key products and services include: market research and financial analysis for prescription and over-the-counter pharmaceutical products in all critical phases of product planning, launch, marketing; sales management information; technology enabled selling solutions; and technology systems and information services that support managed care organizations in easily accessible formats:
- Global MIDAS™ Data which covers the global market place and includes:
- Hospital and retail pharmacy sectors
- Extensive sales, chemical, promotional and medical data.

International links applied to the individual country data allow multi-country comparisons.
MIDAS can be accessed on-line or via software database tools such as Dataview.

IMS produces a series of publications, covering drug intelligence – product **R&D** and lifecycle information, company and market studies – qualitative and quantitative data on global markets and industry players, and chemical products – covering the R&D pharmaceutical pipeline including intermediate/reaction pathways, through market and competitive analysis trend data, quantitative kilogram information and onwards to the provision of patent expiry and new market development data.

Reports on Market Assessment; Customized Forecasting; Company Image; Pharmaceutical sales, therapy and company data pricing; and primary research are all available in hard copy, on CD-ROM or as Lotus Notes, intranet or Web solutions from their website on a pay per view basis.

inactive ingredient
Any drug component other than an **active ingredient**. Substance not therapeutically active, such as starch, added to medicine to provide bulk, flavour, or colour, or for other non-therapeutic purpose.
See also **active ingredient**.

INADA (US)
Investigational New Animal Drug Application (**Food and Drug Administration**).

INAHTA
International Network of Agencies for Health Technology Assessment.

incapacity
Refers to a person's mental status and means inability to understand information presented, to appreciate the consequences of acting (or not acting) on that information, and to make a choice. Often used as a synonym for **incompetence**.
See also **incompetence**.

incidence (Epidemiology)
The rate of occurrence of a disease, **adverse event**, or other event in a given **population**. The rate of occurrence is the number of cases of disease, infection, or some other event having their onset during a prescribed period of time in relation to the unit of population in which they occur. Incidence measures morbidity or other events as they happen over a period of time. Examples include the number of deep venous thrombosis (DVT) cases occurring in women taking oral contraceptives (OCs) in relation to the number of DVT cases in women not taking OCs, or the number of cases of meningitis occurring in a school during a month in relation to the number of pupils enrolled in the school. It usually refers only to the number of new cases, particularly of chronic diseases. Hospitals also track certain risk management or quality problems with a system called incidence reporting.

incidence rate see **incidence**.

incineration
Intentional, controlled burning for the purpose of destroying waste. Some countries have rules stipulating that effective drugs must be incinerated. Incineration is typically performed at high temperatures and with controlled emissions to result in a landfillable ash.

inclusion criteria (Clinical Trials)
Criteria or basis used to select the target patient **population** for a particular **clinical trial**. They are the medical or social reasons why a person may be allowed to enter a trial. All studies have a list of **inclusion criteria** which patients must meet in order to be eligible for entry into a study. In addition, there should also be a list of exclusion criteria and the occurrence of just one of these means that the patient will not be permitted to enter the study even though they met all the inclusion criteria.
See also **exclusion criteria**.

incompatibility, therapeutic
Opposition in therapeutic effect between two or more medicines thus neutralizing their intrinsic effect because they cancel each other.

incompetence
Technically, a legal term meaning inability to manage one's own affairs. Often used as a synonym for incapacity.
See also **incapacity**.

incubation period
The time that elapses between infection (when an infectious organism enters the body) and the appearance of symptoms of a disease. Not the same as the **latent period**.

incurred but not reported (IBNR) (US)
Refers to a financial accounting of all services that have been performed but, as a result of a short period of time, have not been invoiced or recorded. Estimates of costs for medical services provided for which a claim has not yet been filed. Refers to claims which reflect services already delivered, but, for whatever reason, have not yet been reimbursed. These are bills 'in the

pipeline'. This is a crucial concept for proactive providers who are beginning to explore arrangements that put them in the role of adjudicating claims – as the result, perhaps, of operating in a sub-capitated system. Failure to account for these potential claims could lead to some very bad decisions. Good administrative operations have fairly sophisticated mathematical models to estimate this amount at any given time.

incurred claims
All claims with dates of service within a specified period.

incurred claims loss ratio
Incurred claims divided by premiums.

IND see Investigational New Drug

indemnity plan (indemnity health insurance) (US)
Managed care, particularly **Health Maintenance Organization** (HMO) and **capitation**, has evolved away from the indemnity method. Yet, many people are still covered under indemnity plans. It is an insurance programme in which covered person is reimbursed for covered expenses. Health **insurance** benefits are provided in the form of cash payments rather than services. An indemnity insurance contract usually defines the maximum amounts that will be paid for covered services. Indemnity insurance plans may have a **Preferred Provider Organization** option, underwriting and case management features, or include a network or other preferred provider restrictions, but will not have an HMO plan. Indemnity is the traditional form of insurance.

An indemnity plan is a plan which reimburses physicians for services performed, or beneficiaries for medical expenses incurred. Such plans are contrasted with group health plans, which provide service benefits through group medical practice.

Independent Data Monitoring Committee (IDMC) (Clinical Trials)
An independent committee that may be established by the sponsor to assess at intervals the progress of a **clinical trial**, the **safety** data, and the critical efficacy **end points**, and to recommend to the **sponsor** whether to continue, modify, or stop a trial.

Independent Ethics Committee see Ethics Committee.

indication
The disease, sign, symptom, or a condition, presented by a patient, for which a medicinal product has been shown to be effective and for which it may be prescribed or promoted.

Indicative Prescribing Scheme (IPS) see Prescribing Monitoring Documents (PMD).

indicator
A measure of a specific component of a health improvement strategy. An indicator can reflect an activity implemented to address a particular health issue – such as the number of children aged 2 who have received all appropriate immunizations – or it might reflect outcomes from activities already implemented – such as a decline in the number of cases of childhood German measles in any given year.

indirect transmission
Transmission of a parasite through an indirect life cycle.

Individual (Independent) Practice Association (IPA) or Organization (IPO) (US)
An organized form of prepaid medical practice delivery model in which the **Health**

Maintenance Organization (HMO) contracts with the participating physician organization, which in turn contracts with individual physicians. The IPA physicians practise in their own offices and continue to also see their fee-for-service (FFS) basis patients. The HMO reimburses the IPA on a capitated basis; however, the IPA may reimburse the physicians on an FFS or capitated basis. Sometimes thought of as an HMO model in which the HMO contracts with a physician organization that in turn contracts with individual physicians. The IPA physicians provide care to HMO members from their private offices and continue to see their FFS patients.

infectious period

The time period during which the infected are able to transmit an infection to any vulnerable host or vector they contact. Note that the infectious period may not necessarily be associated with **symptoms** of the disease.

Inform–Change–Monitor (UK)

To promote **clinical effectiveness**, the **National Health Service** (NHS) Executive (NHSE) published the booklet titled 'Inform – change – monitor' intended to help Chief Executives of Health Authorities and Trusts to develop ways of promoting greater clinical effectiveness.

The theme of the booklet, Inform – Change – Monitor, is explained as follows: 'Inform' is all about getting the evidence, assessing need and examining clinical and cost effectiveness. 'Change' is to do with policy making, changing practice, concentrating effort and innovating. 'Monitor' examines measuring health benefit, examining outcome indicators and audit.

See also **clinical effectiveness**.

informed consent (IC) (Clinical Trials)

The process of voluntary confirmation of a **subject/patient**'s willingness to participate in a particular trial (after information has been given about the trial), and the documentation thereof in accordance with the current version of the **Declaration of Helsinki**.

IC must be obtained (**participant** should sign the IC Form) from every human subject participating in the **clinical trial**. In general, this signifies that the subject understands the trial and its possible consequences on their health. **Good clinical practice** defines the appropriate elements of informed consent. At a minimum, each subject must be informed of:
1. Purpose/objectives of the study
2. Risks and inconveniences
3. Possible benefits
4. Alternative procedures
5. The subject's rights (e.g. right to not participate) and responsibilities
6. Confidentiality rights
7. Compensation rights if injured
8. Contact person for questions.

If the subject agrees to participate in the study after being informed of all of the above, a proper IC has been obtained. In giving IC, subjects may not waive or appear to waive any of their legal rights, or release or appear to release the **investigator**, the **sponsor**, the institution or agents thereof from liability for negligence.

infusion

The introduction of a substance, such as a **drug**, saline, nutrient, or other solution into the bloodstream (intravenously) or a body cavity for therapeutic purposes.

inhaler

A device used to introduce a powdered or misted drug into the lungs through the mouth, usually to treat respiratory disorders such as asthma.

injection
The use of a syringe and needle to insert a drug into a vein, muscle, or joint or under the skin.

INN see **International Non-proprietary Name.**

inpatient
A patient who has gone through the full admission procedures and is occupying a bed in a hospital, nursing home or other medical or post-acute institution. The term normally does not apply to day care patients, and does not apply to **outpatients** and Accident & Emergency attendances. It is the subject of detailed procedural debate and some flexible interpretation with certain **providers**.
See also **outpatient**.

inpatient care
Care given to a registered bed patient in a hospital, nursing home or other medical or post-acute institution.

inpatient procedure
Medical procedures that require a hospital stay. An example would be any major operation such as renal transplant surgery. In order to improve **cost containment**, many procedures which were once performed on an inpatient basis are now performed on an **outpatient** basis.

in-plan services (US)
Services that are covered under the state **Medicaid** plan and included in the patient's **managed care** contract and/or are furnished by a participating **provider**.

in-process control
Checks performed during production in order to monitor and if necessary to adjust the process to ensure that the product conforms to its specification. The control of the environment or equipment may also be regarded as part of in-process control.

in situ
'In place', often describes a cancer that has not spread.

inspection (Clinical Trials)
Officially conducted audit by relevant authorities or other **competent authority**(ies), at the site of investigation and/or at the **sponsor**'s site in order to verify adherence to **good clinical practice**. It involves conducting an official review of documents, facilities, records, and any other resources that are deemed by the authority(ies) to be related to the **clinical trial** and that may be located at the site of the trial, at the sponsor's facilities, at the contract research organization(s), or at other establishments deemed appropriate by the **regulatory authority**.

instillation
Clinical method involving the administration of a liquid/**medicinal product** drop-by-drop.

Institute of Biology (IOB) (UK)
The body that aims to represent professional biologists in the UK, set standards, and promote education and training. It conducts examinations, organizes local, national and international meetings, publishes books and journals and maintains registers and directories of specialist advisers and consultants. The IOB was founded in 1950 and incorporated by Royal Charter in 1979. Its members are drawn from all fields of life sciences.

Institute of Health Economics (IHE) (Canada)
A non-profit research organization representing a partnership of 16 organizations from

government, industry, a research foundation, and universities. IHE strives to improve health through the advancement of health services research and improved decision-making in health care. It is a unique consortium of academic, government, health industry and other organizations concerned with the **outcomes** associated with the use of pharmaceutical products and other health care interventions who:
- Provide national health policy leadership to secure the adoption of ethical, rational and analytic approaches to the assessment of new and existing drugs
- Provide leading edge expertise in the theory and practice of **pharmacoeconomics** (PE)
- Undertake economic studies of health care interventions initially focusing on PE evaluations
- Support a developing health research capacity
- Collaborate in the training of current and future practitioners in PE
- Bring stakeholders together to leverage their resources for PE research
- Communicate the impacts of economic and outcomes evaluations on health system reform
- Inform and stimulate public dialogue and debate in health care with research-based evidence.

Institute of Health Service Managers (IHSM) (UK)
An institute for those involved in the management of health care.

Institute of Information Scientists (IIS) (UK)
The IIS, founded in 1958, is the UK body for information scientists and information managers. It has 2700 members, about 10% of whom are based outside the UK. IIS members work in all sectors including commerce, industry, science and technology, electronic publishing, finance, law and education. IIS organizes a range of courses, seminars and meetings, as well as holding an annual conference.

Institute of Quality Assurance (IQA) (UK)
A UK leading professional body representing those who regard quality as an essential aspect of their working life. Founded in 1919, IQA has continued to grow and adapt to the needs of its members and the profession. Today it has over 13 000 individual members and nearly 1000 affiliated organizations worldwide. Its mission is:
- To advance the knowledge of quality management and practices, thus to promote the efficiency and international competitiveness of British industry and commerce, and to achieve greater awareness of the importance of quality performance to the national economy and to society in general
- To promote the education, training, qualification and continuing professional development of people with responsibility for quality
- To provide appropriate services for members, industry and commerce and others.

IQA's professional arm constantly monitors all quality management developments, carrying out research projects and supporting higher standards initiatives. IQA also run specialist groups assessing and promoting quality in, for example, pharmaceuticals, process industries, education and the environment.

IQA is a member of a number of professional associations worldwide and ensures that its voice is heard on appropriate committees of the British Standards Institution (BSI), the International Organization for Standardization (ISO) and the **European Committee for Standardization** (CEN). IQA is also represented on:
- The European Organization for Quality (EOQ)

- The UK Accreditation Service (UKAS)
- The Parliamentary and Scientific Committee
- The National Forum for Conformity Assessment and Quality Policy.

Institut für Arzneimittel (Germany)
Institute for Drugs founded on 1 July 1975 as part of the now dissolved Federal Health Office – known as the **BGA**. **BfArM** is the successor to the Institute for Drugs.

institution, medical (Clinical Trials)
As defined by **good clinical practice** is 'Any public or private entity or agency or medical or dental facility where **clinical trials** are conducted.'

Institutional Review Board (IRB) (US)
An independent body constituted of medical, scientific (physicians, scientists), and non-scientific (members of the community, clergy and others) members established at research institutions, hospitals and universities in the US, as required by **HSS** (formerly **HEW**) regulations. The **Food and Drug Administration (FDA)** requires that all **clinical trials** must be approved and overseen by an IRB. The requirements for IRBs are described in the **Code of Federal Regulations** and GLPs. The IRB's responsibility is to ensure the protection of the rights, **safety** and **well-being** of human **subjects** involved in a trial by, among other ways, reviewing, approving, and providing continuing review of trial **protocols** and amendments and the methods and material to be used in obtaining and documenting **informed consent** of the trial subjects. The responsibility of the IRB is, therefore, not only to evaluate the ethical acceptability of the proposed clinical research but also to examine the scientific validity of the study to the extent needed to be confident that the study does not expose subjects to unreasonable risk.

IRB is the American version for the **Ethics Committee**. Other names for such bodies include Independent Review Board, Committee for the Protection of Human Subjects.

See also **Research Ethics Board (REB)**.

instrument qualification (IQ)
IQ defines the functional and operational (or performance) specifications. IQ establishes that the instrument is received as designed and specified and that it is properly installed. Operational qualification (OQ) demonstrates that the instrument will function according to the operational specifications. Performance qualification (PQ) demonstrates that an instrument will function according to a specification appropriate to its routine use.

insufflation
The act of blowing a powder, vapour, gas or air into a body cavity.

insurance
A protection by written contract against the financial hazards (in whole or in part) of the happenings of specified accidental unexpected events.

INT
Interaction, see **drug–drug interaction**.

Integrated Care Pathway (ICP)
A pathway of care devised, for a patient, in such a way that it takes in a whole system approach rather than just one element of care.

Integrated Delivery Systems (IDS) or Integrated Services Network (ISN) (US)
Many different, but similar, definitions exist for IDS. An IDS, as an entity, does not have to abide

by strict regulations as does a **Health Maintenance Organization**. When an IDS offers a health plan, however, it must then abide by the requirements of the State and federal government for health plans, insurance companies or HMOs. Without owning a health plan product, an IDS will usually abide by the regulations that govern its separate businesses, that is, regulations governing hospitals, clinics and physicians. An IDS can be a financial or contractual arrangement between health providers (usually hospitals and doctors) to offer a comprehensive range of health care services through a separate legal entity operating, at least for these purposes, as a single health care delivery system. IDS can be a network of organizations usually including hospitals and physician groups, that provides or arranges to provide a coordinated continuum of services to a defined population and is held both clinically and fiscally accountable for the outcomes of the populations served. IDS can also be a health care provider organization which vertically integrates physician, hospital, and, usually, also health plan businesses in some manner in order to establish a full continuum of care, seamless of delivery of services and the ability to manage care under new reimbursement arrangements.

Also called **accountable health plan**, delivery system, health delivery network, horizontally integrated system, vertically integrated system.

integrated effectiveness
An integrated summary of all available information about the **efficacy** of the **drug product** for the claimed **indication**.

integrated safety
An integrated summary of all available information about the **safety** of the **drug product**.

intellectual property
Intangible property created by the mind. Like tangible real or personal property, the law recognizes the right to own and to control intellectual property. There are four well-recognized types of intellectual property rights: copyrights, trademarks, patents, and trade secrets. They differ significantly in the rights they confer and in how they are obtained and maintained.

'intended purpose'
The use for which the **medicinal product/medical device** is intended and for which it is suited according to the data supplied by the **manufacturer** in the **Summary of Product Characteristics**/instructions, on labelling, in the instruction and/or in promotional materials.
See also **indication**.

Intensified Adverse Drug Reaction Reporting Scheme see Intensive Medicines Monitoring Programme

intensive care
Close monitoring of a **patient** who is seriously ill.

Intensive Medicines Monitoring Programme (IMMP) (New Zealand)
A programme that was established in 1977 as a response to widespread concerns following the **thalidomide** and practolol disasters. The aim of the IMMP is the early identification of unexpected **adverse drug reactions** with selected new medicines. The objective was to undertake **adverse event** monitoring of a small number of drugs in the early post-marketing period. Prescription information was to be supplied by dispensing pharmacists to provide a denominator for calculating rates. The numerator was to be provided by 'intensified' **spontaneous reporting** (SR) and the programme was originally called the Intensified Adverse Drug Reaction Reporting Scheme. The IMMP is part of the Centre for Adverse Reactions

Monitoring (CARM) which is the national centre for drug monitoring and which uses the '**Yellow card scheme**' of SR for all non-IMMP drugs.

See also **Centre for Adverse Reactions Monitoring**.

Intention to Treat (ITT) Analysis (Clinical Trials)

A method of statistical data analysis in which the primary tabulations and companion summaries of all **outcome** data are by assigned treatment, regardless of the subject's suitability or treatment adherence with the study **protocol**. When the results are analysed, **subjects** should be analysed in the group they were originally randomly allocated to. So that if, for example, a subject allocated to receive the control intervention actually received the intervention, they would nonetheless be analysed as if they had not had the intervention. Similarly, if someone allocated to the control intervention did not do so, they would still be counted with the intervention group. If results are not analysed in this way, the whole purpose of the original randomization breaks down: the people in the two groups may then systematically differ from each other and any differences in the results of the two groups could simply be due to this fact. Using ITT analysis only weakens the observed effect of an intervention and does not make an intervention appear effective when it was not. That is to say, it does not undermine any observed association between an intervention and outcome − it makes it more believable.

Also called Analysis by Treatment Administered.

intent to treat group (Clinical Trials)

All subjects administered an **investigational product** and who are receiving at least one efficacy analysis.

interaction see **drug–drug interaction**.

intercurrent illness (Clinical Trials)

Pre-existing disease that a subject, being entered into a clinical trial, has.

Interdoc (South Africa)

Established in response to the need for a Clinical Management System (CMS) that meets the needs of the medical profession while also involving important players such as Medical Aid Administrators and other founders of healthcare. Mission is to develop healthcare products and systems.

interfering variable see **confounding factor**.

interim analysis (Clinical Trials)

An analysis performed before all patients have completed the trial. Reasons for conducting such analysis include the intention to terminate the trial early if the result is favourable or unfavourable. The timing of such analyses should be pre-determined when the study is being planned. They should not be performed too frequently. Termination of studies should be done with due consideration for the study patients.

interim clinical trial report see **interim analysis**.

intermediate product

Partly processed materials that must undergo further manufacturing steps before it becomes a bulk product.

See also **finished product**.

internal assessment

The first part of a **SWOT** analysis is the internal assessment. This consists of an examination of

a company's internal environment and its products. The internal assessment evaluates many factors, including the following:
1. Company environment
2. Company structure
3. Department roles within the company.
4. Product
5. Pricing strategies
6. Promotion
7. Product placement/distribution.

See also **external environment**.

internal audit (Clinical Trials)
Many pharmaceutical companies have a **Clinical Trial Audit** department which undertakes internal trials audit on behalf of the company. The purpose of the audit is to ensure that the clinical research staff are complying with the **standard operating procedures** for the conduct of clinical trials. The audit will also ensure that all the relevant documents are present in the clinical research files for the particular study.

internal consistency
A property of data that does not contradict itself.

internal market (UK)
The **National Health Service** (NHS) system of competition introduced by the Conservative government in 1991, characterized by Purchasers, Providers and contracts.

internal medicine
Generally, the branch of medicine that is concerned with diseases that do not require surgery, specifically, the study and treatment of internal organs and body systems; it encompasses many subspecialties. Internists, the doctors who practice internal medicine, often serve as family physicians to supervise general medical care.

International Agency for Research on Cancer (IARC)
The IARC was established in May 1965, through a resolution of the XVIIIth World Health Assembly, as an extension of the **World Health Organization**, after a French initiative. IARC's founding members were the Federal Republic of Germany, France, Italy, the UK and the US. The IARC's membership is 18 countries. A major goal of the IARC is the identification of causes of cancer, so that preventive measures may be adopted against them.

International Birth Date (IBD)
The date on which the first regulatory authority approved a drug for marketing, i.e. it is the date of the first **marketing authorization** (MA) for a **medicinal product** granted to the MA holder in any country in the world. For medicinal products first authorized in the **European Union** (EU), the **EU Birth Date (EBD)** is the IBD. For administrative convenience, if desired by the MA holder, the IBD may be designated as the last day of the same month.

International Classification of Diseases, Ninth Revision, Clinical Modification (ICD-9-CM)
A classification of disease by diagnosis codified into six-digit numbers. It is the universal coding method used to document the incidence of disease, injury, mortality and illness. It is designed to facilitate the collection of uniform and comparable health information. The ICD-9-CM was

issued in 1979. In the US, this system is used to group patients into **diagnosis-related groups**, prepare hospital and physician billings and prepare cost reports.

See also **coding**.

International Conference on Harmonization (ICH)

A joint endeavour of pharmaceutical regulatory agencies and the pharmaceutical manufacturers' associations in Europe, Japan, and the US which has the goals of reducing redundancy and costs of drug development while hastening the delivery of proven new therapeutic agents to patients. In addition to the regulators from the **European Union**, Japan, and the US, there are official observers from other organizations or countries such as the **World Health Organization** and Canada, and their representation is expected to facilitate a wider acceptance of the expert working group documents. Many aspects of the drug development process were considered in three major areas of quality (designated as Q topics), pre-clinical **safety** (S) and clinical safety (E) to streamline the process, and through the development of consensus expert documents, which if followed, would allow registration of a new product in all three of these global areas. In addition to these three major areas, a fourth was formed after the second conference, which could be applied to all three areas and was designated as the mixed (M) topics.

The ICH process is accomplished in five steps. *Step 1* – A proposal to harmonize some aspects of the drug developmental process is submitted and approved by the steering Committee. *Step 2* – An Expert Working Group (EWG), usually consisting of one representative from each of the six parties involved in ICH, is formed. The EWG (also known as six pack) meets and writes a formal proposal for an ICH guidance including all details for implementation. When completely signed off by the EWG and the Steering Committee, the document (now at Step 2) is published by the regulatory agencies for comments (*Step 3*). After receipt of comments, the EWG reconvenes to make changes deemed necessary and a new document is signed off by the regulators on the Steering Committee and published (*Step 4*). Regulations are often amended and the guidance is implemented at *Step 5*. Since amending regulations is both a legal and political process, Step 5 occurs outside the ICH process. There are three efficacy and two mixed documents which relate to clinical safety surveillance. The **E2A guidance document** entitled 'Clinical Safety Data Management: Definitions and Standards for Expedited Reporting' and the other guidance document is E2B entitled 'Data Elements for Transmission of Individual Case Safety Reports'. The subtopics are handled by the M1 and M2 expert working groups. M1 is the Medical terminology expert working group and M2 is the expert working group for Electronic Standards for the Transfer of Regulatory Information and Data. The E2C document is entitled 'Periodic Safety Update Report'.

See also **E 1–9, Q 1–6, M3** and **S 1–6 guidance documents**.

International Federation of Associations of Pharmaceutical Physicians (IFAPP)

Established in March 1976, amongst its activities, IFAPP acts as a forum for disseminating information on the discipline of pharmaceutical medicine, and holds symposia with themes appropriate to the discipline. Over sixteen countries have medical advisor associations that are affiliated to the IFAPP.

International Non-proprietary Name (INN)

Also called the recommended INN (rINN). This is the name of the medicinal substance as given in the list published by the **World Health Organization**.

International Prescribing Information see Core Safety Data Sheet.

International Society for Pharmacoeconomics and Outcomes Research (ISPOR)

International organization formed in 1995 to promote the practice and science of **pharmacoeconomics** and health **outcomes** assessment.

International Society for Pharmacoepidemiology (ISPE)
A non-profit international professional membership organization dedicated to promoting **pharmacoepidemiology**. ISPE is firmly committed to providing an unbiased scientific forum to the views of all parties with interests in drug development, delivery, use, and effects. Members are employed by the pharmaceutical industry, academic institutions, government agencies, non-profit and for-profit private organizations.

International Society for Quality-of-Life Studies (ISQOLS)
An organization whose members are academic, business, non-profit and government researchers who are interested in **quality of life** studies, can coordinate their efforts to advance the knowledge base and to create positive social change.

International Union of Pharmacology (IUPHAR)
A non-governmental organization in official relations with the **World Health Organization**. It is a voluntary, non-profit association of national organizations presently representing the pharmacologists of member countries and regional associations. It was founded in 1959 as a section of the International Union of Physiological Sciences, and has been independent since 1966. IUPHAR is a member of the International Council for Science (ICSU) and participates in the work of its scientific committees. It receives international recognition, particularly by the United Nations Educational and Scientific Organization (UNESCO). According to its statutes, IUPHAR has full members, i.e. national societies, one from each country, but may also accept associate and affiliate members.

inter-subject variation (Clinical Trials)
In a parallel trial design, differences between subjects are used to assess treatment differences. Also called between-subject variation.

interval estimate (Statistics)
A pair of values for the parameter within which the population parameter is likely to lie. The most common form of interval estimate is the **confidence interval**.

intervention strategy
A generic term used in public health to describe a programme or policy designed to have an impact on an illness or disease. Hence a mandatory seat belt law is an intervention designed to reduce automobile-related fatalities.

intolerance
Allergy to a food, drug, or other substance (e.g. gluten intolerance).

intra-amniotic
Injection into the amniotic cavity.
Compare **extra-amniotic**.

intrabursal
Injection in the bursae and tendons.

intramuscular injection
Putting a fluid into a muscle with a needle and syringe.

intrathecal
Injection of a substance through the theca of the spinal cord into the subarachnoid space.

intrauterine device (IUD)
A device inserted into the uterus that helps to prevent pregnancy.

intravenous injection (IV)
Within or into the veins. Intravenous drugs are injected directly into the veins with a needle and **syringe**.

intravitreal
Injected into the vitreous humour of the eye.

intrinsic
A term used to describe something originating from or located in a tissue or organ.

intrinsic activity
The maximal stimulatory response induced by a compound in relation to that of a given reference compound. The term has evolved with common usage. It was introduced by Ariëns as a proportionality factor between tissue response and **receptor** occupancy. The numerical value of intrinsic activity (alpha) could range from unity (for full **agonists**, i.e., agonist inducing the tissue maximal response) to zero (for **antagonists**), the fractional values within this range denoting **partial agonists**. Ariëns' original definition equates the molecular nature of alpha to maximal response only when response is a linear function of receptor occupancy. This function has been verified. Thus, intrinsic activity, which is a **drug** and tissue parameter, cannot be used as a characteristic drug parameter for classification of drugs or drug receptors. For this purpose, a proportionality factor derived by null methods, namely, relative **efficacy**, should be used. Intrinsic activity − like affinity − depends on the chemical natures of both the drug and the receptor, but intrinsic activity and affinity apparently can vary independently with changes in the drug molecule. Intrinsic activity is not the same as 'potency' and may be completely independent of it. Finally, 'intrinsic activity' should not be used instead of 'intrinsic efficacy'. A 'partial agonist' should be termed 'agonist with intermediate intrinsic efficacy' in a given tissue.
See also **partial agonist**.
Compare **affinity**, **antagonism**, **receptor**.

intubation
The passage of a tube into an organ or body structure; commonly used to refer to the passage of a tube down the windpipe for artificial respiration.

in utero
While in the uterus during early development.

invasive
Describes an entity that spreads throughout body tissues, such as a tumour or micro-organism; also describes a medical procedure in which body tissues are penetrated.

inverse agonist
A **drug** that acts at the same **receptor** as that of an **agonist**, yet produces an opposite effect. Also called negative **antagonists**.

inverse density dependence see **density dependence**.

Investigational Device Exemption (IDE) (US)
Exemptions from certain regulations that apply to **Medical Device** Amendments that allow shipment of unapproved devices for use in clinical investigations. Normally, market approval is needed to distribute a medical device. **Food and Drug Administration** (FDA) can grant a temporary exemption, however, so that a company can conduct **clinical trials**. To receive such

an exemption, a company must file an IDE application with the Center for Devices and Radiobiological Health. If the FDA does not respond to the IDE application within 30 days, the company may distribute its device to clinical investigators and the trials may begin.

Compare **Investigational New Drug**.

investigational medical product

A pharmaceutical form of an **active ingredient** (including biological product for human use), **medical device**, human food additive, colour additive, electronic product or **placebo** being tested or used as a reference in a **clinical trial**, including a product with a **marketing authorization** when used or assembled (formulated or packaged) in a way different from the approved form, or when used for an unapproved **indication**, or when used to gain further information about an approved use.

In the US it is called a 'test article' and defined as any other article subject to regulations under the Act or under sections 351 and 354–360F of the Public Health Service Act (42 USC 262 and 263b–263n)

Every marketed **medicinal product** must go through a lengthy development and approval process which is heavily regulated by the regulatory authorities. Until these authorities grant the licence, the product is considered to be an investigational medical product.

See also **test article**.

investigational new device (US)

A device permitted by the **Food and Drug Administration** to be tested in humans but not yet determined to be safe and effective for a particular use in the general population and not yet licensed for marketing.

investigational new drug (IND) (US and Canada)

The name given to an experimental drug after the **regulatory authority** (**Food and Drug Administration** (US) or the Drugs Directorate of Health and Welfare (Canada)) has agreed that it can be used in clinical trials and tested in humans but not approved for commercial marketing.

See also **investigational medical product**.

Investigational New Drug (IND) application (US)

An application that a drug sponsor must submit to the **Food and Drug Administration** (FDA) before beginning tests of a new drug on humans. From 1963 it has been necessary to inform the FDA before commencing any **clinical trial**, in humans, with an unapproved IND. This notification was called 'A Notice of Claimed Investigational Exemption for a New Drug' or IND. The IND application describes results of pre-clinical studies and is active within 30 days if not delayed by the FDA.

The IND contains the plan for the study and is supposed to give a complete picture of the drug, including its structural formula, animal test results, and manufacturing information. There are two types of INDs:
1. Commercial
2. Non-commercial.

A commercial IND permits the **sponsor** to gather the data on clinical safety and effectiveness that are needed for an NDA. If the drug is approved by the FDA, the sponsor is allowed to market the drug for specific uses. A non-commercial IND allows the sponsor to use the drug in research or early clinical investigation to obtain advanced scientific knowledge of the drug. Before clinical trials can begin, the FDA requires that proposed clinical studies be reviewed both by the FDA and an **Institutional Review Board**.

investigational new drug (IND) exemption application see **Investigational New Drug (IND) application.**

Investigational New Drugs

An interdisciplinary journal for clinicians and scientists with the aim of providing a forum for the development and rapid dissemination of information on new anticancer agents. The papers published are of interest to the medical chemist, toxicologist, pharmacist, pharmacologist, biostatistician and clinical oncologist. It provides the fastest possible publication of new discoveries and results for the whole community of scientists developing anticancer agents.

Investigational New Drug (IND) Safety Report (US)

IND Safety Reports must be submitted by study **sponsors** to the **Food and Drug Administration** (FDA) to document deaths or injuries which occur during **clinical trials**. Serious or unexpected **adverse drug reactions** must be reported to the FDA within 10 days. Detailed reporting requirements are included in 21 **Code of Federal Regulations** 312.

investigational product see **investigational medical product.**

investigator(s) (Clinical Trials)

One or more persons responsible for the practical performance of a **clinical trial** (at the trial site), for the integrity, health and welfare of the subjects during the trial. The investigator is:
- an appropriately qualified person legally allowed to practice medicine/dentistry
- trained and experienced in research, particularly in the clinical area of the proposed trial
- familiar with the background to and the requirements of the study
- known to have high ethical standards and professional integrity.

The legal status of persons authorized to act as investigators may differ between **Member States** of the **European Union** (EU) and between the EU and other countries.

For a multicentre trial, a coordinating (principal) investigator, responsible for the coordination of the investigators at the different centres, may be appointed.

See also **sub-investigator.**

Investigator's Brochure (Clinical Trials)

A collection of all relevant **data** and information, compiled by the company/**sponsor**, consisting of all the relevant information known prior to the onset of a **clinical trial** including chemical and pharmaceutical, toxicological, pharmacokinetic and pharmacodynamic data, in animals and the results of earlier trials. There should be adequate data to justify the nature, scale and duration of the proposed trial. The brochure is given to an investigator to enable him to conduct a trial safely and ethically. The information must be updated during the course of the trial, if new data arise.

in vitro

From Latin meaning in glass; a biological test or process that is carried out in an artificial environment such as a test tube or the equivalent laboratory apparatus.

in vitro assay development

Determination of an *in vitro* system which can be used repetitively and reliably to detect compounds which modulate the activity of a target of interest.

in vivo

Latin for 'in the living body'. *In vivo* refers to biological testing which is performed in living organisms (animals or humans).

IOM (US)
Institute of Medicine.

IoS (UK) see **Item of Service**.

IPA see **Individual (Independent) Practice Association**.

IPO see **Individual (Independent) Practice Association (IPA)**.

IPRO
Independent Pharmaceutical Research Organization.

IPS (UK)
Indicative Prescribing Scheme. Former name for **Prescribing Monitoring Documents**.

IQ
1. Intelligence quotient; a measure of a person's intelligence as determined by specific tests.
2. Installation qualification, see **instrument qualification**.

IRB see **Institutional Review Board**.

IRD
International Registration Document.

ISCB
International Society for Clinical Biostatistics.

ISO
International Standards Organization.

isolator technology
A technology designed and adopted in order to minimize human interventions in processing areas so as to significantly decrease the risk of microbiological contamination, of aseptically manufactured medicinal products, from the environment. There are many possible designs of isolator and transfer devices.

isosteres
Molecules or ions of similar size containing the same number of atoms and valence electrons, e.g., O^{2-}, F^-, Ne.
See also **bioisostere**.

ISTAHC
International Society of Technology Assessment in Health Care.

Item of Service (IoS) (UK)
A provision that a general practitioner gets paid for on an itemized basis.

ITT
Intention to treat, see **Intention to Treat Analysis**.

IUCD see **intrauterine device**.

IUD see **intrauterine device**.

IUPAC
International Union of Pure and Applied Chemistry.

IV
    Intravenous.

IVD
    1. *In vitro* device
    2. *In vitro* diagnostic.

IVF
    in vitro fertilization.

JANET (UK)
Joint Academic Network. A British academic and research network.

JAMA
Journal of the American Medical Association.

Japan Pharmaceutical Association (Nippon Yakuzaishi Kai)
An Association with the objectives of raising the ethical and academic levels of pharmacists and achieving the advancement and development of pharmacology and the pharmaceutical trade to contribute to the improvement of national health and welfare.

The Association was established as a non-profit foundation with a voluntary membership system. The membership of the Association is about 84 500, which is equivalent to about one half of all the pharmacists in Japan, that is, about 176 800. The members of the Association consist of pharmacists engaged in every type of professional (community pharmacists = 56%, pharmacists in general drug stores & pharmaceutical wholesalers = 18%, hospital & clinic pharmacists = 11%, administrative pharmacists = 3.5%, industrial pharmacists = 2.2%, others = 9.3%). The members of the Association automatically become the members of one of the 47 prefectural pharmaceutical associations.

The Japan Pharmaceutical Association is playing an active role in the international pharmaceutical world as a ordinary member of the International Pharmaceutical Federation (FIP) and the Federation of Asian Pharmaceutical Associations (FAPA).

Contact:
Nagai Memorial House 4F,
2-12-15 Shibuya,
Shibuyaku,
Tokyo 150-8389, Japan
Tel: +81-3-3406-1171
Fax: +81-3-3406-1499
Email: webmaster@nichiykau.or.jp.

JCAHO
Joint Commission of Accreditation of Healthcare Organizations.

JCC see **Joint Consultative Committee**.

JCHMT see **Joint Committee on Higher Medical Training of the medical Royal Colleges**.

JCPTGP see **Joint Committee on Postgraduate Training for General Practice**.

Joint Care Planning Team (UK)
A group of health and local authority officers which reports to the **Joint Consultative Committee**.

Joint Committee on Higher Medical Training of the medical Royal Colleges (JCHMT)
A task force of the Faculty of Pharmaceutical Medicine's Education Committee.

Joint Committee on Postgraduate Training for General Practice (JCPTGP) (UK)
The body prescribed by the vocational training regulations (**National Health Service** (NHS) Regulations 1979) of the NHS Act (1977) for the maintenance of national standards. The Committee has the dual role of issuing certificates of experience on completion of training and ensuring that the experience gained is of a reasonable standard throughout the UK. In 1985 the Committee published its Recommendations to regions for the Establishment of Criteria for the Approval and Re-approval of Trainers in general practice.

Joint Finance Initiative (UK)
A special allocation made to health authorities outside their mainstream allocation (Health Act 1977). This allows health authorities to transfer money to local authorities and voluntary organizations for functions clearly linked to the priorities and objectives of community care plans, where better value would be achieved than by equivalent expenditure.
See also **Joint Financing** and **Joint Finance Committee**.

joint financing (UK)
A sum of money taken from the central health **allocation** and given to **health authorities** (HAs) to spend on projects to be jointly agreed with social services departments (SSD). The stipulation is that it should be used for projects which reduce health care costs. Under review and may be withdrawn. It is often the focal point of HAs/SSD relationship.
See also **Joint Finance Committee** and **Joint Finance Initiative**.

Joint Formulary Committee of RPSGB and the BMA (UK)
The committee that represents the views of the **British Medical Association** and the **Royal Pharmaceutical Society of Great Britain** and the **Department of Health**; to decide changes in policy; format or frequency; and to undertake revision of the **British National Formulary**.

JPMA (Japan)
Japan Pharmaceutical Manufacturers Association.

510 (K) (US)
An exemption to the **Food, Drug and Cosmetic Act** which allows **medical devices** to be marketed without the submission of a **Premarket Approval Application** to **CDRH**. This exemption was created to allow new devices which are similar to existing ones a simple path to market. To qualify for a 510(K) exemption, a **manufacturer** must submit a premarket notification to CDRH before the product is introduced for sale.

510(K) Device (US)
A **medical device** that is considered substantially equivalent to one that was or is being legally marketed. A **sponsor** planning to market such a device must submit notification to the **Food and Drug Administration** (FDA) 90 days in advance of placing the device on the market. If the FDA agrees with the sponsor, the device may then be marketed. **510(K)** is the section of the **Food, Drug and Cosmetic Act** that describes premarket notification; hence the designation '510(K) device.'

K_{el} see elimination rate constant.

K_0 see absorption rate constant.

Karnofsky status
A subjective score between 0 and 100 [100% (no symptoms) to 0% (dead)], assigned by a physician to describe a patient's performance status scale, ability to function and perform common tasks.

Karnofsky Performance Status Scale

Karnofsky status	Meaning
100%	No symptoms
90%	Able to carry on normal activity; minor signs or symptoms of disease
80%	Able to carry on normal activity with effort; some signs or symptoms of disease
70%	Cares for self, unable to carry on normal activity or do active work
60%	Requires occasional assistance but is able to care for most of own needs
50%	Requires considerable assistance and frequent medical care
40%	Disabled; requires special care and assistance
30%	Severely disabled; hospitalization indicated although death not imminent
20%	Very sick; hospitalization necessary; active supportive treatment necessary
10%	Moribund, fatal processes progressing rapidly
0%	Dead

See also **ECOG Status**.

Kefauver–Harris Amendment (US)
Amendment to the **Food, Drug and Cosmetic Act** of 1938. It was passed in 1962 to fill gaps in the original 1938 food and drug law. These amendments added a requirement that evidence of **efficacy** of a new **drug product** be submitted to the **Food and Drug Administration** (FDA) as part of the approval process.

See also **Food, Drug and Cosmetic (FDC) Act**.

Kelsey, Francis O.
The **Food and Drug Administration** officer who won the US government's highest honour for civilian employees for keeping the drug **thalidomide** off the market in the US. This prevented

a public health disaster such as the one experienced in Europe, where deformed infants were born to mothers who took the drug during pregnancy.
See also **thalidomide**.

keratolytic
An agent/drug that promotes the softening and peeling/removing of the horny layer (the keratin-containing outer layer) of skin; used to treat skin disorders such as corns, callosities, warts, dandruff, and of chronic scaly lesions especially in psoriasis.

KNMP (Netherlands)
Royal Dutch Association for Advancement of Pharmacy.

Koseisho
Japanese Health Ministry.

label see **labelling**.

labelled use
A US term for use of a **drug product** for its licensed indication, as 'labelled' in its data sheet (Summary of Product Characteristics).
Also called listed.

labelling
The information accompanying a **medicinal product** that, in general, includes drug's name, **indication**, **adverse events**, **contraindications**, etc.

In the **European Union** (EU) the rules governing labelling of medicinal products and leaflets inserted in packages of such products are laid down in Articles 13–20 of **Directive 65/65/EEC** but amended by **Directive 92/27/EEC** (Chapters II and III respectively). The later Directive laid down the rules for labelling and package leaflets of medicinal products marketed in the EU. In accordance with this Directive, all labelling particulars must be consistent with the relevant **product licence**. The product's particulars must be clearly written on the outer packaging or the immediate packaging (if no outer packing is present). Additionally, the Directive made the inclusion of an information package leaflet (in accordance with the **Summary of Product Characteristics**) obligatory unless all the stipulated information and particulars are written on the outer or immediate packaging. The choice of linguistic level is also specified in that it must be deemed understandable by patients. In the US, the **Food, Drug and Cosmetic Act** defines labelling (labeling is the American spelling) as all 'labels and other written, printed, or graphic matter upon any article or any of its containers or wrappers or accompanying such article.' Normally, the term 'labelling' is used to refer to **vial** and carton labels and any inserts (directions for use, etc.) included with a drug, biologic, or **medical device**. When interpreted aggressively by **Food and Drug Administration** (FDA), it can include other items, such as materials displayed in conjunction with a **drug product** at an industry symposium (for example, posters or handouts).

Labelling of **investigational product** samples for **clinical trials** requires, according to **European Community** (EC) guidelines of **good clinical practice**, the following minimal amount of information:
- Name of the **sponsor**
- Pharmaceutical dosage form, route of administration, quantity of dosage units (and name/identifier of the product and strength/potency in case of an open trial)
- The batch and/or code number to identify the contents and packaging operation
- The trial **subject identification number**, where applicable
- Directions for use
- 'For clinical trial use only'
- Name of the responsible physician (**investigator**)
- A trial reference code allowing identification of the trial site and investigator
- The storage conditions
- The period of use (use-by date, expiry date)
- 'Keep out of reach of children' except when the product is for use only in hospital.

For clinical trials of medicinal products for use before and during pregnancy; within the EC, the product has also to be assigned to a certain category that is pre-defined according to the level of knowledge of its potential teratogenicity. For example 'A' denotes 'Product has been assessed, no harmful effects are known' and 'B3' denotes 'Safety not established, animal studies have shown reproductive toxicity' and so forth.

See also **misbranded product**.

laboratory normal range see **normal range**.

LADME System
Deals with the complex dynamic process of liberation of an **active ingredient** from the dosage form, its **absorption** into systemic circulation, its distribution and **metabolism** in the body and the **excretion** of the drug from the body.

L'Agence Française de Sécurité Sanitaire des Produits de Santé (l'AFSSAPS) (France)
The French Agency for the regulation of medicinal products.

lag time
The period which elapses between the time of administration of a drug and the start of absorption or the time a measurable concentration is found in the blood.

larvicide
A preparation used for destroying larvae.

last observation carried forward (LOCF) (Clinical Trials)
Method of assessing the mean effect of a treatment in a clinical trial in which not all the subjects in the group completed the treatment as laid down in the **protocol**. The mean value of the measure being assessed is calculated by including the last recorded value in all subjects in each treatment group, whether or not they completed the treatment, irrespective of the reason for their dropping out of the study.

latentiated drug see **drug latentiation**.

latent period (latency)
Time between action and response, between infection and clinical symptoms, and between drug administration and biological response. For example, it refers to the time between arrival of impulse at a muscle fibre and the contraction of the fibre. It also includes the time from infection to when the individual is infectious to others. In a helminth's infection, it is termed the *pre-patent period*. Not the same as the incubation period.
Compare **time–concentration curve, lag time, quiescence**.

Latin square (Clinical Trials)
A trial design used in cross-over studies. It is commonly used in volunteer studies where a large number of products may be tested by the administration of a single dose of each medication. Each of n patients (or of n groups of subjects) receives n treatments in a randomized order (represented by n times n squares). The volunteers may be dosed at weekly intervals. The Latin square design ensures that the order of the treatments is randomly determined and that each volunteer is dosed with each of the products during the whole of test period.

LD10
Dose that is lethal in 10% of the animals of the species treated.

LDL see **low-density lipoprotein**.

LDLo
Lowest lethal dose (toxicity testing).

lead discovery
The process of identifying active **new chemical entities**, which by subsequent modification may be transformed into a clinically useful **drug**.
See also **drug candidate**.

lead generation
Strategies developed to identify compounds which possess a desired but non-optimized biological activity.

lead optimization
The synthetic modification of a biologically active compound, to fulfil all stereoelectronic, physicochemical, **pharmacokinetic** and toxicological specifications required for clinical usefulness. It is the second phase in the drug design process and comprises the **quantitative structure–activity relationships** developed by the medicinal chemist leading to the optimized drug contender that develops into the prospective novel medication.
See also **drug candidate**.

Lead Researcher (Clinical Trials)
The person with primary responsibility for meeting all ethical, scientific and regulatory requirements for conduct of a study **protocol**, whether or not acting as the **Principal Investigator** for the award that funds the said study.
See also **Investigator**.

lead-time bias (Clinical Trials)
If study patients are not all enrolled at similar, well-defined points in the course of their disease, differences in **outcome** over time may merely reflect differences in duration of illness.

legally acceptable representative (Clinical Trials)
A person authorized either by statute or by court appointment to make decisions on behalf of another person. In human subjects research, an individual or judicial or other body authorized under applicable law to consent on behalf of a prospective subject to the subject's participation in the procedure(s) involved in the research.

legally authorized representative see legally acceptable representative.

legend drug
A, mostly, American term used to describe a **drug** that cannot legally be obtained without a physician's written prescription. In the US, the classification of a drug as a prescription or non-prescription medication is a matter of federal law, and US pharmacists are familiar with the legend, 'Caution: Federal Law prohibits dispensing without a prescription,' found on many products. Hence, the term 'legend drug' is sometimes used to mean **prescription only medicine**.
Compare **prescription only medicine**.

leprostatic
An agent that inhibits the growth of *Mycobacterium leprae*, the causative organism of leprosy.
See also **antileprotic**.

'less suitable' (UK)
A designation, given in the **British National Formulary** (▰), to denote those medicinal products that are considered by the Joint Formulary Committee to be 'less suitable' for prescribing. Although such products may not be considered as drugs of first choice, their use may be justifiable in certain circumstances.

Letter of Intent (LOI) (Clinical Trials) (US)
An **investigator**'s declaration of interest in conducting a **clinical trial** with a specific **investigational product** in a particular disease.

LIF (Sweden)
Läkemedelsindustriföreningen. Swedish Pharmaceutical Industry Association.

life expectancy
Average expected length of life for a group of people (or of individuals in a population) of a particular age, sex, etc., chosen at a particular time.

life-table analysis (Clinical Trials)
A method of analysis that relies on counting of the number of events observed and the time points at which those events occurred, relative to some zero point. The event may be death or some other event. In **clinical trials**, the time to an event for a patient is usually measured from the time of randomization. Treatment effects are assessed by comparing event rates in the different treatment groups.

See also **survival analysis**.

life-threatening
With respect to **serious adverse event** (SAE) reporting, it refers to an event in which the subject was at risk of death at the time of the event; it does not refer to an event which hypothetically might have caused death if it had been more severe.

See also **serious adverse event** (SAE)/**serious adverse drug reaction**.

ligand
A molecular, e.g. hormone or compound, that reacts with another molecule, such as a receptor, to form a complex.

ligand binding domain
The part of the nuclear receptor protein containing the ligand binding pocket.

likelihood ratio
It is the likelihood or the ratio of the probability that a given diagnostic test result would be expected in a patient with the target disorder compared to the likelihood that the same result would be expected in a patient without that disorder.

See also **sensitivity**.

line listing
A format of **drug safety** report required by certain **regulatory authorities** (RAs). It provides key information but not necessarily all the details customarily given and/or on individual cases. However, it does serve to help the RAs identify cases which they might wish to examine more completely by requesting full case reports. The requirement for line listing, summary tabulations, or more detailed report depends on the type or source of the **adverse drug reaction** (ADR).

Marketing authorization (MA) holders are expected to prepare line listings of consistent structure and content for cases directly reported to them (or under their control) as well as those received from RAs. MA holders are also expected to do the same for published cases (usually well documented; if not, a follow-up with the author is expected). Inclusion of individual cases from second- or third-hand sources, such as contractual partners and special registers might not, however, be:
1. possible without standardization of data elements
2. appropriate due to the paucity of information

It might, also, represent unnecessary re-entry/reprocessing of such information by the MAH. Under these circumstances, summary tabulations or possibly a narrative review of these data are considered acceptable by RAs. (CPMP/PhVWP/108/99 corr.)

See also **Periodic Safety Update Report**.

linkage analysis

Represents the first step in identifying the genes responsible for disease. By determining the genetic differences between individuals affected with a disease to those who are not, scientists can associate or link the disease to a specific location within the genetic material. This provides an important road map to finding the precise genetic alterations that contribute to the disease.

lipophilicity

The **affinity** of a molecule or a moiety for a lipophilic environment. It is commonly measured by its distribution behaviour in a biphasic system, either liquid–liquid (e.g. partition coefficient in octan-1-ol/water) or solid–liquid (retention on reversed-phase high performance liquid chromatography (RP-HPLC) or thin-layer chromatography (TLC) system).

See also **hydrophobicity**.

liposome

Microscopic spherical membrane-enclosed vesicle or sac (20–30 nm in diameter) made artificially in the laboratory by the addition of an aqueous solution to a phospholipid **gel**. The membrane resembles a cell membrane (phospholipid bilayers) and the whole vesicle is similar to a cell organelle. They contain aqueous phases between their bilayers. Single-layered liposomes are generally < 0.1–0.2 μm in size and good carriers of water-soluble drugs; their small size generally reduces their rate of elimination; multi-layered vesicles range from about 1 to 5 μm with a higher proportion of lipid to aqueous phases due to multiple lipid bilayers, and are, accordingly, suitable for transporting lipophillic drugs and are more rapidly cleared from the body than the single-layered type. Liposomes can be incorporated into living cells and used to transport relatively toxic drugs into diseased cells, where they can exert their maximum effects. For example, liposomes containing **chemotherapy** can be injected into the patient's blood. The cancerous organ is heated to a temperature, so that when the liposome passes through its blood vesicles the membrane melts and the drug is released.

listed adverse drug reaction

An **adverse drug reaction** whose nature, severity, specificity and **outcome** are consistent with the information in the **Company Core Safety Information** (CCSI) document.

See also **adverse drug reaction**.

liver enzyme tests

Blood tests that look at how well the liver and biliary system are working.

Also called liver function tests.

LL

Läkemedlsindustrins Läkarförening. Swedish Association of Physicians in the Pharmaceutical Industry.

loading dose (D*)

The first dose given, which is larger than the usual dose to ensure that effective drug concentrations (C) in the blood, in the biophase, reach therapeutic levels quicker than would occur only by accumulation of the repeated smaller doses. It is administered in a series of doses, the others of which are smaller than D* but equal to each other. The smaller doses (D) which are given after D* are called 'maintenance doses'. The effect of D* on C becomes relatively less with each succeeding maintenance dose; finally $C_{ss, max}$ and $C_{ss, min}$ are determined by D, and are uninfluenced by D*. The relative sizes of D and D* can be adjusted so that peak plasma concentrations (C_{max}) are the same following every dose, including the first with D*, and all are equal to $C_{ss,\,max}$. The size of the maintenance doses is therefore determined by the rate of elimination of the drug. These conditions are met when $D/D^* = 1\text{-}f$. Examples of drugs given in this way include cardiac glycosides and sulphonamides.

See also **availability, dose, multiple dose regimens, peak plasma concentration**.

local anaesthetic
An agent that inhibits sensation by inducing the loss of feeling in a certain area of the body while the patient remains awake (i.e. without inducing unconsciousness).

LOCF see **last observation carried forward**.

Loi DMOS (France)
A French regulatory law to control the financial incentives that French pharmaceutical companies give to members of the medical profession.

longitudinal data (Clinical Trials)
Data collected from a relatively small number of patients over a long period of time.

longitudinal study (Clinical Trials)
An investigational study in which **data** are collected from a number of **subjects** over a long period of time. If individuals are followed, this is a longitudinal **cohort study**. If individuals are not followed, but classes (usually age classes) are restudied, this is a longitudinal **cross-sectional study (horizontal study)**.

lost to follow-up (Clinical Trials)
A patient who can no longer be followed for the **outcome** of interest, e.g. a patient who is unwilling or unable to return to the clinic for follow-up examinations in the case of a clinical trial using an outcome measured at the clinic, or a patient who cannot be located for subsequent follow-up in the case of a trial involving mortality or some other outcome that can be measured outside the clinic setting.

lot see **batch**.

lotion
A liquid preparation for application to the skin without friction.

lower limit of normal
The lowest value of the normal range for a particular laboratory.

lozenge
A medicated **tablet** or disk intended to be dissolved slowly in the mouth.

LPI (Clinical Trials)
Last patient in.

LPO (Clinical Trials)
Last patient out.

LREC (Clinical Trials)
Local Research Ethics Committee.

LSEQ
Leeds Sleep Evaluation Questionnaire.

M

MA see **marketing authorization**.

MAA
Marketing Approval Authorization.

MAAC see **Medicines Assessment Advisory Committee**.

MAAG see **Medical Audit Advisory Group**.

maceration
The process of steeping a solid substance in a liquid to produce softening and to allow soluble matter to dissolve. The process is used for the preparation of certain tinctures.

MADRS
Montgomery-Åsberg Depression Rating Scale.

MAFF (UK)
Ministry of Agriculture, Fisheries and Food.

MAGE
Mean Amplitude of Glucose Excursions.

magistral formula see **magistral product**.

magistral product
Pertaining to a master; magisterial; authoritative; dogmatic. Commanded or prescribed by a magister, esp. by a doctor; hence, deemed effectual or sovereign (e.g. 'a magistral syrup'). Essentially, it is a **drug product** formulated/prepared extemporaneously in a pharmacy for a specific patient. The **European Union** definition, in **Directive 89/341/EEC**, is 'Any medicinal product prepared in a pharmacy for individual patients in accord with a prescription'.
Compare **official product**.

magnetic resonance imaging (MRI)
A technique that uses magnetic fields and radio waves to create high-quality cross-sectional images of the body's soft tissues without using radiation. The pictures are clearer than X-rays.

MAH
Marketing Authorization Holder (the company).

MAIL see **Medicines Act Information Letter**.

maintenance dose rate
The dose which, given at the stated constant time intervals, would create, but does not exceed, the desired effective drug concentration (EDC). It is calculated as follows:
maintenance dose rate = EDC × clearance rate

$$\text{Clearance} = K_e \cdot V_d \quad \text{or} \quad \frac{0693}{t_{1/2}} \cdot V_d$$

Where K_e = elimination constant
V_d = volume of distribution, and
$t_{1/2}$ = half-life.

major violation (Clinical Trials) see **protocol violation** and **protocol deviation** (minor violation).

MAL see **Medicines Act Leaflet.**

MaLAM see **Medical Lobby for Appropriate Marketing.**

maltodextrin
A sugar which is often used as an **inactive ingredient** in **drug products.**

Managed Behavioral Health Program (US)
A programme of **managed care** specific to psychiatric or behavioural health care. This usually is a result of a '**carve-out**' by an insurance company or **Managed Care Organization** (MCO). Reimbursement may be in the form of sub-capitation, fee for service or capitation.
See also **carve-out.**

managed care (MC)
A broad term and encompasses many different types of organizations, payment mechanisms, review mechanisms and collaborations. In its most basic form, MC refers to the body of clinical, financial and organizational activities designed to ensure the provision of appropriate health care services in a cost-efficient manner. It is a type of health care delivery that emphasizes active coordination and arrangement of health services. Any system of health payment or delivery arrangements where the plan attempts to control or coordinate use of health services by its enrolled members in order to contain health expenditures, improve quality, or both can be called MC. Arrangements often involve a defined delivery system of providers with some form of contractual arrangement with the plan.

MC usually involves three key components: supervision of the medical care given; contractual relationships with an organization of the **providers** giving care; and the covered benefits tied to MC regulations. This concept has been applied to **Managed Care Organization** (MCO)s, which integrate the finance and delivery functions of health care. MCOs include **Health Maintenance Organization** (HMO), **Preferred Provider Organizations, Exclusive Provider Organizations**, PHO, IDS, AHP, **Individual Practice Association**, etc. Usually when one speaks of a MCO in the US, one is speaking of the entity that manages risk, contracts with providers, is paid by employers or patient groups, or handles claims processing.

MC effectively forms a 'go-between', brokerage or third party arrangement by existing as the **gatekeeper** between payers and providers and patients.
See also **Health Maintenance Organization, Independent Practice Association, Managed Care Organization.**

Managed Care Organization (MCO)
The entity which integrates the finance and delivery functions of health care. MCOs are providers that integrate health care finance and delivery, that is, they combine the **payer** arm of the health care system with the provider arm. Generally, this involves contracting with health care **providers** to deliver health care services on a capitated (per-member per-month) basis. MCOs employ **utilization management** (UM) techniques in an attempt to deliver quality care at lower cost than traditional systems. In the US MCOs include **Health Maintenance Organizations** (HMOs) such as Kaiser, FHP and Maxicare, as well as **Preferred Provider Organizations.** MCOs first appeared in the US in the 1960s and they are expected to remain a primary force in the race to control health care costs.
See also **Health Maintenance Organization, Independent Practice Association, Utilization Management.**

managed care plan (US)
A health plan that uses **managed care** arrangements and has a defined system of selected

providers involved in the contracted plan. Enrolees have a financial incentive to use participating providers that agree to furnish a broad range of services to them. Providers may be paid on a pre-negotiated basis.

See also **Health Maintenance Organization, managed care, Preferred Provider Organization**.

Management Services Organization (MSO)

Usually an entity owned by a hospital, physician group, PHO or IDS which provides management services and administrative systems to one or more medical practices. The management services organization provides administrative and practice management services to physicians. An MSO may typically be owned by a hospital, hospitals, or investors. Large group practices may also establish MSOs to sell management services to other physician groups.

management trials

Clinical trials that assess the medical intervention's **effectiveness**.

See also **effectiveness**.

mandated benefits (US)

Benefits that health plans are required by law to provide.

mandated providers (US)

Providers whose services must be included in coverage offered by a health plan. These mandates can be required by state or federal law.

Mann–Whitney test (Statistics)

A non-parametric **hypothesis** test which can be used to compare or analyse two unrelated samples of **data**, from two independent groups, in order to compare two **population medians**.

manoeuvre (Clinical Trials)

Any exposure or treatment that acts upon patients to produce a result (an **outcome**).

MANOVA (Statistics)

*M*ultivariate *AN*alysis *O*f *V*Ariance.

Mantel–Haenzel method (Statistics)

A statistical method for estimating the pooled **odds ratio** and its **confidence interval** across a number of studies or across several strata within a single study.

manufacture

'All operations of purchase of materials and products, production, **quality control**, release, storage, distribution of **medicinal products** and the related controls.' (Crown Copyright)

Compare **production**.

manufacturer

In the **European Union**, a **manufacturer** is defined as 'The holder of the **manufacturing authorization**' (as described in Article 16 of **Directive 75/319/EEC**) on behalf of whom the **qualified person** has performed the specific obligations laid down in Article 22 of the Directive. In the US, a drug manufacturer, as defined in **Food and Drug Administration** (FDA) regulations, is anyone 'who is engaged in manufacturing, preparing, propagating, compounding, processing, packaging, repackaging, or **labelling** of a **prescription drug product**'.

See also **manufacturing authorization, qualified person**.

manufacturing authorization

According to **European Union** pharmaceutical legislative rules, a **manufacturer** of a **medicinal product** must hold a manufacturing authorization (Article 16 of **Directive 75/319/EEC**). The authorization is required for both total and partial manufacture. It is also required for imports from a third country. The requirements for obtaining such authorization are laid down in Article 17 of the same Directive.

manufacturing formula, processing and packaging instructions

Instructions that state all the starting materials used and lay down all processing and packaging operations.

Mapi Research Institute

A source of **quality of life** (QoL) instruments and educational research programmes. Also, information on International Health-related Quality of Life Database (IQOD) and the European Regulatory Issues on Quality of Life Assessment (ERIQA) Project.

MARC see Medicines Adverse Reactions Committee.

Market Basket Index

A common term in the field of economics. In health care business, this refers to a ratio or index of the annual change in the prices of goods and services. Different market baskets exist for PPS based hospital inputs and capital inputs, **diagnosis-related group** exempt facility operating inputs (such as SNF, home health agency and renal dialysis facility).

Also called input price index.

marketing authorization (MA)

The European licensing system which replaced the **product licence** (PL). The legal frame for an MA was first laid down in **Directive 65/65/EEC** which under Article 3 made it a requirement 'for **Member States** (MSs) to issue authorization for medicinal products' and under Article 4 a requirement for documentation and particulars to accompany an application for a MA. A medicinal product may only be placed on the market in the **European Union** when an MA has been issued by the **Competent Authority** of an MS. An MA can be issued by an MS, for marketing only in that MS (**National Authorization**), multiple states (mutual recognition according to **Directives 65/65/EEC** and **75/319/EEC** as amended) or under **Regulation (EEC) No. 2309/92** for the entire Community (**centralized procedure**).

See also **centralized procedure**, **mutual recognition procedure**, **national authorization**.

marketing mix

An evaluation tool used to develop marketing strategies. It is often referred to as the '4 Ps,' since it requires that the following items be determined for each product: (1) Product: strengths, weaknesses, features and benefits; (2) Pricing; (3) Promotion; (4) Placement and distribution.

Marketing Public Relations (MPR)

This is the type of public relations (PR) that is most relevant to health care marketers and is increasingly being utilized as part of the **marketing mix**. Conventionally, MPR is directly controlled by the marketers and PR is controlled by corporate management. In health care, however, MPR can also be said to include lobbying for those products where resourcing has yet to be established or there are governmental constraints on use.

See also **Financial PR**.

Market Research Society (MRS) (UK)
Founded in 1946, it is the largest professional body of its kind with over 8000 members working in organizations currently undertaking market research in the UK and overseas. Membership of the Society is divided into various grades offering a range of associated benefits. A new structure of qualification-based entry was introduced at the beginning of 1997. All members are required to abide by the MRS Code of Conduct when carrying out research, and a Professional Standards Committee meets regularly to review and enforce the Code. The Code incorporates any legislation which may impinge on the conduct of bona fide market research.

market share
A certain percentage of the market area or targeted market population. Usually used to describe a forecasted goal or a past penetration of the market.

masked study designs see **single-blind trial** and **double-blind trial**.

masking see **blinding/masking**.

master cell bank
A culture of (fully characterized) cells distributed into containers in a single operation, processed together in such a manner as to ensure uniformity and stored in such a manner as to ensure stability. A master cell bank is usually stored at $-70\,°C$ or lower.
See also **cell bank**.

Master Patient/Member Index (US)
An index or file with a unique identifier for each patient or member of a health plan that serves as a key to the patient's or member's health record.

matched-pairs design (Clinical Trials)
A type of parallel design of an experiment in which the study subjects are selected so that two subjects with similar characteristics are assigned to a set in pairs (**matching**) according to relevant study factors (who are 'identical' with respect to relevant factors, e.g. weight, smoking habits). One member of the pair receives one study treatment and the other member receives the alternate therapy.
See also **parallel study**.

matching (Clinical Trials)
When confounding cannot be controlled by **randomization**, individual cases are matched with individual controls that have similar **confounding factors**, such as age (**matched-pairs design**), to reduce the effect of the confounding factors on the association being investigated in analytical studies. Most commonly seen in **case–control** studies.

materiovigilance
The **medical device**'s equivalent term to **pharmacovigilance** (for drugs).

mathematical model
A formal framework to convey ideas about the components of a host–parasite interaction. Construction requires three major types of information: (a) a clear understanding of the interaction within the individual host between the infectious agent and the host, (b) the mode and rate of transmission between individuals, and (c) host population characteristics such as demography and behaviour.
Mathematical models can aid exploration of the behaviour of the system under various conditions from which to determine the dominant factors generating observed patterns and

phenomena. They also aid data collection and interpretation and parameter estimation, and provide tools for identifying possible approaches to control and for assessing the potential impact of different intervention measures.

mature minor (Clinical Trials) (US)

Someone who has not reached adulthood (as deemed by law) but who may be treated as an adult for certain purposes (e.g. consenting to medical care). Note that a mature minor is not necessarily an **emancipated minor**.

See also **emancipated minor**.

maximum agonist effect (α)

The preferred term to the old term '**intrinsic activity**'. It is the maximal effect that can be brought about by an **agonist**. It is expressed as a fraction of that produced by a **full agonist** acting at the same **receptors** under the same conditions.

maximum repeatable dose (MRD) study

A toxicity test normally carried out for each species by each route of administration that is planned in the subsequent repeat **toxicity** studies. The objective is to determine the toxicity profile including target organ toxicity and kinetic parameters. Such studies usually involve escalating the dose where increasingly larger doses are administered to the same group of animals each 3–4 days until significant toxicity appears. Escalating doses, however, is not very useful if the target organ toxicity is likely to be dose-limiting or if tolerance to repeated dosing is anticipated. In the latter cases, a fixed dose would prove more meaningful.

maximum residual level (MRL)

The maximum level of an, usually pharmacologically active or toxic, agent in a food-producing animal that is considered to be acceptably safe for human consumption. An example would be steroidal growth hormone levels in cattle.

maximum tolerated dose (MTD)

The highest dose of a therapeutic agent or a combination of drugs that can be given before the number of **adverse reactions** is in excess of an acceptable limit. The MTD is usually investigated in a **dose-escalation** study (a **phase I trial**).

MB

Bachelor of Medicine.

MBIRA (UK)

Member of the **British Institute of Regulatory Affairs**.

MC see **Medicines Commission**.

MCA see **Medicines Control Agency**.

McCarran–Ferguson Act (US)

A 1945 Act of Congress exempting **insurance** businesses from federal commerce laws and delegating **regulatory authority** to the States.

MCO see **Managed Care Organization**.

MCT

Multi-centre trial.

MD

Doctor of Medicine.

M

MDA
1. see **Medical Devices Agency**.
2. see **Medical Device Amendments**.

MDC see **Medical Diagnostic Category**.

MDD
1. Medical Devices Directorate.
2. Medical Device Directives (EU).

MDI
Metered-dose inhaler.

MDIS Data Capture Systems (UK)
A system used by the **Prescription Pricing Authority** to capture prescription information on items submitted monthly by:
- Pharmacy contractors
- Appliance contractors
- Dispensing doctors/practices
- Prescriber doctor/practices.

Once captured, the prescription items are processed by the pricing systems so that payment and reimbursement for a contractor can be calculated.
See also **Direct Payment to Contractors**, **Prescription Pricing Authority**.

MDV
Medical Device Vigilance, see **materiovigilance**.

mean (Statistics)
A measure of the arithmetic average of a sample of observations formed by adding the values/measurements and dividing by the number of observation/measurements.

mean residence time (MRT)
The average time that a pharmacological agent remains in the body following the administration of a single dose. MRT can be calculated by radiolabelling and intravenously administering the agent's molecule and measuring it, at specific time intervals, in the plasma or urine.

MEC see **minimum effective concentration**.

MedDRA see **Medical Dictionary for Drug Regulatory Activities**.

median (Statistics)
Determined by ordering a set of **data** from the smallest to the largest value. For data with an odd number of values the median is the value which lies at the centre of the ordered values. For data with an even number of values, the median is the simple arithmetic mean of the two 'middle' values. In true normal distribution, the mean and the median are the same value.

median time to elimination
The time it takes one half of a drug amount to be eliminated from the body.
See also **half-life**.

media relations
A frequently used approach in all aspects of **public relations** that entails the process of getting newsworthy messages to the media.
Compare **Financial PR**, **public relations**.

Medicaid (Title XIX) (US)

Government entitlement programme of public assistance for the blind, aged, disabled or members of **AFDC** whose income and resources are insufficient to pay for health care. Each state has its own standards for qualification. It is a federally-aided, State-operated and administered programme which provides medical benefits for certain indigent or low-income persons in need of health and medical care. The Act provides matching federal funds for financing state Medicaid programmes, effective 1 January 1966. It does not cover all of the poor, however, but only persons who meet specified eligibility criteria. Subject to broad federal guidelines, States determine the benefits covered, programme eligibility, rates of payment for **providers**, and methods of administering the programme. All States except Arizona have Medicaid programmes.

Medical Advisor see Pharmaceutical Physician.

Medical Audit Advisory Group (MAAG) (UK)

A statutory group, chaired by a general practitioner, which manages a small staff unit that organizes the audit of clinical practice in the district.

Medical Care Evaluation Studies (MCE) (US)

The name given to a generic form of health care review in which problems in the quality of the delivery and organization of health care services are addressed and monitored. A programme based on Mk-Es is recommended as a way of meeting the federal government's requirements for an internal quality assurance programme for federally-qualified **Health Maintenance Organizations**.

medical department

A department in a pharmaceutical company headed by a medically qualified manager (**Medical Director**) and consists of **Regulatory Affairs, pharmacovigilance, Medical Information Department**, statistics and clinical research and **clinical trials** sections.

medical device

Any instrument, apparatus, appliance, material, or other article, whether used alone or in combination, together with any accessories or software for its proper functioning, intended by the manufacturer to be used for human beings in the:
- diagnosis, prevention, monitoring, treatment, or alleviation of disease or injury
- investigation, replacement, or modification of the anatomy or of a physiological process
- control of conception

and which does not achieve its principal intended action by pharmacological, chemical, immunological, or metabolic means, but which may be assisted in its function by such means (**Directive 90/336/EEC**).

The range of products is very wide: it includes aids for the disabled, anaesthetic machines and monitors, apnoea and enuresis monitors, artificial limbs, breast implants, cardiac monitors, CT scanners, defibrillators, incontinence pads, dental equipment, dialysers, endoscopes, pacemakers, nebulizers, physiotherapy equipment, orthopaedic implants, ventilators, contact lenses and condoms; heart valves and hospital beds; resuscitators and radiotherapy machines; surgical instruments and syringes; wheelchairs and walking frames – many thousands of items used each and every day by health care providers and patients.

The **Food, Drug and Cosmetic Act** defines a medical device as 'an instrument, apparatus, implement, machine, contrivance, implant, *in vitro* reagent, or other similar or related article, including a component part, or accessory which is:

- recognized in the official **National Formulary**, or the **United States Pharmacopoeia**, or any supplement to them
- intended for use in the diagnosis of disease or other conditions, or in the cure, mitigation, treatment, or prevention of disease, in man or other animals
- intended to affect the structure or any function of the body of man or other animals, and which does not achieve any of its primary intended purposes through chemical action within or on the body of man or other animals and which is not dependent upon being metabolized for the achievement of any of its primary intended purposes.

See also **active medical device, active implantable medical device, custom-made medical device**.

Medical Device Amendments (MDA) (US)

Amendments to the federal **Food, Drug and Cosmetic Act** of 1938. The amendments were passed in 1976 to regulate the investigational use, registration, distribution as well as **good manufacturing practice** aspects of **medical devices** and diagnostic products. It was based on a classification of the types of devices.

Medical Devices Agency (MDA) (UK)

A British **regulatory authority** concerned with the **safety** and quality of all **medical devices** used in the UK. The MDA (formerly the Medical Devices Directorate) became an Executive Agency of the UK **Department of Health** (DoH) in September 1994. It covers a wide spectrum of devices including pacemakers, bandages, medical laboratory equipment and CT scanners, etc.

The primary task of the MDA is to help safeguard public health by working with users, **manufacturer**s and legislators to ensure that medical devices meet appropriate standards of safety, quality and performance and that they comply with the relevant **Directive**s of the **European Union**. The Agency's activities are organized in a number of business areas, each with a defined responsibility but all interacting with each other across a range of services.

The majority of the MDA's staff are specialists: administrators, medical and nursing staff, professionally qualified technologists and scientists (including biologists, chemists, engineers, toxicologists, pharmacists and physicists); and specialists in **quality assurance**. Many have established international reputations in their fields. Some of these specialists are directly concerned with the testing and evaluation of products in the MDA's own test centres, while other tests are carried out by independent specialists in hospitals and universities. Advice and consultancy is also provided to the UK **National Health Service** (NHS), health care providers in hospitals and the community, as well as to device manufacturers. It has six main activities, many of which are complementary:

- as UK **Competent Authority**: negotiating European Directives and introducing and enforcing UK **Regulations** for medical devices
- investigating adverse incidents associated with **medical devices** and their use, and helping to prevent further incidents by communicating findings to those who make or use the devices
- managing an on-going and independent programme to evaluate medical devices, and provide a range of services, including consultancy advice, published reports and comparative surveys, which enable device users to select equipment suitable for their needs, providing information to purchasers of supplies, and contributing to improved equipment design and performance
- contributing to the preparation of non-statutory safety and performance standards for medical devices in support of the European Directives and international standards

- offering advice to Ministers, the DoH, the NHS and other health care **providers**, device users and their professional bodies, **manufacturers** and other customers, on all aspects of medical devices and their use
- providing support services for the activities above, including: central management; financial; information systems; personnel functions and human resource development; and clinical advice.

The Agency is headed by a Chief Executive, appointed by and accountable to the Secretary of State for Health, and accountable to Parliament on matters concerning the Agency.

The MDA role has changed significantly over the years, partly because of rapid advances in medical devices technology and partly by the development of a world market in device technology and manufacture. The move from voluntary control in the UK to a statutory unified system for Europe has given the MDA a leading position among European regulators of medical devices. The MDA has played a key role in the development of the new European Directives for medical devices.

The MDA's primary objective remains what it has always been: to ensure that medical devices achieve their fullest potential to help health care professionals give patients the high standard of care they have a right to expect.

Medical Diagnostic Category (MDC) (US)

Sub-classifications within the **diagnosis-related group** (DRG) system of codes. In the DRG system, patients are first classified by 23 MDCs, and then they are classified further by more specific diagnoses. There are 467 DRGs in the system. Patients in the same DRG will use roughly the same amount of health care resources.

Medical Dictionary for Drug Regulatory Activities (MedDRA)

MedDRA was designed to incorporate terms that are relevant to all areas of drug regulation. The terminology includes terms relevant to **symptoms**, **signs**, diagnosis, investigations, family and social history and procedures. In addition to facilitating the implementation and compliance with the **European Union** (EU) future Systems **Regulations** and **Directives**, a single dictionary such as MedDRA is aimed to classify data from **clinical trials** and other studies, **spontaneous adverse drug reactions** and **adverse events**, regulatory submissions and product information such as the EU's **Summary** can help to optimize in-house drug assessment.

MedDRA also includes all data entry terms from **WHO-ART** and **COSTART** and hence allow easy transfer of historical data for organizations currently using these terminologies. MedDRA also contains terms from **ICD-9** and its clinical modification **ICD-9-CM** and **ICD-10**. MedDRA terms are classified in a five-level multi-axial hierarchy and it has the facility to flag preferred terms as alert terms for use in in-house signal generation programmes.

Medical Director

The person who heads the **Medical Department** in a pharmaceutical company. **Medical Advisors** report to the Medical Director.

Medical Education Agency

An agency, normally staffed by marketers and communication specialists, employed by the pharmaceutical company to support them with a spectrum of activities such as: the **strategic publication plan** (SPP), satellite symposia, writing of scientific papers, preparation of scientific posters, sole sponsor journals, product monographs, editorial advisory panels, internal staff training, promotional tactics, consensus meetings, audio-visual programmes and multi-media, Internet educational sites, **continuing medical education** programmes, patient support/education programmes, **health economics**, coordination and liaison with opinion leaders. They can bring various extra services to unburden the pharmaceutical marketer and medical department in such areas as: time (speeding up the publication plan), expertise and knowledge of journals and contacts with editorial boards, an external perspective (more objectivity), an intermediary (with opinion leaders, patient associations and editors), extra resource (of writers and medical editors).

Medical Group Practice see Group Practice

medical informatics (MI)

The discipline concerned with the application of information technology and telecommunications techniques in acquiring, processing and disseminating biomedical patient data and clinical knowledge. The optimal use and availability of such information is an essential part of problem solving in clinical practice.

The emergence of medical informatics as a new discipline is due in large part to advances in computing and communications technology and to an increasing awareness that the knowledge base of medicine is essentially unmanageable by traditional paper-based methods. Medical informaticians recognize that the process of retrieving clinical knowledge and making expert decisions is as important to modern biomedicine as the facts based on which clinical decisions or research plans are made. A focus on the IT infrastructure and algorithms needed to manipulate the information separates medical informatics from other medical disciplines, where information content is the focus.

The widespread introduction of computers into clinical practice offers new methods of storing, manipulating and communicating medical information which are more flexible and more powerful than paper based systems. Medical informatics focuses on the following issues:

- Clinical information and decision support systems
- Medical bibliographic information systems
- Medical terminology, coding and classification
- Evaluation of the impact of IT systems on the clinical process, clinical patient outcome, organizations and resources
- Developing methodologies for systems design and evaluation
- Education of health care professionals and informatics specialists
- Objectives, strategies and priorities for IT in health care
- Confidentiality and authentication of electronic patient data.

Medical Information Department (MID)

The Department, in pharmaceutical companies, that deals with enquiries on the company's products. MIDs existed in pharmaceutical companies since at least the 1960s. As from 1994, it has become a legal requirement for companies in the EU to maintain a 'scientific service' to handle product information. Their function is to provide comprehensive, accurate, balanced and relevant information in order to meet ethical, the legal and regulatory requirements. Most enquiries are for information used in making patient care decisions, therefore, responses must be provided rapidly. This is particularly true in the early years of a new product when other sources of clinical information may not be available. Companies, usually, have a second information department for research and development type of information that serves company employees on scientific, chemical or biological but not clinical issues.

Typical functions of a MID usually include:
1. Answering external and internal verbal and written enquiries
2. Maintenance of an internal data collection and, sometimes, the company's library
3. Literature surveillance and current awareness services

4. Receiving and partial processing of **adverse drug reactions** (ADRs) and communicating these to the Pharmacovigilance Department
5. Information support for other departments: Regulatory, Clinical Research, Sales and Marketing
6. Training of the **Medical Representatives** on products and therapeutic areas
7. Proofreading and copy approval of **Patient Information Leaflets** (PILs) and advertising materials
8. Writing product information packs.

The information provided to health professionals and to patients in the EU is ruled by European **Directives**. The **Summary of Product Characteristics** is the basis for this information in the different countries of the **European Community**. Most information professionals in the pharmaceutical industry have a first degree in a biological/biomedical science. Some have an additional MSc in an information related subject (e.g. information science, medical informatics etc.) or scientific PhD. Specialist product information training is normally provided by the employer.

Medical Lobby for Appropriate Marketing (MaLAM)

A consumer organization that keeps an eye on the ethical conduct of multinational drug companies with particular emphasis on their behaviour in developing countries. Their objectives include defending appropriate compassionate scientific medical care, health professionals and the public from marketing malpractices. They also engage in dialogue with bodies involved in health-related marketing, and providing a balance of information and practical opportunities for action, which assist health professionals to act for the benefit of the public.

medically necessary (medical necessity)

Services or supplies which meet the following tests: they are appropriate and necessary for the **symptoms**, diagnosis, or treatment of the medical condition; they are provided for the diagnosis or direct care and treatment of the medical condition; they meet the standards of good medical practice within the medical community in the service area; they are not primarily for the convenience of the health plan member or a plan provider; and they are the most appropriate level or supply of service which can safely be provided.

Medical Management Information System (MMIS) (US)

A data system that allows **payers** and **purchasers** to track health care expenditure and utilization patterns.

Medical Outcomes Trust (US)

The Trust is dedicated to improving health and health care by distributing standardized, high quality instruments that measure health and the **outcomes** of medical care. It was incorporated in 1992 in Massachusetts as a non-profit public service organization. The Trust supports the use of these instruments with membership, education and training, and publications.

Medical Practice Computer System

A PC- or network-based computer system used to manage electronic patient files. Defined by the European Forum for **good clinical practice**, such a system is neither sponsor-supplied nor trial-specific.

Medical Products Agency (Sweden)

The Swedish authority for registration of new drugs. The equivalent to the **Food and Drug Administration**, **Medicines Control Agency** etc.

Medical Representative
An employee of a pharmaceutical company whose job is to call on members of the health profession (prescribers) and their administrative staff for the purpose of the promotion and information on the company's medicines. Companies normally provide their representative with adequate training and medical background in the relevant therapeutic areas so as to ensure that they provide full and accurate information on the products they are promoting. In many countries, medical representatives are required to be trained and only obtain the required qualification from a professional body.

Medical Research Council Act (Canada)
This Act establishes the Medical Research Council responsible for promoting, supporting and conducting research into health science in Canada.

Medical Services Organization (MSO) (US)
An organized group of physicians, usually in one hospital, forming an entity able to contract with others for the provision of services.
See also **Management Services Organization**.

medical underwriting (US)
The federal health benefit programme for the elderly and disabled that covers over 35 000 000 beneficiaries or over 14% of the US with an annual cost of over $120 billion. **Medicare** pays for 25% of all hospital care and 23% of all physician services. This high cost is the source of constant debate in Congress. Medicare is the largest single payer in US.

medicament
A medical substance or agent.

Medicare (Title XVIII) (US)
A US federal government's health **insurance** programme for the elderly and disabled, for persons eligible for social security disability payments for 2 years or longer, and for certain workers and their dependants who need kidney transplantation or dialysis. It is not necessary, as with **Medicaid**, for Medicare recipients to be poor. It was created by the 1965 amendments to the Social Security Act and operates under the provisions of the Act. It is administered by the **Health Care Finance Administration** (HCFA) of the US **Health and Human Services**. Monies from payroll taxes and premiums from beneficiaries are deposited in special trust funds for use in meeting the expenses incurred by the insured. It consists of two separate but coordinated programmes: hospital insurance (Part A) and supplementary medical insurance (Part B). Medicare covers more than 34 million Americans (16% of population) at an annual estimated cost of more than $133 billion.
See also **Medicare Part A** and **Medicare Part B**.

Medicare Economic Index (MEI) (US)
An index that tracks changes over time in physician practice costs. From 1975 to 1991, increases in prevailing charge screens were limited to increases in the MEI.

Medicare Office of Research, Evaluation and Statistics (US)
Provides ongoing statistical data and research analyses of the Old-Age, Survivors and Disability Insurance (OASDI) and Supplemental Security Income (SSI) programmes. Its internet site contains downloadable files such as **Health Care Finance Administration** hospital wage index survey; **diagnosis-related group** (DRG)/ICDM9 file; standardized charges for prospective payment system and many others.

Medicare Part A (US)
The **Medicare** programme that covers **inpatient** hospital stays.

Medicare Part B (US)
The **Medicare** programme that covers physician and outpatient services.

Medicare Provider Analysis and Review (MedPAR) File (US)
A **Health Care Finance Administration** data file that contains charge data and clinical characteristics, such as diagnoses and procedures, for every hospital inpatient bill submitted to **Medicare** for payment.

Medicare risk contract (US)
An agreement by a **Health Maintenance Organization** or competitive medical plan to accept a fixed dollar reimbursement per **Medicare** enrolee, derived from costs in the **fee-for-service** sector, for delivery of a full range of prepaid health services.

Medicare supplement policy (US)
A policy that pays for the cost of services not covered by **Medicare**.

medicinal chemistry
A chemistry-based discipline, also involving aspects of biological, medical and pharmaceutical sciences. It is concerned with the invention, discovery, design, identification and preparation of biologically active compounds, the study of their **metabolism**, the interpretation of their mode of action at the molecular level, the construction of **structure–activity relationships** and chemical synthesis of drug candidates for testing *in vitro* and *in vivo*.

medicinal product
According to the European Union **Directive 65/65/EEC**, a medicinal product is 'any substance or combination of substances presented for treating or preventing disease in human beings or animals. Any substance or combination of substances administered to human beings or animals with a view to making a medical diagnosis or of correcting or modifying a physiological function in human beings or animals'. Former term was **proprietary medicinal product** but Article 1 of Directive 89/341/EEC replaced the old term.

medicine
1. The science or practice of the diagnostics, treatment and prevention of disease.
2. Any drug or preparation used for the treatment or prevention of disease, particularly a preparation that is taken by mouth.

Medicines Act 1968 (UK)
The first Act of Parliament in the UK that gave statutory control over the testing and sale of prescription medicines. It is comprehensive legal framework of control in which the licensing of medicines should be procured and maintained. It is also an 'enabling Act' which lays down the general policies to be followed and leaves the detailed implementation to be dealt with by various Ministers. The Act states 'There shall be established a body called the **Medicines Commission**, appointed by the Ministers of Health after consultation with appropriate organization'.

See also **Medicines Act Leaflets**.

Medicines Act Information Letter (MAIL) (UK)
A formal, bi-monthly, information booklet produced by the **Medicines Control Agency** providing clear information about the legal obligations of marketing authorizations holders and the services they provide. It also covers general news, conferences, publications, and lists contact

points in the Agency. It is circulated to over 3000 organizations including pharmaceutical companies, hospitals, regulatory consultants, and other interested bodies.

See also **Medicines Control Agency**.

Medicines Act Leaflet (MAL) (UK)

An information booklet produced by the **Medicines Control Agency** (MCA), **Department of Health**, or the **Ministry for Agriculture, Food and Fisheries** covering particular aspects of the Medicines Act. It was replaced in 1998 by the MCA Guidance Notes series. Examples include:

MAL 1   Guide to the licensing system
MAL 2   Guidance notes on applications for product licences (1989)
MAL 32 Clinical trials using marketed products
MAL 47 Leaflets supplied with **proprietary medicinal products**.

Medicines Adverse Reactions Committee (MARC) (New Zealand)

An expert committee which is part of the Ministry of Health which may, with the collaboration of **Medicines Assessment Advisory Committee** (MAAC), recommend to the Ministry which drugs to be monitored by the **Intensive Medicines Monitoring Programme**. MAAC may make the recommendation based on signals or problems identified through **spontaneous reporting** in NZ or elsewhere.

See also **Intensive Medicines Monitoring Programme** (IMMP), **Medicines Assessment Advisory Committee**.

Medicines Assessment Advisory Committee (MAAC) (New Zealand)

An expert committee, within the New Zealand Ministry of Health, that is responsible for reviewing applications for the marketing of new medicines. MAAC make the decisions as to what drugs to be monitored by the **Intensive Medicines Monitoring Programme** with or without the collaboration of the **Medicines Adverse Reactions Committee**.

See also **Intensive Medicines Monitoring Programme**.

Medicines Commission (UK)

The only statutory body under the **Medicines Act**, charged with responsibility of seeing that the Act is properly executed. The Commission advises ministers on matters relating to the execution of the Medicines Act, and on medicinal products where the Commission thinks it expedient, or it is requested by the minister. A function of the Commission is to hear appeals against **Committee on Safety of Medicines** (CSM) advice.

Medicines Control Agency (MCA) (UK)

The Executive Agency of the **Department of Health** (DoH). It is the **regulatory authority** in the UK, concerned primarily with safeguarding public health through controlling medicines by ensuring that all medicines, both branded and non-branded, on the UK market, meet acceptable standards of **safety**, quality and **efficacy**. This is achieved through a system of licensing and monitoring medicines after the licence has been granted. The MCA was established by the reorganization of the Medicines Division in April 1989. The delay in granting licences was the prime reason for establishing the MCA but currently is considered to be the fastest licensing authority in Europe. The MCA has separate divisions dealing with licensing, post-licensing, inspection and enforcement of medicines, executive support and finance. It also seeks to apply Citizen's Charter principles by:

- providing information on drug hazards and ways of improving the safe use of medicines through *Current Problems in Pharmacovigilance* bulletins and links with the **British National Formulary**

- providing clear information about the services provided through '**MAIL**', and the publication, 'Towards Safe Medicines'
- undertaking regular consultation and discussion with service recipients
- providing specific Agency telephone contact points, with courteous and efficient staff response
- distribution of 'Controlling Medicines in the UK' to all GP surgeries and retail pharmacists – a leaflet for the public explaining medicines control in the UK in plain language.

Licensing Division
The Division responsible for the assessment of all requests for **marketing authorizations** (MAs) to market drugs in the UK. It carries out the assessment of the medicines safety, efficacy and quality, examining all the research and test results in detail, before a decision is made on whether the product should be granted a MA. Medicines range from high technology medicines, biotechnology products, **new chemical entities** (NCEs), and those active constituents that have previously been evaluated by the MCA (**abridged licensing**). The division is also responsible for the approval and monitoring of all **clinical trials** undertaken in patients within the UK. The assessments are undertaken by multidisciplinary teams of physicians, pharmacists, toxicologists, scientists and statisticians. In carrying out this function, the Division works closely with the Advisory Committees, the **Committee on Safety of Medicines** (CSM) and the **Medicines Commission** who may decide to recommend that an application be refused or granted subject to certain changes being made in the application. The MCA is also a consistent and major contributor to the European licensing system.

The main activities of the Licensing Division are:
- Biotechnology
- NCEs; substances not previously licensed for use in the UK in any dosage form
- Abridged licensing; for products which contain **active ingredients** already licensed in similar or other pharmaceutical forms and for which clinical data is largely established
- European licensing; handling applications for working authorizations, using the **European Medicines Evaluation Agency**
- **Parallel imports**: a scheme under which medicinal products, which hold MAs in any **European Union** (EU) **Member State**, may be imported into the UK for marketing provided that there is a related UK licence
- Clinical trials; to help predict the type of products likely to come to the market
- Licensing registration: this unit initially receives each application for an MA and enters it onto the Agency's licensing database (**PLUS**), ready for assessment. Once a decision is made to grant an MA, the licence is produced automatically from the PLUS system.

Post-Licensing Division
The Division's principal functions include the following units:

1. Pharmacovigilance
This unit monitors medicines as they are used in everyday practice. Information from many different sources is used including the UK's spontaneous **adverse drug reaction** (ADR) reporting schemes (**Yellow Card Scheme**), clinical and epidemiological studies, world literature, **morbidity** and **mortality** databases. The Division works closely with other **European Community** regulatory authorities on **pharmacovigilance** matters. A recent extension of the Yellow Card Scheme is the **HIV Adverse Drug Reactions Reporting Scheme**. The unit also sends out the quarterly bulletin, *Current Problems in Pharmacovigilance*, to doctors and pharmacists. For urgent warnings about drug hazards, letters are sent to all doctors and pharmacists by post or electronic cascade.

2. Post-marketing evaluation

This unit evaluates the changes in experience in clinical use and changes in information on quality, **safety** and **efficacy** of medicines, which need to be reflected in MAs and product information. The functions of this unit include:

(i) Variation of MAs

Responsible for evaluating some 10 000 variations to MAs per year, providing a rapid and efficient means whereby MAs are kept up-to-date by changes, for example in **indications** of use, **formulation**, route of administration, shelf life, packaging and product information. The unit works closely with other EU **Member States** on variations handled through the EU licensing procedures.

(ii) Renewal of MAs

Evaluates renewal applications for each product, every 5 years, taking into account variations authorized over that time and any changes in the manufacture, quality assurance or clinical practice.

(iii) Re-classification of medicines

Evaluates applications for changes in the legal classification and supply of medicines. These may be from **prescription only medicine** (POM) to **pharmacy** (P), or from 'P' to **general sale list** (GSL). Less frequently, medicines previously classified as 'P' are made POM if new risks are identified which require involvement of a doctor in use of the medicine. Alteration of the legal status of any substance requires an amendment to the relevant order, this involves widespread consultation with appropriate bodies and organizations outside the MCA.

(iv) Regulation of product information

Responsible for the policy and regulation on all types of product information. Information on how a medicine should be used is provided to doctors and pharmacists including the **Summary of Product Characteristics**, previously called a data sheet and **Patient Information Leaflets** (PILs). Patient packs for medicines are being introduced to help with the provision of leaflets.

(v) Regulation of medicines advertising and promotion

Responsible for ensuring that advertisements do not give a false or misleading impression or suggest indications for use other than those permitted by the MA. The advertising of medicines is controlled by a combination of statutory measures (with both criminal and civil sanctions), enforced by the MCA and self-regulation through **Association of British Pharmaceutical Industry** (ABPI) **Code of Practice for the Pharmaceutical Industry** (administered by their trade association, the PMCP). The regulations also cover controls over hospitality and inducements to prescribe. The existing legislation applies to advertising and promotion of medicines via all media, including the Internet. The Division monitors advertising and reviews complaints on advertisements to determine what and when action is required.

Inspection and Enforcement Division

1. Inspection

This Division aims to ensure that medicines are not defective through errors or omissions in manufacturing or distribution and comply with requirement of the licensing, through inspections, testing, and legal enforcement. The Inspectorate ensures, by repeated inspections, that the QA arrangements of manufacturers and importerers comply with **good manufacturing practice** and the storage distribution arrangements of wholesalers comply with **GDP**.

The Inspectorate also carries out quality surveillance sampling and testing of all types of medicines from manufacturers, wholesalers, community pharmacies, and other outlets. Any minor problems are resolved with the manufacturer. In the very rare event that a major problem is discovered or reported, urgent assessment and a batch recall may be ordered.

The Division is also concerned with the production or import of unlicensed products to meet the special needs of a patient, borderline products and the operation of various other exemptions from licensing allowed by the **Medicines Act**. The Division also, in collaboration with the British Pharmacopoeia Commission, produces the **British Pharmacopoeia** and makes a major contribution to the production of the **European Pharmacopoeia**.

2. Enforcement

This unit investigates reports of suspected unlawful activities involving medicines and initiates criminal prosecutions in appropriate circumstances.

3. Policy and Standards

The quality of the Division's activities is ensured by internal audit and maintenance of suitable documentation system, including maintaining the Inspectorate registration to ISO 9002. This area advises on medicines exempted by the Medicines Act from licensing and on borderline products. It also develops policy and legislation on good manufacturing practice, good clinical practice and GDP.

Executive Support Division

This Division aims to ensure that the other Divisions in the MCA have at their disposal the infrastructure and support they need to perform their work effectively and efficiently.

European Support and Policy Coordination

- European and other international support: coordinates all major issues affecting licensing in the UK
- Policy coordination: provides advice to Ministers often in collaboration with other parts of the DoH, other Governmental departments and agencies.

Information Management Division

This division, set up on 1 March 2000, is responsible for the development and implementation of an IT strategy. Main activities:

- Strategy: to improve the efficiency and effectiveness by reviewing management systems for internal and external use.
- Existing IT systems: to continue to develop and support the five main business process systems:
  - **PLUS**
  - **ADROIT**
  - BLIS
  - ECS
  - **GPRD**

The unit is also responsible for both **RAMA** and **AEGIS**.

Contact:
Medicines Control Agency
Market Towers
1 Nine Elms Lane
London SW8 5NQ, UK
Tel: +44 (0) 20-7273 0000
Fax: +44 (0) 20-7273 0353
Email: info@mca.gov.uk

Medicines Licence Application 201 (MLA 201) (UK)
The old **Medicines Control Agency** form that an applicant company needs to complete as part of the procedure of applying for a **medicinal product** licence. It has been superseded by the EC form.

Medicines Licence Application 202 (MLA 202) (UK)
The **Medicines Control Agency** form that an applicant company needs to complete, as part of the procedure of applying for a **Clinical Trial Certificate** (CTC), to conduct clinical research on its **medicinal product**.

Medicines Licence Application 221 (MLA 221) (UK)
Old style Variations Application form; superseded by EC form.

Medicines Licence Application 231 (MLA 231) (UK)
Old style Renewals Application form – has been superseded by EC form.

Medicines Monitoring Unit (MEMO) (UK)
A well established and internationally renowned **pharmacoepidemiology** group based at Ninewells Hospital and Medical School, Dundee. MEMO has access to an extensive range of true population based datasets covering the 400 000 people in the Tayside Region of Scotland. In some cases the dataset provides a nearly complete Electronic Health Record. Prescription data for the residents of Tayside are obtained via the Prescription Pricing Division in Edinburgh who sends cashed prescriptions to MEMO. MEMO has the capacity to perform collaborative studies with the Information Statistics Division of the Common Services Agency of Scotland who have access to two key datasets for the whole of Scotland (5 million people) dispensed prescriptions as well as all hospitalizations. MEMO conducts **pharmacovigilance**, **outcomes** and economic studies for government agencies, medical charities, and other peer reviewed funding bodies as well as pharmaceutical companies. All work is undertaken to a strict agreed protocol, governed by appropriate ethics/data protection approval and always published.
Website: www.dundee.ac.uk/memo

Medicines Testing Laboratory (MTL) (UK)
A laboratory run by the **Royal Pharmaceutical Society of Great Britain** to test either routine samples or for certain defects.

Medico-Pharmaceutical Forum (MPF) (UK)
Set up in 1968 to consider matters of joint interest to the pharmaceutical profession and the pharmaceutical industry, to undertake, sponsor or promote studies of problems of mutual interest, and to make recommendations where appropriate. To this end, the Forum has organized many interesting symposia, issued a number of reports and published several booklets on such subjects as postgraduate education, adverse reactions and post-marketing surveillance, academic/industrial relationships, **Ethics Committees** for clinical research and various aspects of medical education.

In 1973 a working party on clinical trials was set up in response to the National Economic Development Office (NEDO) publication 'Focus on Pharmaceuticals' (HMSO 1972). It had the following terms of reference: 'To evaluate and make recommendations upon the organization of clinical trials in the UK, with particular reference to areas of controversy and misunderstanding and to practical points, where errors frequently arise'. The resulting document was welcomed by NEDO and was published by the Forum in 1974.

MEDIF (Denmark)
Pharmaceutical industries association in Denmark.

Medigap (US)
Private health **insurance** plans that supplement **Medicare** benefits by covering some **costs** not paid for by Medicare.

MediSwitch (South Africa)
Through its Virtual Private Healthcare Network (VPHN), MediSwitch provides the South African health care industry with a communication network to facilitate the transfer of pertinent claims-related patient information between service providers and medical aid administrators. MediSwitch connects most major players in the health care industry, such as medical aids, clearing houses, hospitals, clinics, laboratories, doctors, pharmacists, dentists and specialists.

MEDLARS
Medical Literature Analysis and Retrieval System (NLM). The computer on which '**MEDLINE**' and 'AIDS Line' reside at the **National Library of Medicine**.

MEDLINE
A vast source of bibliographic medical information database updated weekly, covering the whole field of medicine, including dentistry, veterinary medicine and medical psychology. Coverage in the database is from 1966 to date. Over 3700 journals from more than 70 countries are regularly indexed. MEDLINE covers clinical medicine, anatomy, pharmacology, toxicology, genetics, microbiology, pathology, environmental health, occupational medicine, psychology, biomedical technology, etc. Author abstracts are provided for about 80% of the records in the database. The database corresponds to the printed publications: Index Medicus, Index to Dental Literature, International Nursing Index and various bibliographies. MEDLINE is produced by National Library of Medicine (NLM) and offered by Knight-Ridder Information on behalf of and in cooperation with the Swiss Academy of Medical Sciences and its documentation Service DOKDI as Swiss National Medlars Center.

Medscape
One of the medical sites on the **Internet**. It offers **MEDLINE**, other databases and several on-line journals.

MedWatch (US)
The **Food and Drug Administration** (FDA)'s programme for **health professionals** to report 'suspected' **serious adverse drug reactions** and problems with **medical products** such as drugs and **medical devices**. Causality is not a prerequisite for MedWatch reporting.

MEFA (Demark)
Association of the Danish Pharmaceutical Industry.

megatrials (Clinical Trials)
Massive **randomized clinical trials** that test the advantages of marginally effective experimental drugs by enrolling 10 000 or more subjects. Synonym: large-sample trials.

Member State (MS)
A country that is a member of the **European Economic Community** (EEC), or **European Union** (EU).

MEMO see **Medicines Monitoring Unit**.

Memorandum of Understanding (MOU) (US)
A MOU between the **Food and Drug Administration** and a regulatory agency in another country allows **mutual recognition** of inspections.

MEP
Member of the European Parliament.

mEq
Milliequivalent.

MeSH Index
Medical Subject Headings Index. Term used by **National Library of Medicine**, and employed in their **MEDLINE** data base.

meta-analysis (Statistics)
A statistical method of grouping the results of many but diverse studies (which may have produced conflicting conclusive results). It is an overview process for pooling data, using quantitative methods, from many clinical trials to summarize the results and glean a clear answer.

metabolism
Alteration (using enzymes) in the character of any substance by chemical or a metabolic process. It is the way cells chemically change a substance/food and it comprises the entire physical and chemical processes involved in the maintenance and reproduction of life in which nutrients are broken down to generate energy (in case of heterotrophic organisms) and to give simpler molecules (catabolism) which by themselves may be used to form more complex molecules (anabolism). It is, therefore, a two-part process. One part is called catabolism – when the body uses food for energy. The other is called anabolism – when the body uses food to build or mend cells. Insulin is, for example, necessary for the metabolism of food.

In **pharmacology**, the term metabolism refers to the **biotransformation** of **xenobiotics** and particularly drugs for the purpose of facilitating their elimination from the body. There are four main patterns of drug metabolism. These are:
1. oxidation
2. reduction
3. hydrolysis
4. conjugation.

The first three are often lumped together as phase I reactions, while the fourth process, conjugation, is called phase II metabolism. A drug may be oxidized, reduced or hydrolysed and then another group may be added in a conjugation step. A common cause of capacity limited metabolism is a limit in the amount of the conjugate added in the conjugation step.

See also **biliary excretion, biotransformation, xenobiotic**.

metabolite
Any intermediate substance or product resulting from **metabolism**. It is the chemical derivative of the original **xenobiotic** (chemical compound that is foreign to a living organism, e.g. drug) produced by a variety of enzymes during metabolism.

metered-dose inhaler (MDI)
An inhaler that gives a specific amount of medication with each use.

'me-too drug'
A compound that is structurally very similar to already known drugs, with only minor pharmacological differences.

MFPM
Member of the Faculty of Pharmaceutical Medicine.

MHW see Ministry of Health and Welfare.

MI (UK)

Medicines Inspectorate, see **Medicines Control Agency**.

MIC

Minimum inhibitory concentration.

micromolar

Term used to express the levels of concentration of a drug: micromolar = 10^{-6} molar.
See also **nanomolar, picomolar**.

Midlevel Practitioner (US)

Nurse practitioners, certified nurse-midwives and physicians' assistants who have been trained to provide medical services that otherwise might be performed by a physician. Midlevel practitioners practice under the supervision of a doctor of medicine or osteopathy who takes responsibility for the care they provide. Physician extender is another term for these personnel.

MIF

Migration inhibition factor.

MIMS see **Monthly Index of Medical Specialities**.

minimal risk (Clinical Trials)

A risk is minimal where the probability and magnitude of harm or discomfort anticipated in the proposed research are not greater than those ordinarily encountered in daily life or during the performance of routine physical or psychological examinations or tests. For example, the risk of drawing a small amount of blood from a healthy individual for research purposes is no greater than the risk of doing so as part of routine physical examination.

minimum concentration (C_{min})

The minimum or 'trough' concentration of a drug observed after its administration. For drugs eliminated by **first-order kinetics** from a single-compartment system, C_{max}, after n equal doses given at equal intervals is given by $C_0 (1 - fn)/(1 - f) = C_{max}$, and $C_{min} = C_{max} - C_0$.

C_{max} = peak plasma concentration, C_0 = initial plasma concentration following intravenous administration, f = fraction of a dose in the system following administration by any route other than intravenous.

See also **accumulation, multiple dose regimens**.

minimum effective concentration (MEC)

The lowest concentration of drug in the systemic circulation at which it can produce a therapeutic effect.

minimum information see **reportable adverse reaction**.

minipill

An **oral contraceptive** containing only the synthetic hormone progesterone (others contain oestrogen and progesterone).

Ministére De La Santé Publique et De l'Environment (Belgium)

Belgian Ministry of Public Health and Environment.

Ministére Des Affaires Sociales et De la L'emploi Direction De La Pharmacie et Du Médicament (France)

Ministry of Social Affairs and Employment, Pharmacy and Medicines Directorate.

Ministry of Health and Welfare (MHW) (Japan)
Responsible for the improvement and promotion of social welfare, social security and public health. One of its nine bureaus is the Pharmaceutical Affairs Bureau within which is the Pharmaceuticals and Cosmetics Division. This Division is responsible for review and licensing of all medicinal products and cosmetics. It acts as the focal point for **International Conference on Harmonization** (ICH) activities.

Affiliated institutions include the National Institute of Health Sciences and academia which carries out research and testing on drugs, vaccines and biologicals. Technical advice on ICH matters is obtained through MHW's regulatory expert groups, with members from NIHS.

Ministry of Health, Directorate-general of the Pharmaceutical Division (Italy) (*Direzione Generale Del Servizo Farmaceutico, Ministero Della Santia*)

minor violation see protocol deviation.

miotic
A drug that causes the pupil to constrict or contract.

misbranded product (US)
The **Food, Drug and Cosmetic Act** defines a misbranded product as 'those drugs or devices with **labeling** which is false or misleading in any manner'.

See also **labelling**.

miscellaneous expenses
Hospital charges, other than room and board (**hotel costs**), such as those for X-rays, drugs, laboratory fees and other ancillary services.

miscible
When two liquids or two gases are completely soluble in each other in all proportions. While gases mix with one another in all proportions, the miscibility of liquids depends on their chemical natures.

mission statement
A statement produced by a company or an organization to describe its areas of expertise and its targets in meeting its customers' needs.

Misuse of Drugs Act (UK)
A British legal Act, created in 1971, which prohibits certain activities in relation to '**controlled drugs**', in particular their manufacture, supply and possession. The penalties applicable to offences involving the different drugs are graded broadly according to the harmfulness attributable to a drug when it is misused and for this purpose the drugs are defined in the following three classes:
- *Class A* includes: alfentanil, cocaine, dextromoramide, diamorphine (heroin), dipipanone, lysergide (LSD), methadone, morphine, opium, pethidine, phencyclidine, and class B substances when prepared for injection
- *Class B* includes: oral amfetamines, barbiturates, cannabis, cannabis resin, codeine, ethylmorphine, glutethimide, pentazocine, phenmetrazine, and pholcodine
- *Class C* includes: drugs related to the amfetamines such as benzftamine and chlorphentermine, buprenorphine, diethylpropion, mazindol, meprobamate, pemoline, piradrol, most benzodiazepines, androgenic and anabolic steroids, clenbuterol, human

chorionic gonadotrophin (HCG), non-human chorionic gonadotrophin, somatotropin, somatrem, and somatropin.
See also **Misuse of Drugs Regulations**.

Misuse of Drugs Regulations (UK)

A British legal Act, created in 1985, which defines the classes of person who are authorized to supply and possess controlled drugs while acting in their professional capacities and lay down the conditions under which these activities may be carried out. In the regulations, drugs are divided into five schedules each specifying the requirements governing such activities as import, export, production, supply, possession, prescribing and record-keeping which apply to them.
See also **Misuse of Drugs Act**.

mitogen

A substance/drug that induces cellular mitosis.

MLA 201 (UK)

Old style Medicines Licence application – a form used to apply for a MA. Superseded by EC form. Available in electronic version.

MLA 221 (UK)

Old style Variations Application form. Superseded by EC form. Available in electronic version.

MLA 231 (UK)

Old style Renewals Application form. Superseded by EC form.

MLD

Minimum lethal dose.

MLSO

Medical Laboratory Scientific Officer.

MLX (UK)

Consultative letters sent out by the **Medicines Control Agency** to interested organizations, companies and individuals when considering proposals to amend the Orders and Regulations made under the **Medicines Act**.

mM

Millimole.

MNLD see **maximum non-lethal dose**.

mode (Statistics)

The most frequently occurring value (observation) obtained in a study. It portrays the peak in the distribution of a set of **data**. A set of data with one mode is accordingly called unimodal, whereas that possessing two modes is called bimodal.

modified community rating

Rating of medical service usage in a given area, adjusted for data such as age, sex, etc.
See also **community rating**.

modified fee-for-service (US)

System that pays providers for services provided, with certain maximum fees for each service.
See also benefits, fee-for-service, **preferred providers**.

modifiers (US)
Codes used in conjunction with **CPT** or **HCPCS** codes to indicate that the service has been changed in some way.

molecular graphics
The visualization and manipulation of three-dimensional representations of molecules on a graphical display device.

molecular modelling
A technique for the investigation of molecular structures and properties using computational chemistry and graphical visualization techniques in order to provide a plausible three-dimensional representation under a given set of circumstances.

monitor (Clinical Trials)
A person appointed by the **sponsor** or **Contract Research Organization** to be responsible, to the sponsor, for the monitoring and reporting on the progress of the trial and for verification of **data**. The monitor must have qualifications and experience to enable a knowledgeable supervision of the particular trial. Trained technical assistants may help the monitor in collection of documentation and subsequent processing.

monitoring (Clinical Trials)
The process of supervising a **clinical trial**, and of ensuring its progress and that it is conducted, recorded, and reported in accordance with the **protocol**, **standard operating procedures**, **good clinical practice**, and **applicable regulatory requirement**(s).

monitoring boundaries (Clinical Trials)
The set of values formed by a line or set of lines (or curves), usually specified before or shortly after the start of patient recruitment, which, if exceeded, indicates the existence of a test-control treatment difference that satisfies certain statistical properties (e.g. has a **P-value** of less than a certain size). The boundaries will be used as a basis for stopping the trial when developed in conjunction with a sequential design, but not necessarily when used in conjunction with a fixed sample size design. Z values larger in absolute values are declared statistically significant. Boundaries are designed to control the overall **type I error**.

monitoring report (Clinical Trials)
A written report from the **monitor** to the **sponsor** after each visit and/or other trial-related communication according to the sponsor's **standard operating procedures**.

monoclonal antibody
Chemically and immunologically homogeneous antibodies produced by a single clone of antibody-secreting cells. Such antibodies will react with only one specific foreign protein. They are used to help diagnose certain kinds of cancer.

Monthly Index of Medical Specialities (MIMS) (UK)
An independently written commercial publication designed as a compact prescribing guide for general practitioners on proprietary **medicinal products**. It contains very concise product monographs comprising information on the product's presentation, price, indication(s), posology, **contraindications** and **side-effects**. MIMS is published by Haymarket Publishing Services Ltd. and it is free of charge to medical practitioners who meet the publisher's criteria.

morbidity
The state or extent of illness, injury, or disability in a defined **population**. It is usually expressed in general or specific rates of **incidence** or **prevalence**.

morbidity rate
  The sickness rate; the number of people who are sick or have a disease compared with the number who are well.

mortality
  The per capita death rate in a **population**, i.e. the number of people who die of a certain disease compared with the total number of people. It is used to describe the relation of deaths to the population in which they occur. The mortality rate (death rate) expresses the number of deaths in a unit of population within a prescribed time and may be expressed as crude death rates (e.g. total deaths in relation to total population during a year) or as death rates specific for diseases and, sometimes, for age, sex, or other attributes (e.g. number of deaths from cancer in white males in relation to the white male population during a given year, infant mortality). Mortality is most often stated as deaths per 1000, per 10 000, or per 100 000 persons in a given period of time, usually a year and usually multiplied by a 10^n population size. These proportions are often broken into cause-specific and age-specific proportions and are often standardized so different groups can be compared and the population at the middle of the time interval is often used as the denominator. The mortality rate is the reciprocal of the population life expectancy.

motility
  The movement of food and drugs through the digestive tract.

MOU see **Memorandum of Understanding.**

mouthwash
  An aqueous solution of a medicament intended for gargling.

MPF see **Medico-Pharmaceutical Forum.**

MPG (Germany)
  Medical Devices Act in Germany. It came into force on 1 January 1995. The **BfArM** deals with **medical devices** matters, such as central recording and assessment of observed and reported risks associated with medical devices as well as coordination of measures where necessary.

MPS (UK)
  Member of the Pharmaceutical Society of Great Britain.

MRA
  1. Medical Research Associate, see **Clinical Research Associate**.
  2. see **Mutual Recognition Agreement**.

MRC
  Medical Research Council.

MRD see **maximum repeatable dose.**

MRFG see **Mutual Recognition Facilitation Group.**

MRI see **magnetic resonance imaging.**

MSF
  Medicins Sans Frontières. Medicine without frontiers.

MSO
  1. see **Management Services Órganization**.
  2. see **Medical Services Organization**.

MSR (Clinical Trials)
Monthly Status Report.

MTC
Minimum toxic concentration.

MTD see **maximum tolerated dose**.

MTL see **Medicines Testing Laboratory**.

MTR (Clinical Trials)
Monitor's Trip Report.

mucilage
A thick aqueous solution of a gum used for suspending insoluble substances in mixtures or to increase the viscosity of the continuous phase of oil-in-water emulsions.

mucolytic
A drug that lessens the sticky quality of phlegm and makes it easier to cough up.

Multi-Agency Group
A group or committee whose membership consists of representatives from different agencies, e.g. **health authority**, **National Health Service**, local authority, voluntary organizations.

multicentre trial (Clinical Trials)
Clinical trial conducted according to one single **protocol** in which the trial is identified as taking place at different investigational sites, therefore carried out by more than one **investigator**, but following the same practical details. The purpose of conducting a multicentre trial is to collect data as rapidly as possible, for unified analysis leading to a single report.

multimodality therapy
The combined use of more than one method of treatment: for example, surgery and **chemotherapy**.

multiple comparisons (Clinical Trials)
A term used to refer to the fact that two or more treatment comparisons, each involving the same **outcome** measure, are made or are to be made at a designated time point in the course of the trial. The comparison may involve all members of the treatment groups or subsets (e.g. as in analyses involving subgroups of patients defined by the presence or absence of some baseline characteristic). Also applies to comparisons among several subgroups and/or use of several **end points**.

multiple dose regimens
The repeated administration of a drug at intervals in order to maintain effective concentrations. The relationships involve assumptions of instantaneous intravenous administration and distribution of a drug which is eliminated by first-order kinetics from a single-compartment system, and is given in equal doses at equal time intervals.
See also **accumulation ratio**, C_{max}, **compartment**, **first-order kinetics**, **infusion kinetics**.

Multiple Project Assurance (MPA) (US)
A formal written agreement with the OPRR (on behalf of the Secretary of **Department of Health and Human Services** (DHHS) and an institution which conducts or supports a large amount of DHHS-sponsored research involving human subjects. The MPA specifies how the institution will implement the DHHS regulations 45 CFR (**Code of Federal Regulations**) 46.

multi-state procedure
An old **European Community** procedure designed to assist companies with a **marketing authorization** in one **Member State** (MS) to extend the licence into two or more other MSs. Now replaced by **mutual recognition procedure**.

multivariate analysis (Statistics)
An analysis where the effects of many variables are considered. Can select a subset of variables that significantly contribute to the variation in outcome.

Munich Convention
A European convention on patents that offered manufacturers a 20-year patent protection.

mutagen
An agent that can increase the rate of abnormalities or causes a permanent inheritable change (i.e. a mutation) into the DNA (deoxyribonucleic acid) of an organism which can lead to cancer.

mutagenicity testing
The bacterial mutagenicity test (Ames Test) that all new drugs are subjected to before being tested in man. An unequivocal positive result would prevent a new drug from being tested in man until further investigations have resolved this situation.

mutual prodrug
The association in a unique molecule of two, usually synergistic, **drugs** attached to each other, one drug being the carrier for the other and vice versa.

Mutual Recognition Agreement (MRA)
Agreement between the **European Union** and third countries to recognize each other's good manufacturing practices.

Mutual Recognition Facilitation Group (MRFG) (EU)
An informal group of **Member State** (MS) representatives established March 1995, which meets monthly at the **European Medicines Evaluation Agency** offices to co-ordinate and facilitate the operation of the **mutual recognition procedure**. Additional *ad hoc* meetings are held as the need arises to consider major issues. The Group is chaired by the country which holds the Presidency of the **European Union**. The group has no formal position in EC legislation, but has established itself as a major player in the new European system. The Group provides a forum where procedural issues can be discussed and problems resolved. It is able to undertake an overview of individual applications. However, scientific discussions relating to individual applications are not discussed within the Group, but rather are handled through 'breakout sessions' which are organized and chaired by the specific reference MS (RMS). If the Group identifies that work is required on further scientific issues, then these will be referred to the **Committee for Proprietary Medicine Products** (CPMP) for the consideration of the establishment of an expert group, or the development of a concept paper or guideline.

The **European Commission** attends the MRFG meetings and this permits many procedural matters to be resolved at the MRFG. The more complex issues are referred formally to the Commission for further work. The Group has played a major role in the ongoing work on the revision of the Notice to the Applicants. A major item of work and discussion over the last 2 years has been the development of a tracking database **Eudratrack**. There is a comparable group in the veterinary sector and a close link has been established between the two groups. Updated information on MRFG is available on the Heads of Agencies web site http://heads.medagencies.com/

See also **Eudratrack, mutual recognition procedure**.

mutual recognition procedure (MRP)
A type of procedure, which became effective as of 1 January 1995, to coordinate the granting of **marketing authorization** (MA) for a **medicinal product** in the **European Union**. The purpose of this type of authorization is to facilitate access to the Community market. A MA holder can achieve this by asking the second or subsequent **Member States** (MSs) to mutually recognize the MA granted by the first MS (called Reference Member State RMS). MSs can mutually recognize the assessment of another MS even in cases where the company has not requested MR with its application. The Reference Member States (RMSs) have a period of 90 days to recognize the application. The legal aspects of MRP are in **Directive 65/65/EEC** and **Directive 75/319/EEC** as amended. Products which have been authorized via the **centralized procedure** (described in Council **Regulation 2309/093**) are not authorized via the MRP. Once MR has been granted, all subsequent Variations to the MA of these products must use the MRP.

In the event of a disagreement between MSs about the quality, the **safety** or the **efficacy** of the medicinal product, a scientific evaluation of the matter should be taken by the **Committee for Proprietary Medicinal Products** (CPMP) for **arbitration** leading to an opinion (that is given to the company) arising from which the Commission would prepare a single decision on the area of disagreement, binding on all the MSs. This decision would be adopted by a rapid procedure ensuring close co-operation between the Commission and the MSs. The procedure to be followed where a MS considers there are grounds for opposing the granting of MA for the product in question, (may present a potential risk to public health) is defined in Articles 13 and 14 of **Directive 75/319/EEC** as amended.

See also **centralized procedure**.

mydriatic
A drug that causes the pupil to dilate (widen).

n (Statistics)
: Overall size of **sample**. Sometimes an upper case is used to represent it, i.e. *N*.

N-of-1 trials
The patient undergoes pairs of treatment periods organized so that one period involves the use of the experimental treatment and one period involves the use of an alternate or **placebo** therapy. The patients and physician are blinded, if possible, and outcomes are monitored. Treatment periods are replicated until the clinician and patient are convinced that the treatments are definitely different or definitely not different.

NABP (US)
National Association of Boards of Pharmacy.

NAD
No abnormality detected.

NADA (US)
New Animal Drug Application (**Food and Drug Administration**).

NAF (US)
Notice of Adverse Findings (**Food and Drug Administration** Post-audit Letter).

NAFTA
North American Free Trade Agreement.

NAHAT (UK)
National Association of Health Authorities and Trusts.

NAI (US)
No Action Indicated (Most Favourable **Food and Drug Administration** Post-inspection term).

named patient basis
An unlicensed drug being supplied to a doctor for use in a particular patient. The drug supply cannot be used for any other patient. The patient should be monitored carefully and a brief report supplied to the drug company. Sometimes the term is also used for supply of a discontinued or unmarketed **drug product** by special request from the patient's doctor either directly, to the company, or indirectly via the pharmacist.

nanomolar
10^{-9} molar.
See also **micromolar**.

NAPH see **National Association of Public Hospitals and Health Systems.**

NAPM (US)
National Association of Pharmaceutical Manufacturers.

narcosis
A drug (or other chemical)-induced drowsiness or stupor.

NAS
New active substance.

NASNR (US)
National Academy of Sciences and National Research.

National Agency for Medicines (Finland)
The Agency works under the Ministry of Social Affairs and Health to maintain and promote safe use of medicines, **medical devices** and blood products. The Agency has three departments: the Pharmaceutical and Pharmacological Departments and the Department of General Affairs. Other units of the Agency are the Secretariat for Marketing Authorizations (MAs), the Drug Information Centre and the Medical Devices Centre. Functions of the Pharmaceutical Department are:
- assessment of quality related to applications for MA of medicinal products (drug applications) and herbal remedies; evaluation of pharmaceutical and chemical documentation
- post marketing **quality control** of medicines
- research relating to quality control activities
- contribution to the **European Pharmacopoeia**.

Functions of the Pharmacological Department
Assessment of documentation related to applications for **marketing authorization** (MA) of **medicinal products** and veterinary medicinal products: evaluation of pre-clinical, toxicological and clinical documentation information concerning medicinal product matters concerning new indications:
- **clinical trials** and **good clinical practice** inspections
- **safety** matters concerning herbal remedies and anthroposophical and homeopathic products
- special marketing licences for non-registered medicinal products
- laboratory monitoring of biological and microbiological **efficacy** and safety of medicinal products
- **good laboratory practice** inspections of toxicological laboratories
- medical and veterinary medical matters concerning **mutual recognition procedures** and those facilitating meetings (MRFG and VMRFG)
- matters concerning members of the **Committee for Proprietary Medicinal Products** (CPMP) and **Committee for Veterinary Medicinal Products** (CVMP).

Functions of the Secretariat for Marketing Authorizations
- regulatory affairs concerning marketing authorizations and procedures (MRFG- and VMRFG-participation)
- validation of MA applications
- coordination of MA procedures
- maintenance of electronic database on national and European MAs
- administrative contacts with **European Union Member States**, **European Medicines Evaluation Agency** and Commission
- **parallel import** of medicinal products
- export certificates
- exemptions from processing and annual fees.

Functions of the Department of General Affairs
- inspection services (pharmaceutical manufacturers, blood transfusion services, wholesale distributors, pharmacies)
- personnel and financial administration
- legal affairs
- personnel and document administration
- information technology

- records management
- information services.

Functions of the Drug Information Centre
- publications on drug information
- **pharmacovigilance**
- drug statistics
- supervision of marketing of medicines.

Functions of the Medical Devices Centre market control of medical devices
- medical devices vigilance
- product control registers
- implant registers
- assessment of applications for clinical investigations of medical devices.

National Association of Public Hospitals & Health Systems (NAPH) (US)

NAPH represents over 100 hospitals and health systems that form the essential infrastructure of urban health systems. NAPH members provide almost 90% of their services to **Medicare**, **Medicaid** and low income uninsured patients. Their website (www.naph.org/) contains legislative and regulatory news, research reports, data and links to NAPH member hospitals.

national authorization (European Union)

A form of authorization for marketing **medicinal products** in the **European Union** where the **competent authority** (CA) of the **Member State** (MS) is that responsible for granting the MA for the product which is placed on the market of that MS, except for products which are authorized under **Regulation (EEC) 2309/93** (see **centralized procedure**).

In order to obtain a National Authorization, an application must be submitted to the CA of the MS. In cases where National Authorizations are requested in more than one MS, an application must be submitted:
- In one MS and once MA has been granted, make applications in other MSs concerned requesting them to mutually recognize the MA already granted (see **mutual recognition procedure**)
- Make parallel applications in each of the MSs concerned and request a national authorization in each MS.

National Center for Health Statistics see National Guideline Clearinghouse.

National Center for Toxicological Research (NCTR) (US)

Investigates the biological effects of widely used chemicals in the US. It is based at Jefferson, Arkansas and operated by the **Food and Drug Administration**.

National Centre for Clinical Audit (UK)

Based at **British Medical Association** (BMA) House, it was set up in 1995 to facilitate best clinical practice in health care by promoting multi-professional clinical audit. It provides advice, information and analysis. Seminars on building teams for clinical audit are organized by the BMA's clinical audit committee and the Royal College of Nursing (RCN).

Contact:
 National Centre for Clinical Audit at BMA head office
 Tel: 0171 383 6451
 Fax: 0171 383 6373
 Email: NCCA@NCCA.org.uk

National Chronic Care Consortium (NCCC) (US, Canada)
A mission-driven organization of leading non-profit health systems in the US and Canada dedicated to transforming the delivery of chronic care services. Each NCCC member provides a full continuum of services, including primary care, hospitals, nursing homes and community-based long-term care.

National Committee for Quality Assurance (NCQA) (US)
An independent, non-profit organization dedicated to assessing and reporting on the quality of **managed care** plans, including **Health Maintenance Organizations**. NCQA is governed by a Board of Directors that includes employers, consumer and labour representatives, health plans, quality experts, regulators, and representatives from organized medicine. NCQA's mission is to provide information that enables purchasers and consumers of managed health care to distinguish among plans based on quality, thereby allowing them to make more informed decisions. NCQA's efforts are organized around two activities, accreditation and performance measurement (report cards), which are complementary strategies for producing information to guide choice. In the future, these activities will be integrated. NCQA can be contacted on the Internet at www.ncqa.org.

National Drug Code (NDC) (US)
Ten-digit codes which uniquely identify every drug product sold in the US. They are often used for billing payers and use the following format: xxxxx-xxx-xx. The first five digits refer to the manufacturer and are assigned by the **Food and Drug Administration**. The last five digits are assigned by the manufacturer and can be used to represent internal product numbers, fill size, etc.

National electronic Library for Health (NeLH) (UK)
An initiative, announced in the Government's Information for Health strategy. The NeLH aims to:
- provide easy access to best current knowledge
- improve health and health care, clinical practice and patient choice

The NeLH's aim is to also link in to a number of virtual branch libraries, focusing on the particular needs of different groups. Other aims include focusing on:
- the outputs of the Research and Development (R&D) Programme and their implementation
- the resources and knowledge required to implement the National Service Framework for Mental Health
- the development of guidelines and quality improvement techniques
- specialist electronic branch libraries for key areas within mental health
  - childhood and adolescence
  - adult psychiatry
  - alcohol and drug abuse
  - mental health in old age
- developing close communication with all **National Health Service** (NHS) Trusts providing mental health services as they develop their own websites with links into local social services.

National Formulary (NF) (US)
A periodically revised book of officially established and recognized drug names and standards. The NF was first published in 1888. Since 1980, both the NF and the **United States Pharmacopoeia** have been issued in the same volume. The NF was originally intended as a list of the official recipes for pharmaceutical formulae; characteristics of those drugs or plants used

in the formulae or that were still recognized as secondary drugs. It also includes the substances needed for the manufacturing of drugs but are not active, like gelatine or pill binders. With the decreased use of tonics and less invasive medications after World War II, the NF became primarily a text defining the inactive substances used in drug manufacturing.

See also **United States Pharmacopoeia**.

National Guideline Clearinghouse (NGC) (US)

A comprehensive database of evidence-based clinical practice guidelines and related documents produced by the **Agency for Health Care Policy and Research**, in partnership with the **American Medical Association** and the AAHP. The NGC mission is to provide physicians, nurses, and other health professionals, health care providers, health plans, integrated delivery systems, purchasers and others an accessible mechanism for obtaining objective, detailed information on clinical practice guidelines and to further their dissemination, implementation and use. Key components of NGC include: Structured abstracts (summaries) about the guideline and its development; a utility for comparing attributes of two or more guidelines in a side-by-side comparison; syntheses of guidelines covering similar topics, highlighting areas of similarity and difference; links to full-text guidelines, where available, and/or ordering information for print copies; an electronic forum for exchanging information on clinical practice guidelines, their development, implementation and use; annotated bibliographies on guideline development methodology, implementation and use. Also called National Center for Health Statistics.

Website: http://www.guidelines.gov/index.asp.

National Health Service (UK)

The NHS was officially established in 1948. It has a workforce of around one million people. The purpose of the NHS is to secure through the resources available the greatest possible improvement in the physical and mental health of the nation by: promoting health, preventing ill-health, diagnosing and treating injury and disease and caring for those with long-term illness and disability.

General Practitioners (GPs) are just one part of the front line of the NHS – the part of the NHS often called 'primary care'. Many other health professionals work as part of this front line team: nurses, health visitors, dentists, optometrists, pharmacists and a range of specialist therapists. Services offered by GP practices are free to patients – although there are flat charges for prescriptions for all patients, children, elderly people, and those on low income receive prescriptions free.

On a national level, the Secretary of State for Health is responsible to Parliament for the provision of health services. The Secretary of State is assisted by the Policy Board and the NHS Executive (NHSE). The Policy Board sets the broad strategic direction of the NHS. It is chaired by the Secretary of State and its membership includes people from the NHS, business people, **Department of Health** officials and ministers. The NHSE deals with operational matters within the strategy set by the Policy Board. It is chaired by the chief executive of the NHS and its membership includes civil servants and people from the NHS and business.

As part of the Health Authorities Act, **Regional Health Authorities** were abolished with effect from April 1996 and replaced by eight regional offices of the NHSE. The regional offices act as outposts of the central NHSE with a particular responsibility for performance management and with a lead role in areas including public health and the NHS research and development programme.

On a local level, most hospital and community services are provided by NHS trusts. Trusts are accountable to health authorities and **primary care groups** (PCGs) for the services they deliver and to the NHSE for their statutory duties. PCGs, comprising all GPs in an area together with other community-based professionals take responsibility for **commissioning** services locally. They work closely with local government social services departments. PCGs are allowed to take a range of forms, including the opportunity to become free-standing primary care trusts, with responsibility for running community hospitals and community health services in addition to their commissioning role. None of these options affects the independent contractor status of GPs. Typically PCGs serve about 50 000–200 000 patients but this varies according to local circumstances.

National Institute for Biological Standards and Control (NIBSC)

A multi-disciplinary scientific establishment whose purpose is to safeguard and enhance public health by standardizing and controlling biological substances used in medicine. Such substances include bacterial and viral vaccines against diseases such as diphtheria and polio as well as products derived from human blood such as clotting factors. Batches of these medicines must be independently assessed before they are released onto the market and NIBSC performs this 'control testing' for the UK and increasingly for Europe. The origins of the scientific work of this Institute date back to 1928 and the activities of **Medical Research Council**'s National Institute for Medical Research situated at Mill Hill in London. In the 1970s the responsibility for the control and standardization part of the work was transferred to the newly established National Institute for Biological Standards and Control (NIBSC).

The quality and validity of the control work undertaken at NIBSC is accredited by the National Measurement Accreditation Service (NAMAS) to comply with the European Standard EN 45001. The Institute is also a **World Health Organization** International Laboratory for Biological Standards and as such prepares and evaluates ampouled biological reference substances that serve the pharmaceutical, regulatory and research communities as International Standards.

National Institute for Clinical Excellence (NICE) (UK)

The NICE (the Institute), brought into being on 1 April 1999, is a special **Health Authority** (HA), which is part of the **National Health Service** (NHS). The Institute aims to systematically appraise new and existing health interventions as formally requested by the **Department of Health** (DoH) and the National Assembly for Wales. The Government believes that NICE is needed to ensure a high quality health service that is available for all and is determined to change the unacceptable variations in the quality of care available to different patients in different parts of the country. The organization comprises a Board which has Executive and Non-Executive members (clinical professions, patients and patient groups, NHS managers and research bodies). It will offer clinicians and managers clear guidance on which treatments work best for patients and which do not. This guidance is aimed to support everyone in the NHS including doctors, nurses, midwives and other health professionals – those who make the complex decisions about the treatment of individual patients.

NICE will take over some existing DoH organizations and bring them together. These include the National Prescribing Centre appraisals and bulletins, **PRODIGY**, the National Centre for Clinical Audit, the Prescriber's Journal, the National Guidelines and Professional Audit Programmes and Effectiveness Bulletins.

The Institute's proposed functions in this context are set out in the Secretary of State's Directions: 'to appraise the clinical benefits and the costs of those interventions notified by the Secretary of State and to make recommendations'.

The Institute will undertake appraisals of new and established technologies comprising:

- pharmaceuticals
- medical devices
- diagnostic techniques

- procedures
- health promotion.

The DoH and National Assembly for Wales will select technologies for appraisal based on one or more of the following criteria:
- Is the technology likely to result in a significant health benefit, taken across the NHS as a whole, if given to all patients for whom it is indicated?
- Is the technology likely to result in a significant impact on other health-related government policies (e.g. reduction in health provision inequalities)?
- Is the technology likely to have a significant impact on NHS resources (financial or other) if given to all patients for whom it is indicated?
- Is the Institute likely to be able to add value by issuing national guidance? For instance, in the absence of such guidance is there likely to be significant controversy over the interpretation of the available evidence on clinical and cost effectiveness?

For new technologies under development the DoH and the National Assembly for Wales would normally expect to provide **manufacturers** or **sponsors** with advance warning (2 years or longer) that their technologies are likely to be the subject of referral to the Institute. In the initial development of the appraisal process, however, shorter periods of such advance warning and formal notice will be inevitable. For such technologies formal notice of referral will usually occur one year before anticipated use by the NHS which, for pharmaceuticals, would be around the time of submission for **marketing authorization**.

For established technologies, manufacturers and sponsors would normally be expected to provide information for appraisal within 3 months of formal notification but the Institute will be prepared to consider a variation to this time-scale, in exceptional circumstances, on the basis of a reasoned application to the Institute's Chief Executive.

Appraisal submissions

The appraisal by the Institute of both new and existing technologies will encompass:
- their clinical effectiveness
- their cost effectiveness
- their wider NHS implications.

Evaluation by the Institute

NICE will also provide guidelines for the management of certain diseases or conditions and guidance on the appropriate use of particular interventions from self-care through to primary care, secondary care and more specialist services.

NICE also aims to develop a range of clinical **audit** methodologies that can be adapted for local use to support the institute's guidance.

Patients and the public will have access to the Institute's information on health and best treatment through the **Internet** (http://www.nice.org.uk) and other emerging public access media.

National Institute of Allergy and Infectious Diseases (NIAID) (US)

One of the institutes of the **National Institutes of Health**, which is part of the US Public Health Service of the federal government.

National Institute of Health (NIH) (US)

One of eight health agencies of the Public Health Service which, in turn, is part of the US **Health and Human Services**. The goal of the NIH's research is to acquire new knowledge to help prevent, detect, diagnose, and treat disease and disability, from the rarest genetic disorder to the common cold.

The NIH conducts research in its own laboratories; supporting the research of non-Federal scientists in universities, medical schools, hospitals, and research institutions throughout the country and abroad; helping in the training of research investigators; and fostering communication of biomedical information. Altogether, about 38 500 research and training applications are reviewed annually through the NIH peer review system. At any given time, the NIH supports 35 000 grants in universities, medical schools, and other research and research training institutions both nationally and internationally.

The Warren Grant Magnuson Clinical Center is NIH's centre for clinical research. Patients come from all over the world to participate in clinical studies here.

National Pharmaceutical Association (NPA) (UK)

The national body of Britain's community pharmacies. It was formed in 1921 to champion the interests of pharmacy owners and promote, improve and protect an essential service to the public. The NPA currently has 5600 members, representing about 11 000 pharmacies – the vast majority of community pharmacies in the UK. It is the voice of its members at local, national and international level and represents them on various bodies which advise the Government on pharmaceutical matters. The national secretariat of the NPA is the administrative body of the Association. It maintains constant contact with members, serving their needs and responding to their problems and interests.

National Pharmaceutical Pricing Authority (India)

An organization created by the government of India for carrying out the functions of fixation and monitoring the prices of medicines marketed in the country.

National Prescribing Centre (NPC) (UK)

A health service organization, formed in April 1996 by the **National Health Service** (NHS) Executive, following a review of centrally funded support for prescribing and medicine use. The NPC's current aim is 'to facilitate the promotion of high quality, cost-effective prescribing through a coordinated and prioritized programme of activities aimed at supporting all relevant professionals and senior managers working in the new NHS'.

The NPC continually reviews its programme to meet the evolving needs of its audience. The change in government in 1997 heralded further positive developments for the NHS and a White Paper – 'The New NHS: modern and dependable' (December 1997) set the broad direction for health services over the next five 5–10 years.

The working environment is constantly changing and the NPC's programme continues to reflect this. In particular, it aims to meet the demands of:

- **Primary Care Groups** (PCGs)
- Health Improvement Programmes
- National Service Frameworks
- **Clinical Governance**
- Managing significant new technologies into routine NHS use
- The **National Institute for Clinical Excellence** (NICE)
- The **Commission for Health Improvement**.

The NPC delivers a wide range of activities across the following five main areas of work:

- Information on Medicines
- Training and Education
- Dissemination of Good Practice
- Information Technology
- Informing Research and Initiatives.

National Primary Care Audit Group (NPCAG) (UK)
: The sole organization representing the interests of **primary care** audit groups. These interests include clinical audit, clinical effectiveness, practice development, education and **clinical governance**.

National Research Register (NRR) (UK)
: A register of ongoing and recently completed research projects funded by the UK's **National Health Service** (NHS). The first release contains information on over 28 000 research projects, as well as entries from the Medical Research Council's Clinical Trials Register, and details on reviews in progress collected by the NHS Centre for Reviews and Dissemination.

natural history of disease
1. The course of a disease when left untreated.
2. The course of a disease when treated with standard modes of therapy.

NBAS
: New Biological Active Substance.

NCAS
: New Chemical Active Substance.

NCE see **new chemical entity**.

NCHGR (US)
: National Center for Human Genome Research (**National Institutes of Health**).

NCHS (US)
: National Center for Health Statistics (In CDC).

NCI (US)
: National Cancer Institute.

NCPIE (US)
: National Council on Patient Information and Education.

NCR paper (Clinical Trials)
: No Carbon Required paper, that does not require carbon to make multiple copies, used in **case record forms** to make three copies.

NCRR (US)
: National Center for Research Resources (**National Institutes of Health**).

NCTR see **National Center for Toxicological Research**.

NCVIA (US)
: National Childhood Vaccine Injury Act (1986).

NDA see **New Drug Application**.

NDA Amendment
: A submission to change or add information to a **New Drug Application** or supplement not yet approved.

NDAB (Ireland)
: National Drugs Advisory Board.

NDC Number see **National Drug Code.**

NDPB
Non-Departmental Public Body.

NDS (Canada)
New Drug Study (Canada's New Drug Application).

nebulizer
A **medical device** that reduces liquid medication to extremely fine cloudlike particles to provide a drug in its misted form through a face mask to deeper parts of the respiratory tract (e.g. into the lungs); used for severe asthma attacks and for children who have asthma but cannot use an **inhaler**.

NEDO (UK)
National Economic Development Office.

NEFARMA (Holland)
Dutch Association of the Innovative Pharmaceutical.

negative binomial distribution (Statistics)
A distribution which is parameterized by a mean m and an aggregation parameter k which is large when aggregation is small; in fact as k becomes large, the negative binomial distribution approximates the Poisson distribution.

negative predictive value (–PV)
The proportion of people with a negative test who are free of disease.
See also **calculating sensitivity, specificity**.

NEI (US)
National Eye Institute (**National Institutes of Health**).

neo-adjuvant treatment
Treatment for locally advanced disease that attempts to reduce the size of the tumour so that it can be completely removed by other means. For example, **chemotherapy** given as the first therapy for a large breast tumour may cause the tumour to shrink to the point where it can be completely removed by surgery, or may permit a less radical operation than would have been needed to remove it before chemotherapy was given.
Compare **adjuvant treatment**.

Netherlandse Farmacopee (Neth. P.)
Netherlands Pharmacopoeia.

neuroleptics see **antipsychotics**.

neurotoxins
Chemicals that attack and damage nerve cells.

neurotransmitters
Chemicals that transfer messages from one nerve cell to another or from a nerve cell to a muscle cell.

New Chemical Entity (NCE)
Any new drug in development or a compound not previously described in the literature.

'New Drug' (US)

A **Food and Drug Administration** (FDA) term for 'A drug first investigated or proposed for marketing after 1938 (when the federal **Food, Drug, and Cosmetic Act** was passed). That is, the drug was not **GRAS**.'

New Drug Application (NDA) (US)

An application to the **Food and Drug Administration** (FDA) requesting market approval for a new **drug product**. It normally takes between 20 and 30 months and costs around $500 000. The application must contain, among other things, data from specific technical viewpoints for FDA review including: chemistry, pharmacology, medical, biopharmaceuticals, statistics, and, for anti-infectives, microbiology.

See also **marketing authorization**, **Pre-market Approval Application**, **Product Licence Application**.

New Molecular Entity (NME) (US)

A molecule which the **Food and Drug Administration** (FDA) considers to be original in nature. Generally, it refers to one that has been synthesized for use as a **drug substance**.

ng

Nanogram.

NGC see National Guideline Clearinghouse.

NGO

Non-governmental organization.

NHB see National Health Board.

NHLI (US)

National Heart and Lung Institute.

NHS see National Health Service.

NHS CCC see NHS Centre for Coding and Classification.

NHS Centre for Coding and Classification (NHS CCC) (UK)

The NHS CCC was established to ensure that the **Read Codes** continued to evolve to serve the needs of the health service. The aim was to facilitate implementation of the recommendation, in 1988, by certain bodies that the Read Codes should be adopted as the basis of a standard classification for use within general practice. These bodies were the technical working party of the Joint Computing Group of the Royal College of General Practitioners and the General Medical Services Committee of the **British Medical Association**. The codes were, accordingly, purchased by the Secretary of State for Health and made Crown Copyright in 1990.

The NHS CCC forms a part of the Information Management Group (IMG) of the Management Executive (ME). Its main functions are to maintain and further develop the Read Codes for use within the **National Health Service** by collaboration with the clinical professions, thus forming a comprehensive Clinical Thesaurus which can form one of the main building blocks of the electronic patient record. More than 2000 clinicians collaborated with the NHS CCC within three major Terms Projects between 1992 and 1995. The output of these projects has formed the basis for Version 3 of the Read Codes.

See also **Read Codes**.

NHS Centre for Reviews and Dissemination (CRD) (UK)

The CRD was established in January 1994 to provide the **National Health Service** (NHS) with important information on the effectiveness and cost-effectiveness of health care interventions. The aim is to identify and review the results of good quality health research and to disseminate, actively, the findings to key decision-makers in the NHS and to consumers of health care services.

The CRD is helping to promote research based practice in the NHS by offering rigorous and systematic reviews on selected topics, a database of good quality reviews and a dissemination service.

Within the NHS Research and Development (R&D) programme, the CRD is the sibling organization of the UK Cochrane Centre. The UK Cochrane Centre is part of an international network, the **Cochrane Collaboration**, committed to preparing, maintaining and disseminating systematic reviews of research on the effects of health care.

The CRD collaborates with a number of health research and information organizations across the world and is a UK member of the International Network of Agencies for Health Technology Assessment.

The functions of the centre are:
1. Undertakes and commissions credible, rigorous reviews of research findings on the effectiveness of health care relevant to the NHS.
2. Liaises with NHS decision makers to prioritize reviews and in particular the questions addressed in reviews.
3. Aims to help raise the general standard of reviews carried out for the NHS.
4. Collaborates in conducting research into methods of reviewing the literature.
5. Disseminates the results of research to NHS decision-makers.
6. Encourages research-based practice in the NHS by networking with health care professionals, particularly nurses and other therapists active in practice and service development.
7. Collaborates in conducting research into ways in which research evidence can be better disseminated and implemented.
8. Maintains databases of abstracts of good quality reviews of health research, abstracts of economic evaluations of health and health technology assessments.
9. Provides an information and enquiry service on reviews and economic evaluations for health care professionals, purchasers and providers, NHS managers, information providers, health service researchers and consumer organizations.
10. Conducts research into providing health service users with research-based information on the effectiveness of health care.

NHS Confederation (UK)

Formed in 1997 when the **National Association of Health Authorities and Trusts** and the **National Health Service** (NHS) **Trust** Federation merged. It is an independent charity managed by a board of trustees which is drawn from the councils. Comprising member representatives, the councils are responsible for the key policy and representational issues. They consist of regional representatives who act as the lynch-pin with the broader membership. The Confederation aims to be the voice of the NHS management through being the only membership body for all NHS organizations. Its membership includes 95% of NHS Trusts and **Health Authorities** in England and Wales; Health Boards and Trusts in Scotland; and Health and Social Services Trusts in Northern Ireland. **Primary care groups** can join as affiliates.

The Confederation is committed to improving health policy and practice by:
- Linking members in the development of policy and ideas

- Creating a range of opportunities for members' views to be heard
- Encouraging agenda setting debate
- Campaigning for change
- Working in partnership with other organizations
- Building awareness and understanding of issues
- Providing a single reference point for expert comment
- Supporting NHS leadership and management.

The NHS Confederation aims to:
- Inform the debate on the wider health agenda and the impact of policy on health. It runs campaigns on priority issues for members and works with policy and decision-makers. The confederation promotes long-term change and does not engage in media activity that undermines the confidence in the NHS or the Confederation
- Promote relations between the NHS and its partners (organizations and individuals interested in promoting better health)
- Lead the debate on the organization of the NHS
- Inform the development of high quality services responsive to the needs of patients
- Improve the governance of the NHS and accountability to citizens
- Promote an understanding of the need for an adequately resourced NHS
- Promote a human resources strategy for the staff of the NHS
- Improve understanding of NHS management and leadership.

NHS Direct (UK)
A 24-hour telephone advice help line, staffed by nurses, for members of the public. It started in March 1998.

NHSE (UK)
National Health Service Executive.

NHS Information Authority (UK)
An information strategy for the UK **National Health Service** (NHS), 'Information for Health', which was published in September 1998. The strategy, a feature to modernize the NHS, was to ensure that the NHS clinicians and managers have the information needed to support the core purpose of the NHS, in caring for individuals and improving public health.

The strategy was aimed to deliver a lifelong electronic health record for every person in the country, on-line 24-hour access to records and information about best clinical practice for all NHS clinicians, full use of the NHS information highway for electronic communication between every general practice and every hospital, increased public access to information and services, through on-line or telephone services, and new ways of delivering services and care through telemedicine or telecare.

The various NHS stakeholders with an interest in the successful implementation of Information for Health are:
- A new Information Policy Unit in the NHS Executive, with overall responsibility for delivery of the strategy
- A new NHS Information Authority, to manage the work programme to develop those products and standards which can best be developed at national level, in order to support local implementation
- Regional Offices providing implementation support to NHS organizations locally, and managing their performance in delivering the national strategy, advising the NHS Information Authority and the Information Policy Unit as appropriate of emerging issues

- Local organizations – including **Health Authorities**, NHS Trusts, **primary care groups** and Social Service organizations – expected to work collaboratively together to develop local plans for the implementation of the national strategy, and then implement those plans.
- Other stakeholders who need to be engaged in advisory roles including the professional and management communities, representatives of patients and the public, suppliers of systems and services and the academic institutions.

The work of the Authority is to progress in partnership with a wide range of NHS professionals, suppliers, academics and others to ensure a better balance between use of in-house and external skills than at present. The new organizational model based on the Information Policy Unit and the new Authority supersedes the previous structure at the NHS Executive for the central management of NHS Information and Technology issues.

NHSnet (UK)
The **National Health Service** (NHS)-wide communication network that was designed to connect all health care professionals to allow clinical information to be securely and reliably shared.

NHST see **NHS Trust**.

NHS Trust (NHST) (UK)
These are self-governing units within the **National Health Service** (NHS). They are hospitals and other units providing patient care who volunteered to become NHSTs. They are run by boards of directors and are accountable to the Secretary of State without any intervention from **Regional** or **District Health Authorities** (RHAs or DHAs). As part of the Health Authorities Act, however, regional health authorities were abolished with effect from April 1996 and replaced by eight regional offices of the NHS Executive. There are no fewer than 152 NHSTs in England. NHSTs have freedom that is not available to directly managed units. In particular, they are able to determine their own management structures, employ their own staff and set own assets, retain surpluses and borrow money subject to annual limits. Each Trust is required to prepare an annual business plan outlining its proposals for service development and capital investment. Like other units, trusts receive their income from contracts with health authorities, **GP fundholders** and other **purchasers**.

NHW (Canada)
National Health and Welfare Department.

NIA (US)
National Institute on Aging (**National Institutes of Health**).

NIAID (US)
National Institute of Allergy and Infectious Diseases.

NIAMD (US)
National Institute of Arthritis and Metabolic Diseases.

NIBSC see **National Institute for Biological Standards and Control**.

NICHD (US)
National Institute of Child Health and Human Development.

NIDA (US)
National Institute on Drug Abuse (**National Institutes of Health**).

NIGMS (US)
National Institute of General Medical Sciences.

NIH see **National Institutes of Health.**

Nippon Yakuzaishi Kai see **Japan Pharmaceutical Association.**

NLM (US)
National Library of Medicine (**National Institutes of Health**).

NLN see **Nordic Council on Medicines.**

NME see **new molecular entity.**

NNT see **number needed to treat.**

noise (Statistics)
The variation from subject-to-subject in the important study **outcome**(s). Usually noise is measured by the **standard deviation** of the **data**.

non-affiliated member (US)
Member of an **Institutional Review Board** who has no ties to the parent institution, its staff, or faculty. This individual is usually from the local community (e.g. minister, business person, attorney, teacher, homemaker).
See also **Institutional Review Board**.

non-classical isostere
Same as **bioisostere**.

non-clinical study
Biomedical studies not performed on human **subjects**.
See also **pre-clinical study**.

non-competitive antagonist
An **antagonist** that stops the effect of an agonist by acting at a site different from that of the **agonist**. It does not combine with the same recognition sites of the **receptors** as the agonist. It may, however, combine, reversibly or irreversibly at an adjoining site, an allosteric site, on the receptor protein.
See also **allosteric binding sites, allosteric interaction**.

non-differential bias (Clinical Trials)
Where opportunities for **bias** are equivalent in all study groups, it biases the **outcome** measure of the study toward the null of no difference between the groups.
See **attrition bias, detection bias, reader bias, recall bias, selection bias**.

non-invasive
A term that is used to describe medical procedures that do not enter or penetrate the body. It also refers to non-cancerous tumours that do not spread to other sections of the body.

non-significant risk device
An investigational **medical device** that does not present significant risk to the patient.
See also **significant risk device**.

non-therapeutic research
Research that has no likelihood or intent of producing a diagnostic, preventive, or therapeutic

benefit to the current subjects, although it may benefit subjects with a similar condition in the future.

non-tropical sprue see **celiac disease**.

Nordic Council on Medicines (NLN)
The NLN was set up in 1975 to promote cooperation among the Nordic drug regulatory authorities and between those authorities and interest groups in the academic world, the pharmaceutical industry and the health care sector. It comprises Denmark, Finland, Iceland, Norway and Sweden.

The NLN takes initiatives in areas where Nordic-wide projects are likely to enable the Nordic countries to make use of the potential savings offered by joint solutions, to influence developments in Europe and/or to promote a transfer of know-how to adjacent areas to the Nordic region. The NLN is an independent organization, uninfluenced by commercial or national interests.

The Board of the NLN consists of two members from each of the Nordic countries. Board members, and their personal deputies, are appointed by the Government of the country concerned. The Board makes policy decisions, makes long-term plans and finalizes the NLN's budget.

The main base for the NLN's work is the Nordic region itself, but the Council also collaborates with the rest of Europe/the **European Union** (EU)/the **European Economic Area** (EEA) and with the Nordic countries' closest neighbours to the east, in particular Estonia, Latvia, Lithuania and the St Petersburg region. Typically, projects are not restricted to specific geographical areas.

A good example of this is provided by the NLN's guidelines on **GCP**, one of a dozen sets of guidelines drawn up by the NLN for the Nordic countries and subsequently widely adopted around the world. The NLN set up a working group to prepare this document in 1987. The results of its efforts were published two years later and adopted as national guidelines in all the Nordic countries except Denmark.

Although the **good clinical practice** guidelines (NLN 28) have no legal status in the Nordic countries following the entry into the EEA Agreement, they are still widely used, since it is the practice of many companies to ensure that every doctor taking part in a clinical trial has a copy.

The focal point of NLN activities is cooperation between different interest groups, centred on three geographical regions:
- The Nordic region
- Cooperation with, and between, the drug regulatory authorities
- Providing a link between interest groups
- Europe/European Union/European Economic Area
- Adjacent areas to the Nordic region
- Cooperation primarily with Estonia, Latvia, Lithuania and the St Petersburg region.

For many years, Nordic guidelines have given drug manufacturers the option of marketing their products in Nordic packages, i.e. packages which provide information in more than one Nordic language and can be sold in more than one Nordic country. This has reduced the number of different variants of drug packages in the Nordic region by almost 10 000. An EC Directive (**Directive 92/27/EEC**) has created the corresponding possibility in the EU/EEA.

As a result of the EEA Agreement and Danish, Finnish and Swedish membership of the EU, it has become increasingly important to ensure that EC directives and guidelines are interpreted and implemented in a uniform manner.

The NLN Secretariat has been chosen by the EC Commission as a 'dissemination point' for EC documents relating to medicinal products. This means that it receives copies of all new guidelines, both drafts circulated for comment and guidelines that have been adopted but have not yet been published.

The NLN cooperates closely with the European Community/European Union. Denmark has acted as a bridge between the NLN and the relevant organs of the EC Commission. The NLN's guidelines on applications for approval of drugs (NLN 24), for example, broadly correspond to the EC's 'Notice to Applicants'.

In 1988 the EC and the NLN agreed on a voluntary exchange of observers between their various working groups and on arrangements to exchange information.

Nord. P.
Nordic Pharmacopoeia.

normal distribution (Statistics)
Data set that has a symmetrical, bell-shaped distribution which is normally assumed in the absence of evidence because it is statistically convenient. It is also referred to as the Gaussian distribution.

normal range
The range of values for a specific (usually laboratory) parameter that are considered clinically normal. These will vary slightly depending on the laboratory and are used as a reference against which individual patient's results are compared.

normal volunteers see **healthy, normal volunteer**.

NORSK (UK)
Old **product licence** and **adverse drug reaction** database at the **Medicines Control Agency**. It was replaced by **PLUS**.

'not approvable' (US)
After a **Food and Drug Administration** (FDA) advisory committee reviews a **drug product**, it will issue an opinion as to whether the drug is **approvable** or not approvable. Although such opinions are not binding on the FDA, the **Agency** will usually follow the advice of its committees and not grant FDA approval to drugs which are deemed not approvable.

Notice of Claimed Investigational Exemption for a New Drug see **Investigational New Drug (IND) application**.

notifiable disease
Diseases, usually of an infectious nature, whose occurrence is required by law to be made known to a health officer or local government authority.

no treatment concurrent control study (Clinical Trials)
A trial where objective measurements of effectiveness are available and **placebo** effect is negligible. This type of trial differs from uncontrolled studies in that the **investigational product** is compared with no treatment and patients are randomly assigned to either the investigational product or no treatment.

NPA see **National Pharmaceutical Association**.

NRB
Non-institutional Review Board.

NRC
Nuclear Regulatory Commission.

NSAID
Non-steroidal anti-inflammatory drug.

NTP (US)
National Toxicology Program.

null hypothesis (H_0) (Statistics)
The proposal that no difference exists between groups or that there is no association between risk indicator and **outcome** variables. It is a postulation about a population which may or may not be rejected as a result of a **hypothesis** test. If the null hypothesis is true then the findings from the study are the result of chance or **random** factors. The purpose of most statistical tests is to determine if the obtained results provide a reason to reject the hypothesis that they are merely a product of chance factors, i.e. to 'reject the null hypothesis'. For example, in an experiment in which two groups of randomly selected subjects have received different treatments and have yielded different means, it is always necessary to ask if the difference between the obtained means is among the differences that would be expected to occur by chance whenever two groups are randomly selected. In this example, the hypothesis tested is that the two samples are from **populations** with the same mean.

Another way to say this is to assert that the investigator tests the null hypothesis that the difference between the means of the populations from which the samples were drawn is zero. If the difference between the means of the samples is among those that would occur rarely by chance when the null hypothesis is true, the null hypothesis is rejected and the investigator describes the results as statistically significant, implying that they are a product of the treatments.

See also **type I error**, **type II error**.

number needed to treat (NNT)
The number of patients who (on average) need to be treated to prevent one bad **outcome** or to produce one additional successful **outcome**. It is reported as a whole number, calculated as 1/**ARR**, rounded to the next highest whole number, and accompanied by its 95% **confidence interval** (CI). 1/ARR = 1/6.8% = 14.7, rounded to 15, with a 95% CI from 9 to 35. Readers can convert this to an NNT for a specific patient by estimating that patient's susceptibility relative to the average control patient in the trial report, expressing it as a decimal fraction, F, and then dividing the reported NNT by F. If a reader's patient is judged to be half as susceptible as the average control patient in the example, F = 0.5 and NNT/F = 15/0.5 = 30.

For example if one is to assess how effective ACE inhibitors are in preventing heart failure for at least 1 year, we need to treat 13 patients by giving them an ACE inhibitor, for one extra person not to have heart failure, i.e. NNT = 13. To calculate NNT one needs to:
a. calculate the percentage of people who have the desired outcome in the treatment group
b. calculate the percentage of people who have the desired outcome in the placebo or control group
c. take (b) away from (a) to give the percentage of people helped by the treatment
d. divide 100 by this percentage to give the NNT.

Example calculation:
1149 out of 6328 patients who were given the ACE inhibitor did not develop heart failure. 893 out of 8380 patients in the control group remained healthy. What is the NNT?

Steps in calculation:
a. 1149 / 6328 = 18.2% (treated people who remained healthy)
b. 893 / 8380 = 10.6% (controls who remained healthy)
c. 18.2 − 10.6 = 7.6 (number of extra healthy subjects / 100 people treated)
d. 100 / 7.6 = 13.2 (NNT).

NNTs are used as a measure of clinical effectiveness because:
1. The NNT gives more information than relative risk because it takes into account the baseline frequency of the outcome, e.g. a drug reduces the risk of dying from a heart attack by 40% (relative risk (RR) = 0.60). In terms of RR this drug has the same 'clinical effectiveness' for everyone. However, if it is given to people with a 1 in 10 annual risk of dying from a heart attack only 25 people need to be treated to prevent one death (NNT = 25). While, if it is given to people whose risk is 1 in 100, the NNT is 250. (If the drug causes serious side effects in 1 in 100 people then we would probably not use it for people with a low risk but it would still be an effective treatment for people with high baseline risk).
2. The NNT helps us estimate how likely the treatment is to help an individual patient, e.g. if the NNT = 25 then a patient has a 1 in 25 chance of the treatment producing the desired outcome (i.e. 4% extra chance).

Nuremberg Code

A code of research ethics developed during the trials of Nazi war criminals following World War II and widely adopted as a standard during the 1950s and 1960s for protecting human subjects.

OAI (US)
Official Action Indicated (Serious **Food and Drug Administration** Post-inspection).

OAM (US)
Office of Alternative Medicine (**National Institutes of Health**).

OB
Ohne Befund. No abnormality detected.

objective measurement (Clinical Trials)
A measurement that cannot be influenced by **investigator bias**; for example, blood glucose levels or ECG tracings.

OBRA see **Omnibus Budget Reconciliation Act**.

O'Brien–Fleming Monitoring Boundary (Clinical Trials)
A set of criteria used to determine how **data** can be looked at during interim analyses, and how much potential error may be caused through looking. It is used in constructing the stopping rules for a trial.
See also **interim analysis**.

observation arm (Clinical Trials)
A group of patients sometimes followed concurrently with a **clinical trial** who are not technically participants in the study, but are being treated in the same fashion as study subjects. The purpose of this group is to gain comparative information when it may not be possible or ethical for patients to be **randomized** to the treatment group.

observational studies (Clinical Trials)
Studies where the allocation or assignment of factors is not under control of an **investigator**. In an observational study, the combinations are self-selected or are 'experiments of nature'. For those questions where it would be unethical to assign factors, investigators are limited to observational studies. Observational studies provide weaker **empirical** evidence than do experimental studies because of the potential for large **confounding factors/biases** to be present when there is an unknown association between a factor and an **outcome**. The symmetry of unknown confounders cannot be maintained. The greatest value of these types of studies (e.g. case series, ecologic, case–control, cohort) is that they provide preliminary evidence that can be used as the basis for hypotheses in stronger experimental studies, such as randomized controlled trials.

OCA (US)
Office of Consumer Affairs (**Food and Drug Administration**).

occupational disease
A disease that occurs as a result of factors in the workplace.

occupational therapy
The treatment of physical and psychiatric conditions by encouraging patients to undertake specific activities that will help them to reach their maximum level of function and independence in all aspects of life. The term is also used to describe the treatment to relearn physical skills lost as a result of an illness or accident.

OCI (US)
Office of Criminal Investigation (**Food and Drug Administration**).

OCPA see **Office of Commissioner for Public Appointments**.

od
Once daily dose regimen.

OD
1. Once daily dose regimen
2. Overdose.

odds
A proportion in which the numerator contains the number of times an event occurs and the denominator includes the number of times the event does not occur. Odds can also be described as a ratio of non-events to events. If the **event rate** for a disease is 0.1 (10%), its non-event rate is 0.9 and therefore its odds are 9:1. Note that this is not the same expression as the inverse of event rate.

See also **event rate, odds ratio**.

odds ratio
A comparison of the presence of a **risk factor** for disease in a sample of diseased subjects and non-diseased controls or the odds of an experimental patient suffering an **adverse event** relative to a control patient. It is a measure of the degree of association; for example, the odds of exposure among the cases compared with the odds of exposure among the controls. The number of people with disease who were exposed to a risk factor (Ie) over those with disease who were not exposed (Io) divided by those without disease who were exposed (Ne) over those without the disease who were not exposed (No). Thus $OR = (Ie/Io)/(Ne/No) = Ie\,No/Io\,Ne$. This measure should be used for case–control studies where we retrospectively look at risks in those with and without disease.

Also known as **exposure odds ratio** and cross-product ratio, relative odds.

ODE (US)
1. Office of Drug Evaluation.
2. see **Office of Device Evaluation**.

OECD
Organization for Economic Cooperation and Development.

OEI (US)
Official Establishment Inventory (**Food and Drug Administration**).

Office for Protection from Research Risks (OPRR) (Clinical Trials) (US)
An office within the **National Institutes of Health**, responsible for implementing **Department of Health and Humans Services** regulations (45 **CFR** Part 46) governing research involving human subjects.

Office of Commissioner for Public Appointments (OCPA) (UK)
The OCPA was created in 1995, following recommendations from the Nolan Committee on Standards in Public Life. The recommendation was that an independent Commissioner should be appointed, their role being to establish a **Code of Practice** for Ministerial appointments to public bodies, and to monitor the appointments process and ensure that all appointments are made on merit after fair and open competition.

The Code of Practice issued by the Commissioner covers all appointments to the **National Health Service** (NHS) bodies and non-departmental public bodies sponsored by the

Department of Health. In line with Government practice, the principles of the OCPA guidance are followed, whenever possible, for other health ministerial public appointments which fall outside the Commissioner's remit. The principles underlying the code include: ministerial responsibility, merit, independent scrutiny, equal opportunities, probity, openness and transparency and proportionality.

Office of Device Evaluation (ODE) (US)

The chief advisor to the Center Director and other **Food and Drug Administration** (FDA) officials on all premarket notification (**510(K)s**), **Pre-market Approval Applications** (PMAs), PDPs, device classifications and **IDEs**.

The ODE
- plans, conducts, and coordinates appropriate Center actions regarding approval, denial, and withdrawal of approval of PMAs, PDPs, IDEs, and makes substantially equivalent decision for 510(K)s, and monitors **sponsors**' conformance with requirements of all programmes
- conducts continuing review, surveillance, and medical evaluation of the labelling, clinical experience, and required reports submitted by sponsors of approved applications
- develops and interprets regulations and guidelines regarding classification, PDPs, IDEs, PMAs, and 510(K)s
- coordinates the Center's classification activities; reviews, or initiates, petitions for reclassification
- provides executive secretariat and other technical support to the medical device advisory panels, including filling vacancies and recommending establishing or restructuring panels as appropriate; and, participates through interaction with appropriate national and international committees in the development of national and international consensus standards and voluntary guidelines.

Office of Health Economics (OHE) (UK)

Founded in 1962 by the **Association for British Pharmaceutical Industry** (ABPI) and supported by an annual grant from the ABPI and by the sale of its publications. Since 1962 the OHE has established an international reputation for its analysis of health economics and statistics and for its booklets, briefings, monographs, compendia and databases. The OHE terms of reference are to:
- commission and undertake research on the economics of health and health care
- collect and analyse health and health care data from the UK and other countries
- disseminate the results of this work and stimulate discussion of them and their policy implications.

The research and editorial independence of the OHE is ensured by a Policy Board. All OHE publications have been peer reviewed by members of its Editorial Board and, where appropriate, other clinical or technical experts independent of the authors.

The OHE provides:
- Objective, policy-orientated analysis
- **Peer-reviewed** publications by expert authors
- OHE Compendium of Health Statistics: the leading one-stop source for health care and health data
- **Health Economic Evaluations Database** (HEED)
- Specialist seminars, lectures, conferences.

The OHE work is in three main areas:
- Health care systems – their finance and organization

- Health technology assessment
- Pharmaceutical industry.

See also **Health Economic Evaluations Database**.

officinal product

As defined under **European Union** rules (Article 1 of **Directive 65/65/EEC**), it is a medicinal product prepared, in a pharmacy, in accordance with the prescriptions of pharmacopoeia and is intended to be supplied directly to the patients served by the pharmacy in question.

off-label (use) (US)

A term (mainly US) for the use of drugs for an unlicensed condition, i.e. not listed in the licence and accordingly the **data sheet** (**Summary of Product Characteristics** (SPC or SmPC). **Food and Drug Administration** regulations allow physicians to prescribe approved medications for other than their intended indications.

Compare **labelled use**.

OGE (US)

Office of Government Ethics.

OHA (US)

Office of Health Affairs (**Food and Drug Administration**).

OHE see Office of Health Economics.

OHMO (US)

The Office of **Health Maintenance Organizations** (HMO).

ointment

A semisolid preparation, usually containing a medicinal substance, for external application to the body.

OJ (European Union)

Official Journal of the European Community.

OLA (US)

Office of Legislative Affairs (**Food and Drug Administration**).

om (OM)

(Latin *Omni mane*), Once daily dose regimen.

Ombudsman or Ombudsperson (US)

An officer of **Food and Drug Administration** who is responsible for mediation of activities and disputes among the various groups within FDA. The Ombudsman is often called in to resolve jurisdiction issues with regard to particular products (for example, should a catheter coated with a **drug product** be regulated as a **medical device** or as a drug?).

The term is also used to describe a person within a **Managed Care Organization** (MCO) or a person outside of the health care system (such as an appointee of the state) who is designated to receive and investigate complaints from beneficiaries about quality of care, inability to access care, discrimination, and other problems that beneficiaries may experience with their managed care organization. This individual often functions as the beneficiary's advocate in pursuing grievances or complaints about denials of care or inappropriate care.

Omnibus Budget Reconciliation Act (OBRA) (US)
The OBRA of 1989 was an act of Congress which established the **Resource-Based Relative Value Scale** (RBRVS) used by **Health Care Finance Administration** (HCFA) to calculate **Medicare** payments. This bill produced major changes in Medicare reimbursement for physicians such as limits on allowable charges, a fee schedule in the future, caps on balance billing, reduction of 'overpriced' procedures.

one-sided alternative hypothesis see **one-tailed alternative hypothesis**.

one-tailed alternative hypothesis (Statistics)
An alternative to the **null hypothesis** that specifies a range of permissible values all of which lie to one side of the null value (e.g. all favouring one treatment).

ONS (UK)
Office of National Statistics.

OPA (US)
Office of Public Affairs (**Food and Drug Administration**).

OPC
One-point-cut (Ampoule).

OPCS (UK)
Office of Population, Census and Surveys.

OPE (US)
Office of Planning and Evaluation (**Food and Drug Administration**).

open arm see **compassionate or open arm**.

open design see **open study**.

open label study (Clinical Trials) see **open study**.

open study (Clinical Trials)
A term used to describe a trial experimental design in which both the patient and the assessor (**investigator**) are aware of the treatment being allocated.
Also called open label study. This may occur in a study involving either one or more treatments.

opinion (European Union)
As applicable to **European Union** law, unlike the legal instruments (**Decisions, Directives, Regulations**), opinions, like **recommendations**, have only persuasive but not binding power.
See also **communications, decisions, directives, recommendations, regulations**.

opinion leaders (OLs)
Clinical experts of integrity and renowned reputation and, thus, leading authority in a particular subject, whose opinion and views are respected by their peers. They are usually invited by a company or a **sponsor** to take part in their **clinical trials** with new compounds. OLs can support drug development at all of its phases, e.g. from pre-clinical through to post-marketing phase IV. Their contribution is particularly useful when they head the advisory board development, **Strategic Publication Plan** (SPP) and participate in **Continued Medical Education** (CME) programmes.

opioid partial agonist
A compound that has an affinity for and stimulates physiologic activity at the same cell receptors as opioid agonists but that produces only a partial (i.e. submaximal) bodily response.

opportunity cost
A complete evaluation of total cost will consider not simply the financial cost of a particular treatment, it will also consider the lost potential of those resources to provide benefits in other ways. This lost potential is known as opportunity cost. For instance, the cost of unnecessary surgical procedures is not only the monetary unit cost of the procedures themselves, but also the opportunity cost of not using those dollars in a way that would be more economically efficient (e.g. to provide childhood vaccinations).

OPRR see **Office for Protection from Research Risks**.

OPSR (Japan)
Organization for Pharmaceutical Safety and Research.

optimum dose
The dose which produces maximal effect in most patients.

ORA (US)
Office of Regulatory Affairs (**Food and Drug Administration**).

oral activity
Refers to the **efficacy** of a drug following oral administration.

oral syringes
A measuring device supplied with oral liquid medicines that are prescribed in doses other than multiples of 0.5 mL. The syringe is marked in 0.5-mL divisions from 1 to 5 mL to measure doses of less than 5 mL. It is provided with an adaptor and an instruction leaflet.

ordinal data (Statistics)
Data that can be ordered or ranked.

Original Medical Record see **source data**.

orphan drug
A term created by the **Food and Drug Administration** (FDA) to describe a drug for which the target population is limited (fewer than 200 patients) or for which the disease it treats occurs rarely. Reasonable recovery of the sponsoring firm's research and development expenditure, for such drugs, is not expected within a reasonable time. The term is also used to describe substances intended for such uses. The licensing duration for such drugs is shortened by the **regulatory authorities** of many countries as an incentive for pharmaceutical companies to develop such drugs. In the UK, the term is used by the **Medicines Control Agency** to refer to new drug applications attracting a reduced licence fee because limited data is available to support their use.

Orphan Drug Act (1983) (US)
A US legislation concerning expedited licensing period for **orphan drugs**. It was intended to act as incentive for pharmaceutical companies to develop such drugs which otherwise would not appeal to the **manufacturers** due to low profit potential.

orthotic
A **medical device** used to correct or control deformed bones, muscles, or joints.

OTC see **over the counter drug**.

OTC Directory (UK)
A listing book of products that patients can buy to treat various conditions. It is produced by the PAGB, the trade association representing manufacturers of **over-the-counter** (OTC) medicines and food supplements. The products include allopathic drugs, herbal products and food supplements. The directory is used to verify treatments taken by patients before they visit their doctor. It is also used to develop shared OTC guidelines between general practitioners, **pharmacists** and nurses. Brief safety information is also supplied in the directory based on publicly documented information and individual **product licences**. The products listed in this directory are supplied by PAGB member companies (manufacturers, distributors). This is estimated to cover 95% of the OTC products marketed in the UK.

otic solution
Ear drops; used to relieve minor ear discomfort by softening of earwax.

ototoxicity
Adverse drug reactions that some drugs have on the organs or nerves in the ears, which can lead to hearing and balance problems.

outcome
1. (Clinical Medicine) An outcome is the result or impact of medical or surgical intervention or non-intervention on the health status of an individual or a population.
2. (Health Economics) Outcomes are the potential consequences, both good and bad, of various interventions (or non-interventions). By associating costs with outcomes in drug therapy, pharmacoeconomic analysis can provide a rational basis for drug decision making.
3. (Clinical Trials) An outcome is an important measure and the basis for comparison between the treatment arms in a clinical trial. Examples of outcomes might be death, number of infections in one year of follow-up, presence of an **adverse reaction** and body temperature.

outcomes-based payment
A system of reimbursement where **providers** receive payment based on improvement of their patients from the treatment provided, or are reimbursed based on success rates of treatment. This creates incentive for the provider to use the most cost-effective therapies and helps payers control costs.

outcomes management
Providers and payers alike wish to find a method of managing care in a way that would produce the best **outcomes** while holding down costs. **Managed Care Organizations** (MCO)s are increasingly interested in learning to manage the outcome of care rather than just managing the cost of care, i.e. to better manage clinical outcomes for their enrolees to increase the satisfaction of patients and payers. It is thought that through a database of outcomes experience, caregivers will know better which treatment modalities result in consistently better outcomes for patients. Outcomes management may lead to the development of clinical **protocols**.

outcomes measurement
System used to track clinical treatment and responses to that treatment. The methods for measuring **outcomes** are quite varied among **providers**. Much disagreement exists regarding the best practice or tools to utilize to measure outcomes. In fact, much disagreement exists in the medical field about the definition of outcome itself.

outcomes research see **health outcomes research**.

outlier (Statistics)
Unusually large or small values compared to the rest of the **data** in a data set. Outliers are often defined as any value larger or smaller than the median plus or minus 1.5 times the interquartile range or any value 2 or more standard deviations from the mean in a large 'normally' distributed data set.

out of area treatments (OATs) (UK)
Payments to health trusts for care for patients from more distant areas. Formerly known as extra contractual referral (ECR).

outpatient procedure
Medical procedures which do not require a hospital stay. An example would be a minor surgery such as cataract removal. In order to improve **cost-containment**, many procedures which were once performed on an **inpatient** basis are now performed on an outpatient basis. The term is also applicable to the patient who is allocated an outpatient treatment.

overdose see **drug overdose**.

over-the-counter drug (OTC)
Any drug that can be sold/bought without a doctor's **prescription** or pharmacist's supervision. Distribution of non-prescription drugs is unrestricted, and they may be sold, for example, in both grocery stores and pharmacies.
    See also **General Sales List (GSL) medicine, legend drug, pharmacy drug, prescription only medicine**.

oxygen free radicals
Active forms of oxygen found in pollution, cigarette smoke, and radiation that can damage cells and are believed to play a role in the ageng process and cancer.

P see **pharmacy drug**.

P450 See **cytochrome P450**.

PA (US) see **Group Practice**.

PAB see **Pharmaceutical Affairs Bureau**.

package insert
A leaflet, produced by the **manufacturer** and approved by the **regulatory authority**(ies) concerned, which is inserted in the pack of a **proprietary medicinal product**. It provides information on **indication, contraindication**, possible **side-effects**, precautions, warnings, etc. The **European Union, Directive 92/27/EEC** lays down the rules governing **labelling** and package leaflets and requires all the information identifying the product be stated on the outer packaging.
See also **Patient Information Leaflet**.

packaging
All operations, including filling and **labelling**, which a **bulk product** has to undergo in order to become a **finished product**.

packaging material
Any material employed in the packaging of a **medicinal product**, excluding any outer packaging used for transportation or shipment. Packaging materials are referred to as primary or secondary according to whether or not they are intended to be in direct contact with the product.

PACT see **prescribing analysis and cost**.

PAHO (US)
Pan American Health Organization.

pairing see **matched-pairs design**.

PAL see **Pharmaceutical Affairs Law**.

palliative
Palliative therapies are those which only relieve the **symptoms** of a disease without curing it.

panacea
A universal remedy; a cure all.

pandemic
Referring to an epidemic disease of widespread prevalence.

Pan European Regulatory Forum (PERF)
PERF is a project that falls within the Regional Programme on Quality Assurance (PRAQ III). The ultimate aim of this programme is the transposition of all technical regulations and European technical acts into the national legislation of central and eastern European countries (CEECs). In this context and in the area of medicinal products, the PERF is designed to establish an internationally open dialogue, design working mechanisms to facilitate adoption of the common technical requirements, ensure effective implementation and identify areas where additional action may be required.

paper trail (Clinical Trials)
Paper records (reports, letters, corrections, etc.) of all of the activities of a **clinical trial**. They are filed as a permanent record of the study should there be, in the future, any need to track the history of any study or part of a study.

parallel imports
Medicinal products purchased in one country, imported into another, often repackaged in the destination country's language, and resold wholesale to pharmacies and other wholesalers at an arbitrage profit. In the UK, the **Medicines Control Agency** has a scheme under which **medicinal products**, which hold **marketing authorizations** in any **European Union Member State**, may be imported into the UK for marketing if there is a related UK licence.

parallel study (Clinical Trials)
A type of **clinical trial** in which two or more treatments are to be compared. The patients are usually **randomized** to different study groups and then followed at the same time. This design is the contrast of **cross-over** studies, in which the patients are treated in sequence.
Compare **cross-over clinical trial**.

parallel track mechanism (US)
A US Public Health Service policy that makes promising investigational drugs for AIDS and other HIV-related diseases more widely available under 'parallel track' **protocols** while the controlled **clinical trials** essential to establish the safety and effectiveness of new drugs are carried out. The system established by this policy is designed to make the drugs more widely available to patients with these illnesses who have no therapeutic alternatives and who cannot participate in the controlled clinical trials.

parallel track trial see **parallel track mechanism**.

parallel trial see **parallel study**.

paramedic
A person trained to give first aid and other emergency medical care.

parametric test (Statistics)
A **hypothesis** test that is based on the assumption that the population distribution of the variable under consideration has a specific shape such as a normal distribution.

parasympathomimetic (cholinergic) agent
Having an action mimicking that produced by stimulation of the parasympathetic nerves.

parent–child report
Report in which the administration of medicines to a parent results in a suspected reaction in a child.

parenteral
The introduction of a substance into the body by any route other than the digestive tract, such as through a vein or muscle.

Parenteral Drug Association (PDA)
A non-profit international association of more than 9500 scientists involved in the development, manufacture, quality control and regulation of pharmaceuticals and related products. The association also provides educational opportunities for government and university sectors that have a vocational interest in pharmaceutical sciences and technology.

partial agonist
An **agonist** that is unable to induce maximal activation of a **receptor** population, regardless of the amount of **drug** applied.
See also **intrinsic activity**.

participant (Clinical Trials)
A patient or subject taking part in a **clinical trial**.

partition coefficient
The ratio of its concentration in the lipid phase to that in the water phase after equilibrium in such a two-phase system. The higher the coefficient the greater its lipid solubility. The higher the lipid solubility of a drug the more rapidly it passes through the lipoprotein matrix of cell membranes. Knowledge of the degree of lipid solubility enables predictions to be made about its pharmacokinetics. This is particularly applicable to drugs crossing the blood–brain barrier (which may be advantageous).

PAS (US)
Public Affairs Specialist (**Food and Drug Administration**).

PASS see **Post-Authorization Safety Study**.

paste
A semisolid preparation, usually for external use, e.g. of a fatty base, a viscous mucilaginous base, or a mixture of starch and soft paraffin.

pastille
A lozenge in which the active ingredient is usually incorporated in a mass of sweetened gum, glycerin and gelatin base intended to be sucked.

patents
There are three different types of patents. Design patents protect novel, non-functional design elements. Plant patents protect asexually reproducible plants. Utility patents, the most common type of patent, are often referred to simply as 'patents'. They provide protection for useful inventions – which may be processes, machines, articles of manufacture, or compositions of matter. A patent permits the patentee to exclude others from making, selling, or using the patented invention or from importing the patented invention or an article made by a patented process into the country. Unlike copyrights, others may be excluded from practising a patented invention whether or not they copied the invention from the patentee. Independent invention is no defence to patent infringement. It is important to realize that a patent by itself does not permit the patentee to do anything with the invention. Patent rights are, for the most part, exclusionary and not permissive rights. This is similar to the rights enjoyed by the owner of other types of property, such as personal property. A patentee may not practise a patented invention if, by doing so, the patent rights of another would be infringed. That may occur, for instance, in the situation where there is a patent for a specific chemical compound but another patent exists that covers the generic class of compounds to which that specific compound belongs.

patient
A person who has a medical condition/a disease, is under treatment for any disease, or under treatment for the prophylaxis of a disease. In the concept of **clinical trials**, it is the person who is receiving treatment (or **placebo**).
See also **human subject**, **healthy**, **normal volunteer**.

Patient Advocacy Groups
Organizations of patients with a particular **disease** or condition. These groups usually include physicians, members of the clergy and political activists. They provide assistance and psychological support for members of the group and often lobby for reforms, research funds and financial assistance for group members.

patient-controlled analgesia (PCA)
A system for administering pain-killing drugs in which the amount of drug delivered is controlled by the patient.

patient file (Clinical Trials)
A file containing demographic, medical and treatment information about a patient or a subject (e.g. hospital file, a consultation record or a special subject file). It may be paper-based or a mixture of computer and paper records. Such files are necessary for the verification of the authenticity of the information presented in the **case record form** and, where needed, the possibility of completing or correcting it, provided that the conditions regulating the use and consultation of such documents are respected.

Patient Identification Number (PID)
A unique identifier number given to all patients participating in a clinical study. It refers to a particular patient, yet preserves confidentiality for record keeping.

Patient Information Leaflet (PIL)
A leaflet (provided by the **manufacturer**) that contains essential information, intended for the patient, on the use of the **drug product**. It is usually contained in the package of a drug product. In most countries, the provision of PILs is obligatory and enforced by the country's health regulatory authorities. In the **European Union**, PILs are now required for all new medicines and for older medicines at the time of renewal of their authorization. Historically many medicines in the UK have been dispensed from bulk, making the provision of patient information leaflets difficult.
See also **Patient Information Sheet**, **Summary of Product Characteristics**.

Patient Information Sheet (Clinical Trials)
An informative sheet given to patients participating in a clinical study. It provides details of the aims, objectives, risks, benefits and any likely inconveniencies of the trial.
See also **Patient Information Leaflet**.

patient number see **Patient Identification Number**.

patient population
The total number of people suffering from a particular condition or disease.

pattern recognition
The recognition of patterns in large **data** sets using suitable mathematical methodologies.

Paul-Ehrlich-Institute (Bundesamt für Sera und Impfstoffe) (Germany)
German regulatory authority for sera, vaccines, allergens and blood products.

PCA
1. see **patient-controlled analgesia**.
2. see **Prescription Cost Analysis**.

PCG see **primary care group**.

PCRF (Clinical Trials)
Patient case record form, see **case record form**.

PCSO see **Pharmaceutical Contract Organization Register**.

PD see **pharmacodynamics**.

PDMA (US)
Prescription Drug Marketing Act (**Food and Drug Administration**).

PDP (US)
Product development protocols (for **medical devices**).

PDQ see **Physician Data Query**.

PDR see **Physicians Desk Reference**.

PDUFA (US)
Prescription Drug User Fee Act (of 1992).

peak plasma concentration (C_{max})
The highest level of drug that can be obtained in the blood usually following multiple doses.

peak plasma drug concentration see **peak plasma concentration**.

pectoral
A medicine used to relieve disorders of the respiratory tract such as a cough mixture or **expectorant**.

pediculicide
An insecticidal drug product used for destroying head/pubic lice.

Peer Review Committee (US)
A committee of physicians within a **Health Maintenance Organization** (HMO) that reviews and establishes guidelines for **capitation** rates.

peer-reviewed
Peer-reviewed articles are those which appear in scientific journals and have been inspected by members of the scientific community before publication.

Peer Review Organization (PRO) (US)
An organization in which practising doctors assume responsibility for reviewing the suitability and quality of health care services provided under **Medicare** and **Medicaid**.

PEM see **Prescription Event Monitoring**.

peptidomimetic
A compound containing non-peptidic structural elements that is capable of mimicking or antagonizing the biological action(s) of a natural parent peptide. A peptidomimetic does not have classic peptide characteristics such as enzymatically scissile peptidic bonds.
See also **peptoid**.

peptoid
A **peptidomimetic** that results from the oligomeric assembly of N-substituted glycines.

per capita rate
A rate which is proportional to the number of individuals in a population.

percentage method
A method used to calculate the corresponding paediatric dose for commonly prescribed drugs that have a wide margin between the therapeutic dose level and the toxic one.
See also **body surface area**.

percutaneous
A procedure that is carried out through the skin, such as an injection.

per diem
Per day.

per protocol analysis
A term used to describe the act of including all patients treated, according to the **protocol**, in the analysis.

PERF see **Pan European Regulatory Forum**.

PER Scheme see **Pharmaceutical Evaluation Report Scheme**.

Periodic Safety Update Report (PSUR)
A report, produced by the **marketing authorization** (MA) holders, intended to provide an update of the worldwide safety experience of a **medicinal product** to the **competent authorities** (CAs) at defined times post-authorization. At these defined times, MA holders are expected to provide succinct summary information together with a critical evaluation of the benefit to risk balance of the product in the light of new or changing post-authorization information. This evaluation should ascertain whether further investigations need to be carried out and whether changes should be made to the MA, the **Summary of Product Characteristics** (SPC), **Patient Information Leaflet** (PIL), or product advertising. (CPMP/Ph V WP/108/99 corr.)

Once a medicinal product is authorized in the **European Union** (EU), even if it is not marketed, the MA holder is required to submit a PSUR. PSURs are normally required: immediately upon request, at 6-monthly intervals for the first two years following the medicinal product's authorization in the EU (i.e. its **EU birth date** [EBD]), annually for two years, at the first renewal, and then 5-yearly at renewal thereafter. There may, however, be exceptions where the cycle may be re-started or an exemption to the requirement for 6-monthly and annual PSURs is granted. **Data lock** points may be set according to the EBD of a medicinal product or its **International Birth Date** (IBD). For administrative convenience, if desired by the MA holder, the IBD may be designated as the last day of the same month.

Each PSUR should cover the period of time since the last update report and should be submitted within 60 days of the last data lock point. The MA holders should submit the renewal application at least three months before the date of the MA in the EU. This may be submitted earlier in order to facilitate coordination with the regular cycle of the PSUR. MA holders should lock their data not more than 60 days before submitting the application for renewal.

For medicinal products authorized under the **centralized procedure** PSURs should be submitted to the competent authorities of all **Member States** and the **European Medicines Evaluation Agency** (EMEA) in accordance with Council **Regulation (EEC) No. 2309/93** Articles 21 and 22, and Commission **Regulation (EC) 540/95** Articles 2 and 3.

For products authorized by mutual recognition or national procedures, PSURs should be submitted to the competent authorities of the Member States in accordance with **Directive 75/319/EEC** Articles 29c and 29d.

PSURs should incorporate the following sections:

1. Introduction:
   Definition of the medicinal product and brief details so as to place the product in perspective relative to previous reports and circumstance.

2. World-wide MA status
   Cumulative information, usually as a table, for all countries where a regulatory decision about marketing has been made related to the following:
   - Dates of MA, and subsequent renewal
   - Any qualifications surrounding the authorization, such as limits to indications if relevant to safety
   - Treatment indications and special populations covered by the MA, when relevant
   - Lack of approval, including explanation, by **regulatory authorities** (RAs)
   - Withdrawal by the company of an authorization application submission if related to **safety** or **efficacy**
   - Dates of launch
   - Trade name(s).

3. Updates of RA or MA holder actions taken for safety reasons
   This section should include details on the following types of actions relating to safety that were taken during the period covered by the report and between data lock-point and report submission:
   - MA withdrawal or suspension
   - Failure to obtain an MA renewal
   - Restrictions on distribution
   - Clinical trial suspension
   - Dosage modification
   - Changes in target population or indications
   - Formulation changes.

   The safety reasons that led to these actions should be described and documentation appended when appropriate; any communication with the health care professionals (e.g. Dear Doctor letters) as a result of such action should be described with copies appended.

4. Changes to reference safety information
   The version of the **Company Core Data Sheet** (CCDS) with its **Company Core Safety Information** (CCSI) in effect at the beginning of the period covered by the report should be used as the reference. It should be numbered, dated and appended to the PSUR and include the date of the last version.

   Changes to the CCSI, such as new **contraindications**, precautions, warnings, **adverse drug reactions** (ADRs), or interactions, already made during the period covered by the report, should be clearly described, with presentation of the modified sections. The revised CCSI should be used as the reference for the next report and the next period. With the exception of emergency situations, it may take some time before intended modifications are introduced in the product-information materials provided to prescribers, pharmacists, and consumers. Therefore, during that period the amended reference document (CCDS) may contain more 'listed' information than the existing product information in many countries.

   When meaningful differences exist between the CCSI and the safety information in the

EU SPC (or the official data sheets/product information documents approved in a country), a brief comment should be prepared by the MA holder, describing the local differences and the consequences on the overall safety evaluation and on the actions proposed or initiated. This commentary may be provided in the cover letter or other addendum accompanying the local submission of the PSUR.

5. Patient exposure

Where possible, an estimate of patient exposure should cover the same period as the interim safety data. While it is recognized that it is usually difficult to obtain and validate accurate exposure data, an estimate of the number of patients exposed should be provided along with the method used to derive the estimate. An explanation and justification should be presented if the number of patients is impossible to estimate. In its place, other measures of exposure, such as patient-days, number of prescriptions or number of dosage units are considered appropriate; the method used should be explained. If these or other more precise measures are not available, bulk sales (tonnage) may be used. The concept of a defined daily dose may be used in arriving at patient exposure estimates. When possible and relevant, data broken down by sex and age (especially paediatric vs. adult) should be provided.

When a pattern of reports indicates a potential problem, details by country (with locally recommended daily dose) or other breakdown (e.g. indication, dosage form) should be presented if available. When ADR data from clinical studies are included in the PSUR, the relevant denominator(s) should be provided. For ongoing and/or blinded studies, an estimation of patient exposure may be made.

6. Presentation of individual cases histories

- *General considerations* Follow-up data on individual cases may be obtained subsequent to their inclusion in a PSUR. MA holders should monitor standard, recognized medical and scientific journals for safety information literature relevant to their products. Published cases may also have been received as spontaneous cases, be derived from a sponsored clinical study, or arise from other sources. Care should be taken to include such cases only once. Medically unconfirmed reports should be submitted as addenda line listings and/or summary tabulations only when requested by the RAs.
- *Cases presented as line listings* The following types should be included in the listing. Attempts should be made to avoid duplicate reporting of cases from the literature and RAs:
  - All serious reactions, and non-serious reactions, from the literature
  - All serious reactions from RAs

  Collection and reporting of non-serious, listed ADRs may not be required in all EU countries. Therefore, a line listing of spontaneously reported non-serious listed reactions that have been collected should be submitted as an addendum to the PSUR only when requested by the RA.
- *Presentation of the line listing* This should include each patient only once regardless of how many ADR terms are reported for the case. If there is more than one reaction, they should all be mentioned but the case should be listed under the most serious ADR (sign, symptom, or diagnosis), as judged by the MA holder.
- *Summary tabulations* These usually contain more terms than patients. Breakdown, by 'serious' vs. 'non-serious', 'listed' vs. 'unlisted', and 'source', is deemed helpful by the authorities.

- *MA holder's analysis of individual case histories* Brief comments on the data such as discussion presented on particularly serious unanticipated findings.
7. Studies
   All completed studies (non-clinical, clinical, and epidemiological) yielding safety information with potential impact on product information, studies specifically planned or in progress, and published studies that address safety issues, should be discussed:
   - Newly analysed studies.

   All relevant studies containing important safety information and newly analysed during the reporting period should be described, including those from epidemiological, toxicological or laboratory investigations. The study design and results should be clearly and concisely presented with attention to the usual standards of data analysis and description that are applied to non-clinical and clinical study reports. Copies of full reports should be appended only if deemed appropriate.
   - Targeted new safety studies.

   New studies specifically planned or conducted to examine a safety issue (actual or hypothetical) should be described. When possible and relevant, if an interim analysis was part of the study plan, the interim results of ongoing studies may be presented. When the study is completed and analysed, the final results should be presented in a subsequent PSUR.
   - Published studies.

   Reports in the scientific and medical literature, including relevant published abstracts from meetings, containing important safety findings (positive or negative) should be summarized and publication reference(s) given.
8. Other information; including
   - Efficacy-related information. For a product used in prevention or to treat serious life-threatening diseases, medically relevant lack of efficacy reporting, which might represent a significant hazard to the treated population.
   - Late-breaking information. Examples include significant new cases or important follow-up data.
9. Overall safety evaluation
   The MA holder should provide a concise analysis of the data presented, taking into account any late-breaking information and followed by the MA holder's assessment of the significance of the data collected during the period.
10. Conclusion
    The conclusion should:
    - Indicate which safety data do not remain in accord with the previous cumulative experience, and with the reference safety information, the CCSI.
    - Specify and justify any action recommended or initiated.

    See also **E2C guidance document**.
    Source: (CPMP/PhVWP/108/99 corr.). The author wishes to thank the European Medicines Evaluation Agency (EMEA) for their contribution, assistance and cooperation.

person appointed
Independent assessor(s) appointed by the Licensing Authority to hear an appeal against a proposed licensing action.

PERT chart
Programme Evaluation and Review Technique. An analysis developed in the 1960s in the US and used widely in complex engineering and construction applications. It is applied also to management of projects in other disciplines such as clinical research.

pessary
A medicated vaginal suppository.

pesticide
A preparation used for destroying pests of any kind; the term embraces insecticides, larvicides, molluscicides, rodenticides.

Pfeiffer's rule
Pfeiffer's rule states that in a series of chiral compounds the **eudismic** ratio increases with increasing **potency** of the **eutomer**.

PFU
Prescription follow-up.

pH
A measure of the acidic or basic character of a substance.

PHARMAC see **Pharmaceutical Management Agency Limited**.

pharmaceutical
Any **medicinal product**. It is normally a **drug** derived from an organic or inorganic chemical and used to treat a wide range of medical conditions.

Pharmaceutical Affairs Bureau (PAB) (Japan)
A department within the **Ministry of Health and Welfare**. The PAB is responsible for the administration of the approval procedure. It is supported by expert bodies such as the Central Pharmaceutical Affairs Council, the National Institute of Hygienic Sciences and National Institute of Health.

Pharmaceutical Affairs Law (PAL) (1960) (Japan)
The Japanese legislative law on authorizing medicinal products to be marketed in Japan. It was issued on 10 August 1960 and revised on 2 December 1983.

pharmaceutical alternates see **pharmaceutical alternatives**.

pharmaceutical alternatives
Drug products that contain the identical therapeutic moiety or its precursor and contain the same amount(s) of same **active ingredient**(s) (i.e. erythromycin ethyl succinate and erythromycin palmitate; ampicillin suspension and ampicillin capsule), but not necessarily in the same amount or dosage form or as the same salt or ester. Each such drug product individually meets either the identical or its own respective compendial or other applicable standard of identity, strength, quality, and purity, including potency and, where applicable, content uniformity, disintegration times and/or dissolution rates.
Compare **pharmaceutical equivalence**.

Pharmaceutical Benefits Manager (PBM) (US)
A company that manages and administers the prescription benefit for health plan sponsors.

Pharmaceutical Committee (European Union)
The committee established by a Council **Directive 75/320/EEC** of 20 May 1975 to assist the **European Commission** in its pharmaceutical work. It is one of three committees set up by the Commission (the other two are the Regulatory Committee and the **GMP** Group). It is chaired by a senior representative of the **Commission of European Community**, and its membership consists of 'senior experts in public health matters from the **Member States** (MSs)'. It formally

consists of one representative from each MS, but each member is also allowed one deputy who is allowed to participate in the meetings of the committee. In the Council Decision, it is indicated that the committee is to be consulted on any new proposals for Directives on **proprietary medicinal products** (and in particular any amendments to Council **Directive 65/65/EEC**), and should examine any question relating to the application of the Directives and any other question on medicinal products which is brought to it by its chairman or a representative of a MS.

Pharmaceutical Contract Organization Register (PCSO Register) (US)
A register that was developed to provide recognition for the many companies supporting the development and management of the new drug development process.

pharmaceutical equivalence
The situation where two medicinal products are pharmaceutically equivalent in that they contain the same quantity of **active ingredient**(s), have the same dosage form, meet the same or comparable standards. The colour, flavour, shape, inert ingredients, shelf life and packaging could however be different. Pharmaceutical equivalence does not necessarily imply **bioequivalence**.
Compare **bioequivalence, pharmaceutical alternative**.

pharmaceutical equivalent
Drug products that contain identical amounts of the identical active **drug ingredient**, i.e. the salt or ester of the same therapeutic moiety, in identical dosage forms, but not necessarily containing the same inactive ingredients, and that meet the identical compendial or other applicable standard of identity, strength, quality, and purity, including potency and where applicable, content uniformity, disintegration times and/or dissolution rate.
Compare **bioequivalence, pharmaceutical alternatives**.

Pharmaceutical Evaluation Report (PER) Scheme
A scheme for the mutual recognition of evaluation reports on pharmaceutical products which was started on 13 June 1979 with Austria, Norway, Finland, Sweden and Switzerland as the founding members. The aim of the scheme is to ease the trade in pharmaceutical products by eliminating, through the exchange of evaluating reports, the unwarranted reassessment of data for registration. The scheme operates by the regular quarterly circulation of lists of new active substance products approved in the **Member States**.

Pharmaceutical Inspection Convention (PIC)
A European organization which mutually recognizes inspection reports on manufacturers. It is an agreement between the health authorities of the **European Union Member States** that they will, on request, with the agreement of the manufacturers, exchange information during their own national inspections of the manufacturing sites.

Pharmaceutical Inspection Cooperation Scheme (PICS)
A scheme closely affiliated to the **Pharmaceutical Inspection Convention** (PIC) with identical aims except mutual recognition. It was created for **European Community** members who were previously with PIC.

Pharmaceutical Journal, The (UK)
The official journal of the **Royal Pharmaceutical Society of Great Britain**, with a circulation of about 45 000, which was founded by Jacob Bell in 1841 and has been published weekly since 1870. The journal covers all aspects of pharmaceutical practice and science worldwide as well as technical articles and reviews.

Pharmaceutical Management Agency Limited (PHARMAC) (New Zealand)
The company that manages the New Zealand Pharmaceutical Schedule on behalf of its owner – the Health Funding Authority (HFA). PHARMAC aims to get the best health care value from the New Zealand Government when recommending which drugs are subsidized, and at what level of expenditure on pharmaceuticals. PHARMAC's decisions incorporate a balanced view of the needs of both prescribers and patients. The PHARMAC Board with input from independent medical experts on the Pharmacology and Therapeutics Advisory Committee (PTAC) and its specialist sub-committees, and PHARMAC's managers and analysts make decisions on listing, subsidy levels, and prescribing guidelines and conditions.

Pharmaceutical suppliers may apply to PHARMAC to have a medicine listed on the Pharmaceutical Schedule for subsidy, following Ministry of Health registration of the product. PHARMAC's decisions are made by having regard to PHARMAC's Decision Criteria.

The core activity of PHARMAC is review and publication of regular updates of the Pharmaceutical Schedule. This involves continual assessment of drug performance and cost, usually by reviewing trends within defined groups of drugs (therapeutic group reviews). PHARMAC sets its review priorities by taking into account the reports of the National Health Committee, known patient needs, the size of the therapeutic group relative to total drug usage, and cost trends within that therapeutic group.

pharmaceutical medicine (PM)
In essence, it is the medical discipline specializing in the discovery, research, and development of new **drugs**, vaccines, **medical devices** and diagnostics, monitoring their **safety**, teaching their appropriate and safe use and supporting their ethical promotion. It deals with basic research, pharmaceutical development, **clinical pharmacology** (**pharmacokinetics**, **pharmacodynamics** and **toxicology**), clinical research, patient care, **pharmacoeconomics**, **pharmacoepidemiology**, **pharmacogenetics**, **pharmacogenomics**, **pharmacognosy**, **pharmacometrics**, **pharmacodiagnosis**, **pharmacovigilance**, **Regulatory Affairs**, **biostatistics** and, of course, clinical medicine.

See also **pharmaceutical physician**.

pharmaceutical physician
It is only during the last 10 years that the term Pharmaceutical Physician has begun to replace the broader term **Medical Advisor** in the pharmaceutical industry, although the designation was originally suggested by Dr Eric Snell in 1970 for the doctor who stands at the interface between the industry and the many clinical problems that **R&D** entail. With the enormous growth of pharmaceuticals, particularly in the 1950s, the larger companies begun to employ full time doctors to reflect sound medical opinion, to help with various aspects of pharmaceutical research (in particular the scope, design, organization and interpretation of clinical trials) and to support their marketing activities. Pharmaceutical physicians are responsible for providing medical input into clinical trials, marketing, regulatory affairs, sales activities, and medical expertise for one or more therapeutic areas. They often also play a major role in the evaluation of **adverse events** (AEs) and **adverse drug reactions** (ADRs). The most important educational role for pharmaceutical physicians is to ensure that accurate knowledge about the drug is widely disseminated within the medical profession.

Pharmaceutical Quality Group (UK)
A group for professional qualified practitioners within the pharmaceutical industry. The group is incorporated within the UK's Institute of Quality Assurance (IQA). They organize regular meetings on **quality assurance** and **good manufacturing practice** within the pharmaceutical

industry. It maintains close liaisons with other UK organizations such as the **Association for the British Pharmaceutical Industry** and the **Medicines Control Agency** (MCA). A series of monographs on pharmaceutical quality assurance have been published and have received wide acclaim and usage in the industry throughout the world. The group have also published pharmaceutical codes of practice to ISO 9000.

The Group's objectives are:
1. To promote the open exchange of information and experience concerning pharmaceutical quality matters.
2. To promote the development of a consistent approach to pharmaceutical quality and good manufacturing practices.
3. To promote the status of, and to represent, **qualified persons** and other pharmaceutical quality professionals.
4. To promote education and training in the achievement of pharmaceutical quality, in line with the current requirements for continuing professional development (CPD).

To meet these objectives, the Group's activities include organizing meetings on subjects of special interest, submitting members' comments on proposed changes to guidelines and regulations relating to the industry, arranging training courses, developing **Codes of Practice** for pharmaceutical suppliers and publishing monographs on QA aspects of pharmaceutical manufacture membership.

Pharmaceutical Research and Manufacturers of America (PhRMA) (US)

Formerly known as the Pharmaceutical Manufacturers Association (PMA), it is an industry group which supports and lobbies on behalf of the pharmaceutical manufacturing industry. The Association has a membership of sixty-seven companies which are involved in the discovery, development and manufacture of prescription medicines. There are also 24 research affiliates which conduct biological research related to the development of drugs and vaccines. PhRMA coordinates its technical input to **International Conference on Harmonization** (ICH) through its Scientific and Regulatory Section. Special committees have been set up, of experts from PhRMA companies, to deal with ICH topics.

Pharmaceutical Sciences Group (UK)

Established in 1992 to provide a forum for pharmaceutical scientists working in industry, academia, government departments and research organizations. It is part of the **Royal Pharmaceutical Society of Great Britain**. Aims of the group include providing a forum for the dissemination of knowledge and the promotion of the pharmaceutical sciences through the activities of its members. Additionally the group seeks to be active in the process of consultation on strategies for science within the UK and to influence the opinion and policy in government to the advantage of pharmaceutical sciences and society as a whole.

Pharmacist reporting (UK)

A pilot scheme that was started in April 1997 to evaluate the reporting of **adverse drug reactions** by hospital pharmacists. Pharmacists have been asked to report directly to the **Medicines Control Agency** (MCA) through the **Yellow Card Scheme**.

pharmacodiagnosis

The employment of drugs in the diagnosis of diseases.

pharmacodynamics (PD)

The science concerned with the measurement of the total value of particular courses (mechanism of action) of pharmaceutical therapy. More specifically, it is the study of effects of the drug, its mechanism of action, and relationship between drug concentrations at the site of action (**receptor**) and intensity of effect (pharmacological, biochemical, physiological, or immunological). It is what the drug does to the body. It is based on the principle that every clinical intervention produces a change in the health status of a patient, which has an intrinsic, measurable value impacting the patient's future use of the health care system and productive output to society.

Compare **pharmacology, pharmacogenetics, pharmacokinetics**.

pharmacoeconomic analysis

An analysis carried out to improve public health through better and rational decision-making, to establish relative values among alternative therapies and to allow **costs** and consequences of alternative drug therapies to be evaluated using a systematic approach that takes into account medical care and pharmaceutical variables as well as the value and perception of 'health.'

The data can be used by clinical and administrative decision-makers, including pharmacists, physicians, formulary committee members, and organization administrators. However, the value of a drug therapy is best determined by considering a combination of clinical and administrative factors and conducting a complete analysis of all costs and potential outcomes.

In the US, drugs have traditionally been evaluated for **safety** and **efficacy** prior to **Food and Drug Administration** (FDA) **Approval** and later for effectiveness in the broader population. As a result of increasing concern over rising health care costs, evaluations of drug efficiency have become more common. Although there are no regulatory requirements in the US for economic evaluations, pharmaceutical companies are beginning to commission **cost-effectiveness** and **cost–benefit analyses** of their products, primarily in response to the requirements of **Managed Care Organization** (MCO)s. Economic evaluations are increasingly incorporated into **phase III clinical trials**, although questions remain as to the overall applicability of such analyses. The number of pharmacoeconomic evaluations appearing in the literature is also growing.

The basic requirements of a pharmacoeconomic analysis are the selection of a perspective; the identification, measurement, and comparison of all categories of costs and consequences of alternative interventions; specification of a study type; and a determination as to whether an incremental or average analysis is appropriate.

Direct costs related to providing medical services (such as hospital care, physician fees, and drug costs) are always a part of pharmacoeconomic analyses. Other costs, such as indirect costs (such as loss of work and unpaid caregivers' time) may be included, but they are more difficult to value. Humanistic benefits, which represent the optimal target of any health care goods and services, may be evaluated to assign a value to indirect and intangible costs (such as pain and suffering!).

The four types of pharmacoeconomic analysis most commonly referred to in the literature differ in that they measure different benefits or outcomes and in the terms of the consequences of selecting particular pharmaceutical goods or services for each alternative under comparison. The **cost–benefit analysis** (CBA) is strictly a comparison of the monetary value of alternative uses of resources. The **cost-effectiveness analysis** (CEA) compares the costs of alternatives in terms of a natural unit or health outcome such as life-years gained or reduction in blood pressure. A **cost-utility analysis** (CUA) typically measures consequences in terms of life-years gained or lost adjusted by a quality factor based on patient preference or on the quality of the health care outcome. A **cost-containment** or -identification or -minimization analysis (CCA, CIA or CMA) compares costs when consequences are assumed to be equal. CEA and CUA are most frequently used in comparing alternative drug therapies.

See also **cost–benefit analysis, cost-containment analysis, cost-effectiveness analysis, cost-utility analysis.**

pharmacoeconomics
Branch of economics that applies **cost–benefit, cost-effectiveness, cost-minimization** and **cost-utility analyses** to compare the economics of different pharmaceutical products or to compare drug therapy interventions to other treatments. It involves research that identifies, measures, and compares the costs (i.e. resources consumed) and consequences of use of various pharmaceutical products and services. Pharmacoeconomics relates the monetary unit alternative treatments to consequences; these consequences may be described in monetary terms or in terms such as lives saved, hospitalizations averted, operations prevented, or some measure of the quality of life enhanced.

pharmacoepidemiology
Application of epidemiological techniques to study the use, **effectiveness**, value, and **safety** of medicinal products.

pharmacogenetics
The science that seeks to identify and characterize polymorphic genes, encoding drug metabolizing enzymes, drug receptors and drug transporters in man and animals. It studies the effect of their expression on the disposition and metabolism of foreign chemicals, together with the cellular and clinical responses they evoke. It also focuses on the understanding of genetic mechanisms of species differences in foreign compound metabolism and responsiveness, and to the regulation of drug-metabolizing enzymes and their genes.
Compare **pharmacodynamics, pharmacology.**

pharmacogenomics
An emerging science which uses genetic information to predict the responses of individuals to drugs. It is the study of how genes and gene variations affect the discovery, development, **toxicology**, and use of drugs. By identifying who is and who is not going to respond to a drug, pharmacogenomics can be used to:
- Predict efficacy in the population
- Individualize dosages and avoid inappropriate medications
- Avoid drug toxicity in a population
- Reduce the cost of drug development
- Improve outcomes with drug therapy
- Rescue drugs that have failed to reach, been withdrawn from, the market because of toxicity in a small number of patients.
- Find new applications for older drugs.

Compare **pharmacogenetics.**

pharmacognosy
The branch of **pharmacology** which studies natural drugs and deals with the identification/analysis of biological, biochemical, chemical components, economic features and botanical sources.

pharmacokinetics (PK)
A science and study (or kinetics) of the factors and processes of bodily **absorption, distribution, metabolism,** and **excretion (ADME)** of agents/drugs. Simply put, it is what the body does to the drug. The processes of drug distribution and elimination (metabolism and excretion) are also known as drug disposition. Pharmacokinetic measures determine the amount

of chemical agents at their sites of biological effect, at various times, after administration/ application of the agent/drug to biological systems.

Compare **biotransformation, half-life, pharmacodynamics, pharmacology, volume of distribution**.

pharmacology

(Gr. *Pharmakon* = drug, and *Logy* = study) The science of drug action on biological systems. In its entirety, it embraces knowledge of the sources, chemical properties, biological effects and therapeutic uses of drugs. It is a science that is basic not only to human medicine, but also to pharmacy, nursing, dentistry and veterinary medicine. In the context of drug development, the discipline is devoted to establishing systems which confirm the activity of potential drug compounds. Pharmacological studies range from those that determine the effects of chemical agents upon sub-cellular mechanisms, to those that deal with the potential hazards of pesticides and herbicides, to those that focus on the treatment and prevention of major diseases by drug therapy. Pharmacology therefore encompasses **pharmacodynamics**, **pharmacokinetics** and **toxicology**. Pharmacologists are also involved in molecular modelling of drugs, and the use of drugs as tools to investigate aspects of cell function.

Compare **pharmacodynamics, pharmacogenetics, pharmacokinetics, toxicology**.

Pharmacology and Therapeutics Advisory Committee (PTAC) (New Zealand)

An organization whose primary purpose is to provide **PHARMAC** with independent advice on the pharmacological and therapeutic consequences of proposed amendments to the Pharmaceutical Schedule. PTAC is a committee of 8 senior medical specialists and general practitioners nominated by professional medical bodies such as the New Zealand Medical Association, the Royal New Zealand College of General Practitioners, the Royal Australasian College of Physicians, and the Australasian Society of Clinical and Experimental Pharmacologists and Toxicologists. PTAC members are appointed by the PHARMAC Board.

PTAC considers and makes recommendations on the medical implications of:
- All significant applications by drug companies for inclusion on the Pharmaceutical Schedule, or amendments to it, where there are clinical issues to consider
- Requests by PHARMAC for de-listing
- The management of the Pharmaceutical Schedule; and the need for reviews of specific drugs, or groups of drugs.

pharmacometrics

The comparative evaluation of drug activity, distinguished from **bioassay** in that substances with differing chemical constituents are compared.

See also **bioassay**.

pharmacon

A **drug**.

pharmacophore (pharmacophoric pattern)

The ensemble of steric and electronic features that is necessary to ensure the optimal supramolecular interactions with a specific biological target structure and to trigger (or to block) its biological response. The term is also used to describe a preliminary compound on which chemical modifications can be made to develop a potential 'lead' compound or **drug candidate**.

A pharmacophore does not represent a real molecule or a real association of functional groups, but a purely abstract concept that accounts for the common molecular interaction capacities of a group of compounds towards their target structure. The pharmacophore can be considered as the largest common denominator shared by a set of active molecules. This definition discards a misuse often found in the **medicinal chemistry** literature which consists of naming as pharmacophores simple chemical functionalities such as guanidines, sulfonamides or dihydroimidazoles (formerly imidazolines), or typical structural skeletons such as flavones, phenothiazines, prostaglandins or steroids.

pharmacophoric descriptors
Used to define a **pharmacophore**, including H-bonding, hydrophobic and electrostatic interaction sites, defined by atoms, ring centres and virtual points.

pharmacopoeia
A compendium containing (with descriptions) a list of drugs, chemicals, and medicinal preparations. It is issued by an officially recognized authority. The purpose of a pharmacopoeia is to serve as a standard for determining identity, purity and formulae.

pharmacotherapeutics
The broad term used to describe the study of the use of drugs in the diagnosis, prevention, and treatment of disease states.

pharmacovigilance
The process of (a) monitoring medicines as used in everyday practice and in clinical research to identify previously unrecognized changes in the patterns of their adverse effects; (b) assessing the risks and benefits of medicines in order to determine what action, if any, is necessary to improve their safe use; (c) providing information to users to optimize safe and effective use of medicines; (d) monitoring the impact of any action taken.

In the **European Union** (EU), the **marketing authorization** holder of a product has to comply with the EU **Directive 65/65/EEC** and **Directive 75/319/EEC** to:

- Employ a **qualified person** (QP) responsible for pharmacovigilance
- Establish a pharmacovigilance system
- Report serious **adverse drug reactions** (ADRs) within 15 days
- Provide the regulatory authorities with **Periodic Safety Update Reports** (PSURs)
- Provide benefit–risk analyses
- Take the necessary actions to improve safety of its products.

Pharmacovigilance Working Part (PhVWP) (European Union)
A working party of the **Committee for Proprietary Medicinal Products** (CPMP) which deals with the safety issues relating to medicines authorized through European procedures (centralized and mutual recognition) and through national procedures. It consists of two delegates from each **Member State** and is chaired by a CPMP member. Secretariat functions are undertaken by the **European Medicines Evaluation Agency** (EMEA).

Member States (MSs) may refer drug safety issues to the PhVWP where they consider there is a Community interest. Matters may also be referred by the CPMP and the **Commission**. A **rapporteur** is assigned to assess the issues and prepare a report for discussion. There may be more than one rapporteur for major issues involving multiple drugs. If a product has an authorization granted through a European procedure, the lead member state usually acts as rapporteur for the PhVWP but this does not have to apply. The rapporteur circulates an assessment report prior to the meeting, which is then discussed and a position reached. The MSs then decide how and if they wish to implement the recommendations individually for national authorizations, but for centralized or mutual recognition authorizations this is taken

forward by rapporteur or reference member state (RMS) respectively.
See also **Committee for Proprietary Medicinal Products** (CPMP).

pharmacy
The science of preparing, compounding and dispensing medicines.

pharmacy analysis see prescription cost analysis.

Pharmacy and Therapeutics Committee (P&T Committee)
A Committee in hospitals and **Managed Care Organization** (MCO)s which determines the appropriateness of particular medical products, based on **safety**, **efficacy**, **cost** and **cost-effectiveness** data. This committee usually controls the **formulary** for the hospital or MCO.

Pharmacy Assistant (UK)
A journal published quarterly, by the **Royal Pharmaceutical Society of Great Britain**, for community pharmacy staff.

pharmacy drug (P) (UK)
A drug that may only be obtained from a pharmacy, where they are supplied under the supervision of a pharmacist, who may ask questions to ensure that, if a medicine is necessary, the patient gets the best one suited to their needs.
See also **controlled drug**, **general list medicine**, **prescription only medicine**.

pharmacy margin see subsidy.

pharmacy network (US)
The term used when referring collectively to all the pharmacies throughout the US and Puerto Rico that participate in a particular PCS plan.

Pharmacy World & Science
An official journal of the Royal Dutch Association for the Advancement of Pharmacy (KNMP), the European Society of Clinical Pharmacy (ESCP), and the United Kingdom Clinical Pharmacy Association (UKCPA).

phase I clinical trial
The initial phase of the clinical development process in which primarily the safety of a new therapeutic is examined either in a set of normally **healthy**, **normal volunteers** or a group of diseased subjects.

It is the study in which primarily the safety of a new **medicinal product** is examined and is carried out in 50–1000 usually **healthy**, **normal volunteers** (who do not have the condition under investigation) but sometimes in severely ill patients, for example, those with cancer or AIDS, under the close supervision of the **investigator**. Its main purpose is to identify the dose-related **adverse drug reactions** (ADRs) but it also establishes the dose range tolerated, dose regimen, **pharmacokinetics** and **pharmacodynamics** of the therapy. Initial doses will be as low as possible to produce an expected effect; this will often be the same as the expected therapeutic dose, or the dose will be gradually increased to the expected therapeutic dose. Pharmacokinetic trials are usually considered phase I trials regardless of when they are conducted during a medicine's development.

Despite the relatively small number of individuals in these studies, a well conducted phase I trial will accumulate a large volume of valuable information which is essential for the development programme to go forward to the next phase. However, before any further studies can be undertaken, a submission must be made to the local regulatory authority for permission to carry out phase II trials. In the UK, for example, this permission is in the form of a **Clinical Trials Certificate** (CTC) or a **Clinical Trial Exemption** (CTX).

See also **clinical trial, phase II clinical trial, phase IIa clinical trial, phase III clinical trial, phase IV clinical trial.**

phase II clinical trial

The second phase of the clinical development process and it is the first time the potential medicinal product is given to selected populations (of about 100–300) of patients (and frequently only to men if there is a lack of information on the product's effects on reproductive function) with the actual condition that the compound is intended to treat. In order to ascertain the correct dosage levels for therapeutic effects and unwanted side effects, the drug is given to different groups of patients at different dosages. The purpose of phase II studies is to gather **efficacy** and **safety data** specific to an indication or disease, and also to establish dosages to be employed in phase III. This phase may sometimes be further subdivided into two types of studies **phase IIa** (the early therapeutic) and **phase IIb** (later therapeutic) **clinical trials**.

See also **clinical trial, phase II clinical trial, phase IIa clinical trial, phase III clinical trial, phase IV clinical trial.**

phase IIa clinical trial

Pilot clinical trials to evaluate **efficacy** and **safety** in selected populations of about 100–300 patients who have the disease or condition to be treated, diagnosed, or prevented. Often involve hospitalized patients who can be closely monitored. Objectives may focus on dose-response, type of patient, frequency of dosing, or any of a number of other issues involved in safety and efficacy.

phase IIb clinical trial

Well-controlled trial to evaluate **safety** and **efficacy** in patients who have the disease or condition to be treated, diagnosed, or prevented. This trial usually represents the most rigorous demonstration of a medicine's efficacy. It is sometimes also called the pivotal trial although this term is mostly reserved for **phase III trials**.

phase III clinical trial

The third and most important phase of the clinical development process in which the **efficacy** and **safety** of the intervention is studied under carefully controlled conditions, often in a double-blinded randomized fashion. It is carried out after satisfactory completion of **phase II study**. In order to assess the effects statistically, usually 3000 (or more) patients, for whom the medicine is eventually intended, are treated. Ideally the circumstances of the trials should be close to normal conditions of use for the new drug. All **adverse events** (AEs) are closely monitored, with the emphasis placed on severity, duration, etc. A local independent **Ethics Committee** must study the clinical trial **protocol** and approve the trial before it can start. Trials are also conducted in special groups of patients or under special conditions dictated by the nature of a particular medicine and/or disease.

Once the study is complete and the trials have been statistically analysed, the company can decide whether it wishes to collate the data to submit a **marketing authorization** application to a regulatory authority for the medicinal product in a given country. Thus, these studies will determine the fate of the drug and are often referred to as 'pivotal' or 'proof-of-principle' trials. Phase III trials often provide much of the information needed for the package insert and **labelling** of the medicine.

See also **phase I clinical trial, phase II clinical trial, phase IIa clinical trial, phase IIb clinical trial, phase IIIb clinical trial, phase IV clinical trial.**

phase IIIb clinical trial
In the US, this term is applied to trials conducted after submission of a **New Drug Application** (NDA), but before the product's approval and market launch. Phase IIIb trials may supplement or complete earlier trials, or they may seek different kinds of information (for example, **quality of life** or marketing). Phase IIIb is the period between submission for approval and receipt of **marketing authorization**.

phase IV clinical trial
The last phase of the clinical development process that is usually conducted after marketing of the **medicinal product** in order to gain additional **safety** and **efficacy** information on the product in particular patient populations in **indications** for which it is licensed. They may be used to evaluate **formulations**, dosages, durations of treatment, medicine interactions, and other factors. Patients from various demographic groups may be studied. An important part of many Phase IV studies is detecting and defining previously unknown or inadequately quantified adverse reactions and related risk factors. Phase IV studies that are primarily observational or non-experimental are frequently called **post-marketing surveillance**.

phase V clinical trial
This is an interchangeable term for **post-marketing surveillance** (PMS).

phase I metabolism see metabolism.

phase II metabolism see metabolism.

phases of clinical trials
Clinical trials are generally categorized into four (sometimes five) phases. An investigational medicine or product may be evaluated in two or more phases simultaneously in different trials, and some trials may overlap two different phases.

See also **phase I clinical trial, phase II clinical trial, phase IIa clinical trial, phase IIb clinical trial, phase IIIb clinical trial, phase IV clinical trial**.

Ph Eur see European Pharmacopoeia.

Ph F
Pharmacopée Française (French Pharmacopoeia).

PhINTO (UK)
Pharmaceutical Industry National Training Organization, see **Association of British Pharmaceutical Industry**.

PHL
Public Health Laboratory.

PHLS see Public Health Laboratory Service.

PHO
Provider Health Plan.

phosphorylation
The process of adding phosphate (a unique combination of phosphorus and oxygen atoms) molecular groups to a compound.

photosensitivity
Abnormal reactivity of the skin to sunlight, leading to erythema, rash, blisters, etc. Some drugs (e.g. benoxaprofen) and other chemicals (e.g. porphyrins) may cause such a reaction.

pH–partition theory
For a drug to cross a membrane barrier it must normally be soluble in the lipid material of the membrane to cross that membrane. Also it has to be soluble in the aqueous phase as well to get out of the membrane. Most drugs have polar and non-polar characteristics or are weak acids or bases. For drugs which are weak acids or bases the pKa of the drug, the **pH** of the gastrointestinal tract fluid and the pH of the bloodstream will control the solubility of the drug and thereby the rate of absorption through the membranes lining the gastrointestinal tract.

Brodie *et al.* (in 1957) proposed the pH–partition theory to explain the influence of gastrointestinal pH and drug pKa on the extent of drug transfer or drug absorption. Brodie reasoned that by suggesting that when a drug is ionized it will not be able to get through the lipid membrane, but only when it is non ionized and therefore has a higher lipid solubility.

PhRMA see **Pharmaceutical Research and Manufacturers of America**.

PHS see **Public Health Service**.

PhVWP see **Pharmacovigilance Working Party**.

physiatrist
A doctor who specializes in the diagnosis and management of injuries and diseases causing pain, loss of function and disability. Treatment plans often include the use of exercise, massage, heat, electricity (TENS), relaxation techniques, splints and braces, and local injections to relieve pain.

Physician Data Query (PDQ) (US)
An on-line database which makes state-of-the-art treatment, directory, and protocol information available to **primary care** physicians. This database is maintained by the International Cancer Research Data Bank Branch, International Cancer Information Center (ICIC), and the **National Cancer Institute**.

Physician's Desk Reference (PDR) (US)
Listing of pharmaceutical products on sale in the USA, in the form of a book, produced by American companies. The PDR contains the data sheets for the drug products. It is equivalent to the **ABPI Compendium and Data Sheets and SPCs** in the UK.

Physicians' GenRx (US)
Drug index, that is unique in that it includes **Health Care Finance Administration** (HCFA) reimbursement codes, **Food and Drug Administration** (FDA) **approval** date, patent expiration, FDA's evaluation of new molecular entities, and relative sales volumes.

PI
1. see **Principal Investigator**.
2. see **parallel import**.

PIC see **Pharmaceutical Inspection Convention**.

picomolar
10^{-12} molar.
See also **micromolar**.

PICS see **Pharmaceutical Inspection Cooperation Scheme**.

PIL see **Patient Information Leaflet**.

pill see **tablet**.

pilot study (Clinical Trials)
A mini-study/**clinical trial** conducted in advance of the main experiment, usually to obtain information and assess feasibility (work out logistics and management). A pilot study is deemed necessary for further trials. Phase II are sometimes referred to as pilot studies.

pINN
proposed International Non-proprietary Name.

pivotal trial see **phase IIb clinical trial**.

PK see **pharmacokinetics**.

PL (PI)
Product Licence (parallel import).

PLA see **Product Licence Application**.

placebo (Clinical Trials)
(Latin; *Placere* = to please or satisfy). A product that looks identical to the investigational medicinal product but without the **active ingredients**. Its use is intended as a negative control in a **bioassay** or to negate the psychological effects that receiving or not receiving the drug may bring in a clinical study. A placebo may be compared with a new drug in double-blind trials. It is well recognized that the use of placebo is unethical in trials involving a disease for which there is no known effective therapy or in a trial involving a **life-threatening** disease.

Placebos are also used as a wash-out instrument before or between treatments in order to standardize the baseline. They are also used as additions to existing therapy when a test drug is being added to a comparative group or even as a sole therapy in order to define the **placebo effect**, especially when the assessment of **efficacy** is subjective.

See also **placebo concurrent control study, placebo effect**.

placebo concurrent control study (Clinical Trials)
A trial in which an investigational product is compared to an inactive preparation (i.e. **placebo**).

placebo effect
A patient's positive or negative clinical response whilst receiving **placebo** treatment. It is caused by a person's expectations of a drug rather than the drug itself.

placement
The placement is one of the variables included in the **marketing mix**. It refers to how a product is positioned in the market, and includes the concept of how a product is delivered to the patient (hospital versus home health care, for example).

PLAG (UK)
Post-Licensing Assessment Group – used to be a part of Post-Licensing Division at the **Medicines Control Agency**.

plan sponsor (US)
The company or organization that assumes financial responsibility for an insured group.

plasmapheresis
A procedure for removing unwanted substances from the blood in which blood is drawn, its plasma is separated and replaced, and the cleansed blood is returned to the body.

PLR see **Product Licence of Right**.

PLUS see **Product Licence User System**.

PMA (US)
1. Pharmaceutical Manufacturers' Association.
2. see **Pre-market Approval Application**.

PMCPA see **Prescription Medicines Code of Practice Authority**.

PMS see **Post-Marketing Surveillance**.

poison
Any substance which, when ingested, inhaled or absorbed into the body may cause damage, by its chemical action, to the organs or tissues of the body and so impair or destroy life.

polygenic
A term used to describe diseases that are caused by changes in more than one gene. Most common human diseases are considered polygenic (e.g. asthma, diabetes, obesity, osteoporosis, etc.).

polymer
A molecule formed by the joining of many smaller molecules; a protein, for example, is a polymer of **amino acids**.

POM see **prescription only medicine**.

POM to P switch (UK)
This is the process of changing the legal status of a drug product from being a **prescription only medicine** (POM) to a **pharmacy drug** (P). This can be allowed by the **regulatory authority** if they are satisfied that the ingredient(s) fulfil certain **safety** criteria. There are two routes for changing the legal classification if applied for by the **marketing authorization** (MA) holder; by **variation**, or by a new application. In addition to the licence holder, other interested parties (such as professional bodies, consumer groups) can also request such reclassification. The products must also satisfy the requirements of all **over-the-counter** (OTC) drugs of appropriate indication, dosage, duration, and clear label instructions.

In general, to confirm that a drug/product is suitable for switching from POM to P, the following criteria must all apply:
- The indication(s) for the drug are suitable for self-medication including self-diagnosis of the condition which may be recurrent attack of a condition which requires a physician aided diagnosis on first attack/episode
- The drug has an acceptable margin of safety, in the doses recommended, during unsupervised use including safety in overdose or following accidental misdiagnosis of the condition by the patient
- The drug does not have an abuse/dependence potential
- The drug is not for parenteral use.

The **Medicines Control Agency** (MCA) process the application in the following manner:
1. Receipt of request and supporting data
2. Assessment and consultation of the **Committee on Safety of Medicines** (CSM)
3. External consultations (including public considerations, consumer groups, etc.)
4. Consideration by **Medicines Commission** of responses. Minister's approval sought

5. Ministerial/Parliamentary approval
6. Statutory Instrument into effect.

The whole approval process takes about a year.

If the CSM recommends that a request for reclassification be refused, the originator of the proposal will be notified as to which POM criteria have been considered to apply and the reasons for refusal.

population (Clinical Trials)

The universe of subjects to which the results of a **clinical trial** should be applicable to. The definition of the study population is always described in detail in the study **protocol**.

porphyria

A group of rare, inherited blood genetic disorders. When a person has porphyria, cells fail to change chemicals (porphyrins) to the substance (haem) that gives blood its colour. Porphyrins then build up in the body. They show up in large amounts in stool and urine, causing the urine to be coloured blue. They cause a number of problems, including rashes brought on by exposure to sunlight, reactions to certain drugs, and strange behaviour. Porphyria is a contraindication for many drugs.

positive predictive value (+PV)

The proportion of people with a positive test who have disease.

posology

The branch of medical science concerned with dosage of drug therapy.

post approval (Germany)

The **marketing authorization** that is also needed for the so-called 'old products', i.e. products that had already been on the market before the **AMG** came in force. This process, which is still ongoing, is referred to as post-marketing authorization, or, shorter, post approval.

Post-Authorization Safety Study (PASS)

A pharmacoepidemiological observational study, or a **clinical trial** carried out in accordance with the **Summary of Product Characteristics** (SPC), conducted with the aim of identifying or quantifying a **safety** hazard related to an authorized **medicinal product**. Any study where the number of patients to be included will add significantly to the existing safety data for the product will also be considered a PASS. PASS and other formal safety studies are deemed necessary particularly in the confirmation, characterization, and quantification of possible hazards identified at an earlier stage of product development or during the marketed stage. They are also useful in identifying previously unsuspected reactions or in confirming the safety profile of a product under marketed conditions. The guidance on **good clinical practice** (GCP) does *not* apply to observational pharmacoepidemiological studies. Designs of these studies can be any of the following:

1. Observational cohort. The population studied should normally be as representative as possible of the general population of users, and be unselected unless specifically targeted by the objectives of the study (e.g. a study in children). Where the product is used outside the indications of the SPC at the discretion of the prescribing doctor, the European regulatory authorities require that such patients be included in the analysis of the study findings. **Exclusion criteria** should be limited to the **contraindications** stated in the SPC. In prospective studies, the doctors involved in the study should be provided with the SPC for all products to be used.
2. **Case–control**. Retrospective comparison is made between the product exposure of

'cases' with the disease/event of interest and appropriate controls without the disease/event.
3. **Case-surveillance**. Marketing authorization (MA) holders are expected, by European regulatory authorities, to liase closely with them to determine the most appropriate arrangements for the reporting of cases.
4. **Clinical trials**. Specific clinical trials are sometimes necessary to determine the mechanism of **adverse drug reactions** (ADRs) and to identify the means of prevention. Exclusion criteria should normally be limited to those in the SPC unless they are closely related to the particular objectives of the study. These should adhere to GCPs.

In the **European Union** (EU), the MA holder carrying out a PASS has responsibility to:
- Submit the protocol to the **regulatory authorities** (RAs) before the onset of the study
- Inform the RA when the study starts
- Comply with the ADRs reporting regulations (e.g. expedited, etc.)
- Publish the study findings.

See also **post-marketing surveillance, post-authorization study**.

post-authorization study (PAS)

Any study conducted within the conditions of the approved **Summary of Product Characteristics** or under normal conditions of use. A post-authorization study may sometimes also fall within the definition of a **PASS**. In reference to **adverse drug reaction** reporting and **PSUR** requirements, reference to a post-authorization study means any post-authorization study of which the **marketing authorization** (MA) holder is aware.

See also **post-authorization safety study, post-marketing surveillance**.

post hoc analyses

Analyses conducted after the results are available that were not defined before the start of the trial. Such analyses are particularly prone to **false-positive** claims or **type I error**.

post-marketing surveillance (PMS)

A term used to describe sections of the **regulations** requiring the collection and monitoring, and evaluation of **safety** and **efficacy** information about a **drug product** or **device** after it is approved and marketed. These are **phase IV studies** involved in the close observation of drug effects in a large number of patients following the granting of a **Product Licence**. The purpose of PMS studies is to evaluate the drugs as they are used to treat a wide spectrum of patients. Additional data on efficacy will be obtained and more information on the unwanted effects associated with long-term use of a drug may also occur to identify 'new signals', or to test hypotheses. Many PMS studies are conducted with 10 000 or more patients.

See also **phase IV clinical trial**.

potency

The amount of drug required to produce a particular magnitude of response. Potency is a comparative rather than an absolute expression of drug activity. Drug potency depends on both **affinity** and **efficacy**. Thus, two agonists can be equipotent, but have different intrinsic efficacies with compensating differences in affinity. Potency also refers to the concentration of an agent (drug) at which it inhibits an enzyme to a defined extent, e.g., $IC50$ is the concentration at which an inhibitor blocks the activity of an enzyme 50 percent.

Compare **bioassay, dose–effect curve, equipotent, intrinsic activity, sensitivity**.

powder

A mixture of two or more dry substances in the form of fine particles, usually intended for internal use.

power (Clinical Trials)

The probability of detecting the expected difference between two treatments or between a treatment and a **control group**, if such a difference exists (i.e. a true positive). It is the probability of demonstrating that an effective treatment works in the confines of the study. Power is a function of study **sample size**, the biological **variability** in the **population**, the desired proportions of false positives (alpha) and false negatives (beta), and the type of statistical test used. A well-designed study with a sufficient **sample size** is considered to be properly powered. The power of a study is the opposite of **type II error**. For a statistician, the power of a test is the probability that the test will reject the hypothesis tested when a specific alternative hypothesis is true.

To calculate the power of a given test it is necessary to specify alpha (the probability that the test will lead to the rejection of the hypothesis tested when that hypothesis is true) and to specify a specific alternative hypothesis. In such calculation, one must also specify the size of the difference. For example, a paper describing a **clinical trial** with a new hypertension medication may contain the following statement: 'the study had a power of 80% to detect a difference of 5 mmHg in diastolic blood pressure between the treatment and control groups'. The aim of any trial is to have a power of at least 80%. Higher powers require larger study sizes. The concept of power is extremely important because the lack of it (i.e. the sample size was too small) can lead to statistical insignificance in the presence of biological significance. Power $= 1 - \beta$, where β is the probability of a type II error.

See also **beta error, false negative, producer's risk, type II error**.

PPA see **Prescription Pricing Authority**.

PPI
1. Patient Package Insert.
2. See **Patient Information Leaflet** (PIL).
3. Patient Pack Initiative (UK).

ppm
Parts per million.

PPO see **Preferred Provider Organization**.

PPRS see **Prescription Pricing Regulation Scheme**.

PR see **Public Relations**.

precaution
An alert to the prescriber or **principal investigator** (Clinical Trials) to exercise special care in particular circumstances to ensure safe and effective use of the study drug.

precision (Statistics)
The range in which the best estimates of a true value approximate the true value.
See also **confidence interval**.

pre-clinical development see **pre-clinical study**.

pre-clinical study
A study which tests biological activity and toxicity of a **drug product** or **medical device** in animals to collect data in support of **safety** claims that in turn support **phase I** safety and **tolerance** studies. Pre-clinical studies are, therefore, required before **clinical trials** can be initiated. It usually also involves extensive laboratory testing and must comply with **good**

laboratory practice (GLP). Because many animals have much shorter life spans than humans, preclinical studies can provide valuable information about a drug's possible toxic effects over an animal's life cycle and on its offspring.

pre-clinical testing see pre-clinical study.

pre-determined specifications

The specifications against which the performance of the equipment is verified. Validation activities start with the definition of these specifications. Acceptance criteria must be defined before testing.

predictive value

In screening and diagnostic tests, the probability that a person with a positive test is a true positive (i.e. does have the disease), or that a person with a negative test truly does not have the disease. The predictive value of a screening test is determined by the **sensitivity** and **specificity** of the test, and by the prevalence of the condition for which the test is used.

pre-existing condition

Any medical, obstetrical or psychiatric condition that exists before the activity in question. As applied to medical insurance, it is the condition that a policy holder has at the time their **health insurance** becomes effective. Treatment of the condition may be limited by a 'pre-existing condition clause'.

preferred provider

Some insurance plans now use preferred providers to help control costs. These plans are based on the same principle as traditional indemnity (fee for service) plans, except that each beneficiary is encouraged (through financial incentives such as minimal co-payment) to use providers which have contracted with the payer at a pre-arranged fee schedule.

Preferred Provider Organization (PPO)

Based on the same principle as **indemnity** (fee for service) plans, each beneficiary is encouraged (through financial incentives such as minimal co-payment) to use 'preferred providers' contracted with the payer at a pre-arranged fee schedule.

pregnancy

The period of time from confirmation of implantation of a fertilized egg within the uterus until the fetus has entirely left the uterus (i.e. has been delivered). Implantation is confirmed through a presumptive sign of pregnancy such as missed menses or a positive pregnancy test. This 'confirmation' may be in error, but, for research purposes, investigators would presume that a living **fetus** was present until evidence to the contrary is clear. Although fertilization occurs a week or more before implantation, the current inability to detect the fertilization event or the presence of a newly fertilized egg makes a definition of pregnancy based on implantation necessary.

Pre-IND (Investigational New Drug Application) Meeting (US)

Before an **Investigational New Product** is filed with the **Food and Drug Administration** (FDA), it is wise to hold a pre-IND meeting with the Agency. These meetings, which are described in the **Code of Federal Regulations**, can be used to finalize study **protocols** to help the manufacturer determine what information the FDA is seeking and prevent misunderstandings which would be expensive to resolve once **clinical trials** are underway.

Pre-Market Approval application (PMA) (US)

An application to the **Centre for Devices and Radiological Health** (CDRH) group at the

Food and Drug Administration (FDA) requesting approval to manufacture and distribute a **medical device** (such approval is required by the law in the US).
See also **New Drug Application** (NDA), **Product Licence Application**.

pre-marketing clinical trials
Clinical trials designed to signal **efficacy, safety**, etc. Generally considered to comprise phases I, II, and III.

pre-market notification (US)
An application a manufacturer must submit to the **Center for Devices and Radiological Health** (CDRH) to qualify for a **510(K)** exemption for a **medical device**.

premature termination (Clinical Trials)
The situation where a subject/patient does not complete the trial, as they should have done according to the **protocol**.

premedication
Drugs, usually painkillers and/or sedatives, taken 1–2 hours before surgery.

Prescribing Analysis and Cost (PACT) (UK)
One of four major information systems, provided by the **Prescription Pricing Authority** (PPA), that give prescribers a broad spectrum of prescribing information including regular information on their prescribing habits and costs.

The objective is that prescribers use PACT to:
- Improve their prescribing habits and costs
- Improve their service to patients
- Develop and monitor prescribing formularies
- Compare themselves with other prescribers.

The PACT Standard Report contains an analysis of the prescribing which has taken place during the quarter. This document is available at the following levels:
- GP/Practice
- Health Authority
- Regional Office
- National.

Information provided includes a summary of prescribing costs, followed by a breakdown of prescribing e.g.:
- The 20 leading drugs and their costs
- Number of prescriptions written
- The average cost per prescription item
- The top 40 **British National Formulary** sections.

In addition, each quarter of the year, the centre pages of the report provide an article discussing a different drug-related issue. This article is written by the Medical and Pharmaceutical Management of the PPA. The PACT catalogue complements the PACT Standard report by providing a full inventory of the prescriptions issued for the period required. A catalogue is available, on request, for prescribing information over the previous 24 months. A catalogue is available at the same levels as for the PACT Standard Report. Following the introduction of nurse prescribing, the Prescription Pricing Authority implemented the PACT Nurse Formulary Report. This report is available at the following levels:
- Health Authority
- Regional Office
- National.

It provides information on community nurse, practice nurse and general practitioner prescribing for the quarter, i.e. total cost, number of items and average cost. To support the PACT Nurse Formulary Report, a PACT Catalogue is also available for:
* An individual nurse
* All practice nurses prescribing within a practice, health authority, regional office or nationally.
* All community nurses prescribing within a Community Trust
* All prescribing for a community nurse showing a breakdown for all practices where the nurse has prescribed.

See also **Electronic Prescribing Analysis and Cost, Prescription Pricing Authority, Prescribing Monitoring Documents.**

Prescribing Monitoring Documents (PMD) (UK)

Formerly known as the Indicative Prescribing Scheme (IPS). The PMD provide financial statements to:
* General practitioners
* Community units
* Health authorities
* Regional offices
* **Department of Health.**

Reports are issued every month and show cumulative expenditure throughout the financial year. This information is also provided electronically via the **ePACT** system. The purpose of PMD is to:
* Make precribers aware and therefore more accountable for the cost of drugs being prescribed.
* Monitor prescribing that may be wasteful or unnecessarily expensive.
* Increase the involvement of **primary care groups** and health authorities in monitoring prescribing habits.

Figures are based on the 'actual' cost; the **Prescription Pricing Authority** calculates a national average discount percentage (this is to account for different discounts received by pharmacists from their suppliers). This is then deducted from the basic price of the prescription items. An allowance for the containers in which the drugs are dispensed is then added back.

See also **electronic prescribing analysis and cost, prescribing analysis and cost, Prescription Pricing Authority.**

Prescribing RatiOnally with Decision-support In General-practice studY (PRODIGY) (UK)

A computer software system designed to support the UK General Practitioners in making decisions about management of patients. It aims to provide the support immediately after a doctor made the initial diagnosis, by presenting a prescribing recommendation on the condition diagnosed. It provides advice on pharmaceutical prescribing and also suggests options for non-drug treatments. The project was commissioned in 1995 by the **National Health Service** (NHS) Executive, which has contracted the Sowerby Centre for Health Informatics (SCHIN) at the University of Newcastle, to carry out an independent evaluation of the system. The system has been trialled in two phases in nearly 200 GP practices across England. Five GP clinical computer system suppliers have been involved in the project – EMIS, Globalsoft, TOREX Medical, AAH Meditel and Reuters.

PRODIGY is the first national prescribing system in the world. During a consultation, GPs can type the patient's diagnosis into the PRODIGY system, which then suggests an appropriate medicine and course of treatment. All recommended treatments have been validated by a national panel, and chosen on the basis on clinical effectiveness and **safety**.

PRODIGY will provide a platform for disseminating guidance from the **National Institute for Clinical Excellence** (NICE) and will be a basis for prescribing audits. As it will manage updating needs, NICE will bear most of the costs of the system.

The guidance on PRODIGY has been produced by a multidisciplinary team, including doctors, pharmacists and researchers, choosing treatments on the basis of effectiveness, safety and appropriateness. Drug cost is considered where more than one drug with similar clinical effect exists, or where the benefits of one drug over another are marginal.

Prescribing Toolkit (UK)

An on-line system which is available to authorized users via the **Prescription Pricing Authority** (PPA) website (www.ppa.nhs.uk). The system consists of the following three reports, which run twice a year. Data is reported at **primary care group** (PCG) and health authority (HA) level.

- Potential generic savings report – this report shows the potential savings of prescribing generically as opposed to proprietary products
- Specialists drugs report – this report shows costs for a pre-defined list of drugs.
- Prescribing indicators report – this report shows performance according to pre-defined indicators.

The system is used by the following organizations for performance management purposes:
- Prescribing Support Unit
- National Prescribing Centre
- National Health Service (NHS) Executive
- Regional Offices
- HAs
- PCGs.

See also **cost, prescribing analysis, prescribing analysis and cost, Prescribing Monitoring Documents, Prescription Pricing Authority**.

prescription

The written direction from a doctor to a pharmacist for the preparation of **medicinal product** or **medical device** in a suitable form for administration to a particular patient. Each country has its own rules and conventions of writing prescriptions. In the UK for example, they have to be written and signed (by the prescriber) in ink, should be dated, should state the full name and address of the patient and should, legally, have the age of the patient (if under 12) when prescribed a **prescription only medicine**.

Prescription Cost Analysis (PCA) (UK)

A report on all prescriptions dispensed in England in the Community by:
- Community pharmacists
- Appliance contractors
- Dispensing doctors.

This includes prescriptions:
- For items personally administered by general practitioners
- Written by a dentist or hospital doctor and dispensed in the community
- Written in Wales, Scotland, Northern Ireland and the Isle of Man but dispensed in England.

The purpose of the PCA system is to provide:
- An analysis of drug prices

- A national forecasting information
- Data for monitoring new products
- Data for monitoring **adverse drug reactions** for the **Committee on Safety of Medicines**
- Claims made according to patient exemption categories
- Flexibility for *ad hoc* analysis
- Potential for research
- Possible fraud indications or irregularities.

The following are the four categories of report, which are produced on a monthly, quarterly or annual basis.

Drug analysis
This information relates to cost and number of items dispensed. It provides lists of individual drug products, which are produced by class of preparation (proprietary or generic) within **British National Formulary** therapeutic classification.

Pharmacy analysis
This provides information on:
- Number of establishments
- Size
- Group
- Type of ownership
- Type of fees claimed.

The reports also include the corresponding number of prescriptions dispensed and the total cost.

Dispensing doctor analysis
This provides information on the number and cost of prescriptions:
- Written by dispensing doctors
- Personally administered by prescribing and dispensing doctors.

Miscellaneous analysis
This is a facility to meet specific user requests for information.

See also **Prescription Pricing Authority**.

prescription drug benefit (US)
A benefit normally included with a medical plan that allows prescription medicine to be obtained using a benefit card. The member normally pays only a small copayment or coinsurance amount for each prescription obtained.

Prescription Event Monitoring (PEM) (UK)
An initiative, pioneered by Professor W. Inman at the Drug Safety Research Unit (DSRU) in Southampton, UK, which relies on information obtained from the **Prescription Pricing Authority** (PPA) in order to monitor and provide information on **Adverse Events** (AE) in patients receiving pre-selected drugs in general practice. It is independent of the **Medicines Control Agency** (MCA)/**Committee on Safety of Medicines** (CSM)'s reporting scheme. The method (real life cohort observational) determines the incidence of side effects associated with a particular drug with scores given to each AE. The score given, called 'incidence density', is then calculated taking into account patients' exposure to the drug in terms of 'patients' months exposure' which forms the denominator in such a calculation. PEM is particularly useful immediately post-marketing when the drug enters general practice.

The **FP10** prescription forms are used to gather data on doctors, patients, and drugs. All prescriptions issued under the **National Health Service** (NHS) pass through PPA whose task it is to provide information about quantity and cost of drugs through the health services for the purpose of remunerating pharmacists for the medicines they dispense. Doctors who had used the drug in question are identified by the PPA and are asked to complete one of two green forms giving basic demographic data about the patient and information on any adverse events, associated with the drug, which are already recorded in the patient's records. The PPA supplies, in confidence, a copy of every prescription written for the new drugs, which are being monitored, by PEM, as well as information about drugs that are prescribed concurrently to the same patient. The first green form (questionnaire) is used to generate hypothesis about the adverse event occurring during and after treatment with the drug. The second green form is used to test a proposed hypothesis. Response to PEM ranges from 50 to 70%. About 10–12 drugs are selected for evaluation at a time, with evaluation periods lasting 2–3 years.

The drawbacks of PEM, however, include:
- Data limited to those from UK only
- The percentage on non-respondents (i.e. 30–50%) is large and it is difficult to establish whether these doctors' patients are different from those whose doctors who responded.
- Confounding by indication may also pose a problem.

Prescription Medicines Code of Practice Authority (PMCPA) (UK)

Established by the **Association of British Pharmaceutical Industry** (ABPI) on 1 January 1993 to operate the **ABPI Code of Practice for the Pharmaceutical Industry** independently of the ABPI itself. The Code of Practice has been regularly revised since its inception in 1958 and is drawn up in consultation with the **British Medical Association**, the **Royal Pharmaceutical Society of Great Britain** and the **Medicines Control Agency** (MCA). Compliance with the Code is obligatory for ABPI member companies and, in addition, more than 50 non-member companies have voluntarily agreed to comply with the Code and to accept the jurisdiction of the Authority. The Code regulates the advertising of medicines for prescription to health professionals and administrative staff and also covers information about such medicines made available to the general public.

Complaints

The Constitution and Procedure for the PMCPA includes complaints procedure. Complaints submitted under the Code of Practice are considered in the first instance by the Code of Practice Panel which consists of the Director, Secretary and Deputy Secretary of the Authority, acting with the assistance of independent expert advisers where appropriate. Both the complainant and the respondent company may appeal to the Code of Practice Appeal Board against rulings made by the Panel. The Code of Practice Appeal Board is chaired by an independent legally qualified chairman and includes independent members from outside the industry. Details of its composition can be found in the Constitution and Procedure. Reports on completed cases and comments on matters of current concern are published quarterly in the Code of Practice Review.

Copies of the Code of Practice for the Pharmaceutical Industry, the Code of Practice Review and the Annual Report are available from PMCPA.

prescription only medicine (POM)

A drug that can only be dispensed by a pharmacy upon receipt of a prescription from a practising physician. In the **European Union** (EU), the prescription criteria are laid down in **Directive 92/26/EEC** which states that medicinal products shall be classified as POM where they:
- Are likely to present a danger either directly or indirectly, even when used correctly, if utilized without medical supervision
- Are frequently and to a very wide extent used incorrectly, and as a result are likely to present a direct or indirect danger to human health

- Contain substances or preparations of the activity and/or **side-effects** which require further investigation
- Are normally prescribed by a doctor to be administered parenterally.

Although the prescription criteria apply to all EC **Members States** (MS), the procedure for assigning prescription classification remains the responsibility of each individual MS. In the US, the classification of a drug as a prescription or non-prescription medication is a matter of Federal Law, and US pharmacists are familiar with the legend, 'Caution: Federal Law prohibits dispensing without a prescription,' found on many products. The **Food and Drug Administration** (FDA) is charged with this responsibility. This came about as a result of the **Durham-Humphrey Amendment** of 1951. Note that, in the US, the term '**legend drug**' is sometimes used to mean POM.

See also **controlled drug, general list medicine, legend drug, pharmacy drug (P)**.

Prescription Pricing Authority (PPA) (UK)

A special **health authority** (HA) within the **National Health Service** (NHS) Executive (NHSE), its roots go back to 1913. In 1999 the Authority processed over 484 million prescription items, with a total cash value of over £4.5 billion and the annual growth in prescription volume was approximately 3%.

The PPA has four main functions:
- Scrutinize pricing and payment to contractors for the dispensing of NHS prescriptions
- Provision of prescribing and dispensing information to the NHS (excluding hospital dispensing)
- Management of the NHS low-income scheme
- Prevention of prescribing and dispensing fraud within the NHS.

Information is provided in a variety of formats to prescribers and other groups. This includes the **Department of Health**, NHS Executive (NHSE), Regional Offices of the NHSE (ROs), HAs, hospitals, medical and pharmaceutical advisers, **NHS Trusts** (NHSTs), dispensers, police, auditors, Home Office and research groups.

There are four major information systems that provide a broad spectrum of prescribing information. These systems are:
- **Prescribing Analysis and Cost (PACT)**
- **Indicative Prescribing Scheme (IPS)**
- **Prescribing Monitoring Documents (PMD)**
- **Prescription Cost Analysis (PCA)**
- **electronic PACT (ePACT)**.

The Authority designed three drug coding systems in 1981 that all the projects revolve around. For high-speed data capture operators use a simple velocity drug code of two to five digits. The more popular the drug, the shorter the code used to identify the drug. The velocity code is converted to a structured code especially designed for the pricing of drug items in accordance with the drug tariff. This structured code is a nine-digit code which links all packs and presentations of the same drug together. Several commercially available practice computer systems use the PPA's structured coding system.

The third coding system reflects the **British National Formulary** (BNF). This groups drugs for analysis purposes and enables all like drugs, or chemical substances, to be identifiable under the same therapeutic classification. All PPA information service reports on prescribing are based on this coding system and an agreement has been reached with the authors of the BNF to keep the two standards in step. Both the Welsh and Scottish Office have adopted the Authority's coding standards for their prescription pricing and information services.

NHS prescriptions are dispensed by community pharmacies, dispensing general (GPs) and appliance contractors under contract to the local HAs. These are collectively known as **dispensing contractors**. Prescriptions are also received from prescribing GPs for items that have been administered to the patient by the GP. For example, influenza vaccines are usually referred to as personal administration items.

Dispensing contractors are required to despatch their prescriptions to the PPA no later than the fifth working day of the month following the month in which the drug was issued. Remuneration and reimbursement paid to dispensing contractors for prescriptions dispensed varies according to contract type and is detailed in the Drug Tariff. Dispensing contractors receive reimbursement for the following:

- The total price of the drugs, appliances and chemical reagents supplied, less a deduction from the discount received by the contractors, the professional fees for each item dispensed and, an allowance for containers and measuring devices.
- Prescription charges that have been collected from patients by the pharmacy contractor are deducted from the payment. The PPA calculates the payment from all the dispensing contractors in England, approximately 16 000. The PPA also calculates payments on an agency basis for the Isle of Man, Jersey and Guernsey.

Prescription Pricing Regulation Scheme (PPRS) (UK)

A UK system introduced in the 1950s as the 'Voluntary Price Regulation Scheme' (VPRS). The name was then changed to PPRS in the mid 1970s. The scheme aims, in general, to ensure that the **National Health Service** (NHS) obtains safe and effective medicines at affordable prices while promoting support and reward for the pharmaceutical research industry. The scheme applies to all companies supplying the NHS with medicinal products prescribed by physicians excluding private prescribing. It also excludes generics and **over-the-counter** medicines.

preservative

A substance or preparation added to a product for the purpose of destroying or inhibiting the multiplication of micro-organisms.

pre-study visit (Clinical Trials)

A visit made to a potential investigating site to determine whether the centre has the experience, equipment and resources to undertake a proposed clinical study. Such a visit must be documented and appears as part of the study records. Sites with deficiencies should not be recruited to take part in a clinical study.

pre-treatment sign or symptom (Clinical Trials)

Any unfavourable and unintended sign (including an abnormal laboratory or vital sign finding), symptom, or disease that occurs after a subject has been enrolled in the clinical trial (i.e. the subject is listed on the Master Subject Log) but before the administration of the **investigational product** (i.e. the start of the investigational product on Day 1).

pre-trial data

Animal toxicity and pharmaceutical data.

prevalence

The proportion or total number of persons that are affected by a particular disease within a given population at a given time.

price ex-supplier see subsidy.

price to wholesaler see subsidy.

PRIM&R (US)
Public Responsibility In Medicine and Research.

primary disease
A disease that began in the affected location.

primary care
Basic health care that would be delivered by a general practitioner, dentist, pharmacist and optician from whom an individual has an ongoing relationship and who knows the patient's medical history. Primary care services emphasize a patient's general health needs such as preventive services, treatment of minor illnesses and injuries, or identification of problems that require referral to specialists. Traditionally, primary care physicians are family physicians, internists, gynaecologists and paediatricians.

In the US, **Managed Care Organizations** (MCOs) often use primary care physicians as 'gatekeepers' to control which patients are treated by specialists. Since specialists usually command higher fees than primary care physicians, this helps payers control **costs**.

primary care group (PCG) (UK)
A grouping to bring together general practitioners, community nurses, a lay member, a social services representative and a member of the health authority. Typically, PCGs serve about 50000–200000 patients but this varies according to local circumstances. They take responsibility for **commissioning** services locally. They work closely with local government social services departments. PCGs are allowed to take a range of forms, including the opportunity to become free-standing Primary Care Trusts, with responsibility for running community hospitals and community health services in addition to their commissioning role. None of these options affects the independent contractor status of GPs. They contribute to the **Commission for Health Improvement Programme** (CHImP) and health service planning and have a budget reflecting their population's share of cash for hospital and community health services, the general medical services cash limited budget and prescribing.

See also **commissioning**.

primary care providers
Health care professionals capable of providing a wide variety of basic health services. They include practitioners of family, general, or internal medicine; paediatricians and obstetricians; nurse practitioners; midwives; and physician's assistant in general or family practice.

primary containment
A method of **containment** which prevents the escape of a biological agent into the immediate working environment. It involves the use of close containers or safety biological cabinets along with secure operating procedures.

See also **clean/contained area, contained area, containment**.

primary drug resistance (PDR)
Resistance of bacteria or other pathogens to drugs which exists prior to the beginning of treatment.

primary source
The information source that is derived directly from fully described (or referenced) formal observation, procedures or experiments performed with valid, scientifically accepted methods. In its strongest form, this material is usually (but not only) a paper in a refereed scientific publication.

1. *Scientific refereed journal*: A journal that has a mission of publishing and storing primary scientific evidence. By convention primary sources include: evidence published in such a journal is subjected to anonymous review by several experts (referees) in the field prior to publication and is published only once. The methods used to acquire the evidence must be described (or a primary reference cited) with sufficient detail that a person knowledgeable in the discipline can critically appraise the study and could replicate it if they so desired. *Note that although the review process is the best we have for assuring evidence integrity, a significant proportion of such papers contain serious flaws in methods and interpretation, some of which render the study invalid.* The presence of these flaws is one of the primary reasons why literature assessment is a critical skill for clinicians. Repetition of the study by another research group, either in whole or in part, may support or refute a previous study. The critical reader looks for these additional studies.
2. *Scientific proceedings*: A compilation of current research reports, typically presented as short abstracts, from a scientific meeting. These are a much weaker form of a primary source than is a full scientific journal article because the selection of the abstracts, which are of varying quality, is based on a much more cursory review, the reports are usually incomplete, and much of the work is in-progress. As such, these represent a form of 'pre-primary' source.

priming dose see loading dose.

Principle Investigator (PI)
Physician in charge of a **clinical trial**, responsible for supervising the scientific, technical and administrative conduct of the personnel involved at a site, and reporting the findings to the **sponsor**.
See also **investigator**, **lead researcher**.

prn
pro re nata. Administer medicine as/when needed.

PRO see Peer Review Organization.

probe library
In the context of **combinatorial chemistry**, a probe library is used to represent as much structural diversity as possible in a given set of compounds and to find new structural motifs that will aid in the design of new drugs.

probability (P) (Statistics)
The likelihood (e.g. of 5% or less) that an observed difference could have arisen by chance.

procedures
A communication instrument to give directions for performing certain operations (e.g. cleaning, clothing, environmental control, sampling, testing, **recalls**, **validation**, and equipment operation) to be carried out, the precautions to be taken and measures to be applied directly or indirectly related to the manufacture of a **medicinal product**.
See also **standard operating procedure**.

PRODIGY see Prescribing RatiOnally with Decision-support In General-practice studY.

prodromal
Pertaining to symptoms indicating the onset of a disease. May include symptoms prior to those adequate for accurate diagnosis.

prodrug
Any compound that undergoes **biotransformation** before exhibiting its pharmacological effects. Prodrugs can thus be viewed as drugs containing specialized non-toxic protective groups used in a transient manner to alter or to eliminate undesirable properties in the parent molecule.
See also **double prodrug**.

producer's risk
The risk of error incurred when an effective product is improperly considered to be ineffective as a result of a **clinical trial**. It is referred to as producer's risk, since the producer (**manufacturer**) would suffer from a failure to introduce an effective therapy.
See also **beta error, false negative, type I error**.

production
All operations involved in the preparation of a **medicinal product**, from receipt of materials, through processing and **packaging**, to its completion as a **finished product**.

product liability
This is a concept addressing the question of who has responsibility for the product.

Product Licence (PL)
A licence that authorizes the holder, in relation to the product in question to:
- Sell, supply, or export
- Procure the sale, supply or export
- Procure the manufacture or assembly of the product for sale, supply or export
- Import.

Applications for PLs are made to the licensing authorities who base their decision on satisfactory data on pharmaceutical quality, safety, and efficacy of the proposed medication.

Product Licence Application (PLA)
The submission of all the relevant data pertaining to a drug in order to obtain a product licence. All the clinical studies which have obtained regulatory approval must be included in the submission. The Regulatory affairs department, in a pharmaceutical company, are responsible for submitting these data to the relevant **regulatory authority**.
In the US, a PLA is an application to the **Committee for Biologics Evaluation and Review** group at the **Food and Drug Administration** (FDA) requesting approval to manufacture and distribute a biological product.
See also **New Drug Application**, and **Pre-marketing Approval Application**.

Product Licence of Right (PLR) (UK)
A licence granted for all medicines which were already on the market when the **Medicines Act** of 1968 came into effect.
See also **Committee on Review of Medicines**.

Product Licence User System (PLUS) (UK)
A database at the Licensing Division of the **Medicines Control Agency** (MCA). This unit initially receives each application for a **marketing authorization** (MA) and enters it onto the PLUS ready for assessment. Once a decision is made to grant an MA, the licence is produced automatically from the PLUS system.
See also **Medicines Control Agency**.

product listing (US)
A process dictated by **Food and Drug Administration** (FDA) requiring submission of a short

form, on an annual basis, which lists all **drug products** marketed by a **manufacturer** for that time period.

product specification file
Reference file containing all information necessary to draft detailed written instructions on processing, packaging, quality control testing, batch release and shipping.

prognosis
A doctor's probable forecast of the effects, duration, and outcome of a particular disease and its response to medical treatment.

prognostic factors
Factors used to forecast the course or **outcome** of a disease or injury and its response to medical intervention. They include demographic, disease-specific, or co-morbid characteristics associated strongly enough with a condition's outcomes to predict accurately the eventual development of those outcomes. Neither prognostic nor **risk factors** necessarily imply a cause and effect relationship.
Compare **risk factor**.

Project Manager
As applied to the **centralized procedure**, this is a member of staff of the Human Medicines Evaluation Unit of the **European Medicines Evaluation Agency** (EMEA) appointed (by the EMEA) to coordinate the validation of application submitted and monitor compliance with the time-frame provided for processing the application using the EMEA Application Tracking System. The manager also provides assistance to the **rapporteur** and **co-rapporteur**, organizes any expert meeting, prepares the opinion of the **Committee for Proprietary Medicinal Products** (CPMP) in all official languages of the EU and coordinates (with the Rapporteur and Co-rapporteur) the preparation of the **Assessment Report** and its transformation into **EPAR**.

prokinetic drugs
Medicines that cause muscles in the gastrointestinal tract to move food. An example is cisapride.

Promoting Action on Clinical Effectiveness (PACE) (UK)
This initiative, run from the King's Fund in London, works through a network of sixteen demonstration projects to achieve clinical change for effective health care. A progress report is available from their site.
Website: http://www.kingsfund.org.uk/pace/evidence.htm

proof of principle
Achieved when a compound has shown the desired activity *in vitro* that supports a **hypothesis** or concept for use of the compound.

proof-of-principle trial see **phase III clinical trial**.

prophylactic
Anything used to prevent disease.

proportional reporting ratio (PRR)
A tool used in signal generation from spontaneous **adverse drug reaction** data. It is the proportion of all reactions to a specific drug which are the particular medical condition of interest (e.g. hepatitis), compared to the same proportion for all drugs in the database. The PRR is a/a + b divided by c/c + d as in the following two by two table:

	All other reactions	Reactions(s) of interest
Drug of interest	a	b
All other drugs in database	c	d

The expected or null value for a PRR is one and the numbers generated are measures of association, which reflect strength of the signal. Measures of statistical association for each value may be calculated using standard methods such as 95% **confidence intervals** and the **chi-squared** test. Judgement about whether or not there is a signal, and its strength, may then be made based on three key pieces of information, i.e. the PRR, value of chi-squared and the absolute number of reports. A minimum signal would be a PRR of at least 2, chi-squared of at least 4 and three or more cases.

proprietary drugs
Drugs whose formulations are associated with an active **patent**.

proprietary medicinal product (PMP)
As defined in Article 1 of **EU Directive 65/65/EEC** is 'Any ready-prepared **medicinal product** placed on the market under a special name in a special pack'. This definition was later broadened and became medicinal product.

See also **medicinal product**.

prospective, randomized, double-blind trial (Clinical Trials)
A **clinical trial** in which the method for analysing data has been specified in the protocol before the study has begun (prospective), the patients have been randomly assigned to receive either the study drug or alternative treatment, and in which neither the patient nor the physician(s) conducting the study know which treatment is being given to the patient.

prospective study (Clinical Trials)
Studies designed to observe outcomes or events that occur subsequent to the identification of the group of subjects to be studied. They are the studies where one or more groups (**cohorts**) of individuals who have not yet had the outcome event in question are then followed up at subsequent times and monitored for the number of such events which occur over time. Prospective studies need not involve manipulation or intervention but may be purely observational or involve only the collection of data.

protectant
A topical drug that remains on the skin and serves as a physical barrier to the environment.

protocol (Clinical Trials)
The formal detailed plan of design of a drug trial or research activity which is submitted to the **Ethics Committee (Investigational Review Board** in the US) for review. The protocol states the rationale, purpose, objective(s), a description of the research design or methodology to be employed, drug dosages, length of treatment, how the drug is given, inclusion and exclusion criteria for prospective subjects and controls, the proposed methods of analysis that will be performed on the collected data and how those running the trial will determine if the trial was a success or a failure.

protocol amendment (Clinical Trials)
A written description of a change(s) to or formal clarification of a **protocol** during the course of the study.

protocol annexures (Clinical Trials)
Documents attached to the protocol, such as **case record forms** or informed consent.

Protocol Chair (US) (Clinical Trials)
The scientific coordinator of the study who is responsible for developing and monitoring the study as well as analysing, reporting and publishing its results.

protocol deviation (Clinical Trials)
A divergence from full **compliance** with the **clinical trial's protocol** when no **protocol amendment** has been submitted and approved. Also called minor deviation.

protocol violation (Clinical Trials)
An event taking place in a study which is not in agreement with and constitutes a divergence from full compliance with the **protocol**, when no adjustment or a **protocol amendment** has been submitted and approved leading to the exclusion of the subject/patient from the per-protocol group. The commonest protocol violation involves the recruitment of patients outside the **inclusion criteria** specified. Also called major deviation.

See also **protocol deviation**.

provider
A **National Health Service Trust** (hospital, community unit or ambulance service) or independent health care organization from which care is purchased. Usually used when talking about doctors, but also can refer to pharmacies, nurses and other health care professionals.

PRR see **proportional reporting ratio**.

PSA
Prescription Sequence Analysis.

PSNC (UK)
Pharmaceutical Services Negotiating Committee.

psoralens
Drugs that contain chemicals derived from plants; used to treat the skin disorders such as psoriasis and vitiligo.

PSUR see **Periodic Safety Update Report**.

psychodelic
A drug inducing hallucinations or perceptual distortion.

psychopharmacological agent see **psychotropic drugs**.

psychoplegic agents
Same as neuroleptics or **antipsychotics**.

psychotropic drugs
Any agent which exerts a psychological effect on the higher parts of the central nervous system.

P&T Committee see **Pharmacy and Therapeutics Committee**.

PTAC see **Pharmacology and Therapeutics Advisory Committee**.

PTO see **United States Patent and Trademark Office**.

P to GSL Status (UK)
The procedure of changing the legal status of a medicinal product from a Pharmacy only

medicine (P) to **General Sales List (GSL)** product according to Section 51 of the Medicines Act of 1968. Such change can take place if the product can, with reasonable safety, be sold or supplied otherwise than by, or under the supervision of, a pharmacist. The definition of reasonable safety was elaborated by the Medicines Commission in 1973 to mean that:
1. the hazard to health is small
2. the risk of misuse is small
3. the need to take special precautions in handling is small
4. the wider sale would be a convenience to the purchaser.

public affairs
A term frequently applied to corporate relationships; lobbying is a sub-discipline used to influence legislative decisions by government.

publication policy (Clinical Trials)
A policy, that is agreed internally within the company, covering the publication of trials' data and results. Such policy is normally incorporated in the study protocol.

Public Health Laboratory Service (PHLS) (UK)
An organization whose focus is on detecting, diagnosing, and monitoring communicable diseases. It provides evidence for action to prevent and control infectious disease. The evidence comes from expert analysis and assessment of data generated from the PHLS's own epidemiological investigations, microbiological testing of specimens, surveillance, research, evaluation and training and education and from many other sources.

Its customers include local, regional, national and international clinicians and public health professionals and policy-makers. Its products include advice on effective management of infected patients, advice on policy development for population-based interventions, support for incident and outbreak control, and application of new technologies and improved methods.

The PHLS integrates microbiology and epidemiology at every level within a national organization comprising a network of Public Health Laboratories organized into nine groups in England and Wales, the Communicable Disease Surveillance Centre, including the regional epidemiology service, and the Central Public Health Laboratory based with the PHLS Headquarters in Colindale, north London.

Public Health Service (PHS) (US)
A part of the **Department of Health and Human Services** and is responsible for the public health of the American people. It administers several government agencies including **Food and Drug Administration** (FDA), **National Institutes of Health** and **Centers for Disease Control**.

public relations (PR)
On the most general level, public relations is a subset of marketing that specializes in media relations working with editors who write about technology products, trends and issues. In the high tech industry, the mission of PR is to educate and communicate. While any company with good financial base can pay for advertising, a positive story on the benefits of a particular technology or an outstanding review lends a third party credibility that the best advertisement cannot achieve.

PR companies make sure that the company spokespeople interact effectively with the press, and that the message being delivered is believable and compelling. They also work with editors to make sure they understand their client's key messages, and that they have access to any people, information, artwork and materials they need to publish their stories.

Compare **financial PR, media relations**.

pulmonary excretion
The lung is the major organ of excretion for gaseous and volatile substances. The breathalyzer test is based on a quantitative pulmonary excretion of ethanol. Most of the gaseous anaesthetics are extensively eliminated in expired air.

purgative
A drug that promotes defaecation to bring about emptying of the bowels (Greek: *kathartikos*, making completely clean). Some purgatives work by causing irritation along the whole length of the intestine and increase peristalsis.

Also called aperient.

purchaser (UK)
A health authority, **GP Fundholder** or **Total Purchasing Group** responsible for assessing the needs of their local populations or patients and for purchasing the best possible care for them.

Compare **commissioning**.

See also **Commissioner, contracts, purchasing intelligence.**

PUVA
A form of phototherapy that combines the use of **psoralens** and ultraviolet light to treat skin disorders.

P-value (Statistics)
The probability of obtaining as big a difference between the treatments as that observed if in reality there is no difference. The smaller this probability the greater is the likelihood that the effects of the two treatments are different. The *P*-value is the lowest level of significance at which a given **null hypothesis** can be rejected; that is, the necessary criterion for determining that the result probably did not happen by chance. It is not the probability that a given result is wrong or right, the probability that the result occurred by chance, or a measure of the clinical significance of the results, i.e. that the **outcome** was due entirely to chance **variability** of individuals or measurements alone. A very small *P*-value cannot compensate for the presence of a large amount of systematic error (bias). If the opportunity for bias is large, the *P*-value is likely to be invalid and irrelevant. Some introductory texts seriously mis-define this term.

Conventionally, *P*-values are interpreted as follows:

$P > 0.05$ is regarded as not significant (symbolized as NS)

$P < 0.05$ is regarded as significant (symbolized as *)

$P < 0.01$ is regarded as highly significant (symbolized as **)

$P < 0.001$ is regarded as very highly significant (symbolized as ***)

A $P < 0.05$ indicates that the probability of the result occurring by chance is 1 in 20 whereas when $P < 0.01$, the chance is 1 in 100 and likewise if $P < 0.001$, the chance is 1 in 1000.

See also **statistical significance**.

Q

Q1

International Conference on Harmonization (ICH) guidance document on Stability.
See also **Q1A guidance document, Q1B guidance document, Q1C guidance document**.

Q1A guidance document

An **International Conference on Harmonization** (ICH) guidance document on Stability entitled 'Stability Testing of New Drug Substances and Products'.
See also **Q1B guidance document, Q1C guidance document**.

Q1B guidance document

An **International Conference on Harmonization** (ICH) guidance document on Stability entitled 'Stability Testing: Photo-stability Testing of New Drug Substances and Products'.
See also **Q1A guidance document, Q1C guidance document**.

Q1C guidance document

An **International Conference on Harmonization** (ICH) guidance document on Stability entitled 'Stability Testing for New Dosage Forms'.
See also **Q1B guidance document, Q1A guidance document**.

Q2 guidance document

An **International Conference on Harmonization** (ICH) guidance document on Analytical Validation.
See also **Q2A guidance document, Q2B guidance document**.

Q2A guidance document

An **International Conference on Harmonization** (ICH) guidance document on 'Analytical Validation' entitled 'Text on Validation of Analytical Procedures'.
See also **Q2B guidance document**.

Q2B guidance document

An **International Conference on Harmonization** (ICH) guidance document on 'Analytical Validation' entitled 'Validation of Analytical Procedures: Methodology'.
See also **Q2A guidance document**.

Q3 guidance document

An **International Conference on Harmonization** (ICH) guidance document on 'Impurities'.
See also **Q3A guidance document, Q3B guidance document, Q3C guidance document**.

Q3A guidance document

An **International Conference on Harmonization** (ICH) guidance document on 'Impurities' entitled 'Impurities in New Drug Substances'.
See also **Q3B guidance document, Q3C guidance document**.

Q3B guidance document

An **International Conference on Harmonization** (ICH) guidance document on 'Impurities' entitled 'Impurities in New Drug Products'.
See also **Q3A guidance document, Q3C guidance document**.

Q3C guidance document
An **International Conference on Harmonization** (ICH) guidance document on 'Impurities' entitled 'Impurities: Guideline for Residual Solvents'.
See also **Q3A guidance document, Q3B guidance document**.

Q5 guidance document
An **International Conference on Harmonization** (ICH) guidance document on 'Biotechnology quality'.
See also **Q5A guidance document, Q5B guidance document, Q5C guidance document, Q5D guidance document**.

Q5A guidance document
An **International Conference on Harmonization** (ICH) guidance document on 'Biotechnology quality' entitled 'Viral Safety Evaluation of Biotechnology Products'.
See also **Q5B guidance document, Q5C guidance document, Q5D guidance document**.

Q5B guidance document
An **International Conference on Harmonization** (ICH) guidance document on 'Biotechnology quality' entitled 'Quality of Biotechnological Products: Analysis of the Expression Construct in Cells Used for the Production of r-DNA Derived Protein Products'.
See also **Q5A guidance document, Q5C guidance document, Q5D guidance document**.

Q5C guidance document
An **International Conference on Harmonization** (ICH) guidance document on 'Biotechnology quality' entitled 'Quality of Biotechnological Products: Stability Testing of Biotechnological/Biological Products'.
See also **Q5A guidance document, Q5B guidance document, Q5D guidance document**.

Q5D guidance document
An **International Conference on Harmonization** (ICH) guidance document on 'Biotechnology quality' entitled 'Quality of Biotechnological Products: Derivation and Characterization of Cell Substrates Used for Production of Biotechnological/Biological Products'.
See also **Q5A guidance document, Q5B guidance document, Q5C guidance document**.

Q6 guidance document
An **International Conference on Harmonization** (ICH) guidance document on 'Specifications'.
See also **Q6A guidance document, Q6B guidance document**.

Q6A guidance document
An **International Conference on Harmonization** (ICH) guidance document on 'Specifications' entitled 'Specifications: Test Procedures and Acceptance Criteria for New Drug Substances and Products: Chemical Substances'.
See also **Q6B guidance document**.

Q6A guidance document
An **International Conference on Harmonization** (ICH) guidance document on

'Specifications' entitled 'Specifications: Test Procedures and Acceptance Criteria for New Drug Substances and Products: Chemical Substances'.
See also **Q5B guidance document**.

Q6B guidance document
An **International Conference on Harmonization** (ICH) guidance document on 'Specifications' entitled 'Specifications: Test Procedures and Acceptance Criteria for Biotechnological/Biological Substances'.
See also **Q5A guidance document**.

QA see **quality assurance**.

QALY see **quality adjusted life year**.

QC see **quality control**.

qd
Quaque die. Every day.

qds (QDS)
Four times daily dose regimen.

QID
Quars (or quarter) in die. Four times daily. A dose regimen used in writing a **prescription**.

QL see **quality of life**.

QM Committee see **Quality Management Committee**.

QoL see **quality of life**.

QSAR see **quantitative structure–activity relationships**.

Quackwatch (US)
A member of Consumer Federation of America, it is a non-profit corporation whose purpose is to combat health-related frauds, myths, fads and fallacies. Its primary focus is on quackery-related information that is difficult or impossible to get elsewhere.

qualification
Action of proving that any equipment works correctly and actually leads to the expected results. The word '**validation**' is sometimes broadened to incorporate the concept of qualification.

qualified person (QP)
According to **European Union** (EU) law, 'all holders of **manufacturing authorization** or wholesale dealer's (import) licenses are required to have available a QP, who must be named on their licence' (**Directive 75/319/EEC**). No **batch** of **medicinal product** may be released to the market within the **European Community** unless a nominated QP has certified that it has been manufactured and checked in compliance with the laws in force. According to **Directive 75/319/EEC**, the QP must have certain academic, professional, and actual practical experience. In the UK, for example, 'when considering a nomination, the Licensing Authority regularly takes into account the assessment of the nominee's eligibility made by the joint assessment panel of the Institute of Biology, the **Royal Pharmaceutical Society of Great Britain** (RPSGB) and the **Royal Society of Chemistry**.' (Crown Copyright).

For veterinary products, the equivalent directive is **Directive 81/851/EEC**. In a similar spirit, the wholesalers are required to appoint a QP who has the knowledge and responsibility to ensure that correct procedures are followed during distribution.

Compare **responsible person**.

qualitative variable

One that cannot be measured numerically (race or sex, for example).

See also **quantitative variable**.

quality

As pressure mounts to reduce the **cost** of health care, there is increasing concern that the quality of care will suffer, as has happened in many countries with single-payer or government subsidized health care systems.

quality adjusted life year (QALY)

A standardized method of assessing health care on the basis of **cost** and benefit which takes into account both life expectancy and **quality of life**. QALY is a year of life adjusted for its value or quality. For instance, a year in perfect health would be considered equal to 1 QALY. However, a year in ill-health must be discounted accordingly to the **utility** of that health state. Thus a year bedridden might have a value equal to 0.3 QALY.

See also **quality of life**.

quality assurance (QA)

1. 'A wide ranging concept which covers all matters which individually or collectively influence the quality of the product. It is the sum total of the organized arrangements made with the object of ensuring that medicinal products are of the quality required for their intended use. QA therefore incorporates **good manufacturing practice** (GMP) plus other factors. The system of QA appropriate for the manufacture of medicinal products should ensure that medicinal products are designed and developed in a way that takes account of the requirements of GMP and **good laboratory practice**.' (Crown Copyright)

2. (Clinical Trials)
Systems and systematic processes established to ensure that the trial is executed and the data are produced in compliance with **good clinical practice** including procedures for ethical conduct, **standard operating procedures**, the **applicable regulatory requirements**, reporting personal qualifications etc. This is validated through in-process quality control and in- and post-process auditing, both being applied to the clinical trial process as well as to the data.

Personnel involved in QA audit activities must be independent of those involved in managing a particular trial.

See also **quality control** (QC), **quality management**.

quality control (QC)

1. Concerned with sampling, specifications and testing as well as the organization, documentation and release procedures which ensure that the necessary and relevant tests are carried out, and that materials are not released for use, nor products released for sale or supply, until their quality has been judged satisfactory. QC is not confined to laboratory operations, but must be involved in all decisions that concern the quality of the product. The independence of QC from production is considered fundamental to the satisfactory operation of QC.

2. (Clinical Trials) The operational techniques and activities undertaken within the system

of **quality assurance** to verify that the requirements for quality of the trial have been fulfilled.

QC activities concern all members of the investigational team, including the staff of the sponsor or **contract research organization** involved with planning, conducting, monitoring, evaluating and reporting a trial including data processing, with the objective of avoiding trial subjects being exposed to unnecessary risk, or false conclusions being drawn from unreliable data.

quality management

The broad discipline comprising **quality assurance**, **quality control**, and incorporating **good manufacturing practice**.

Quality Management Committee (QM Committee)

A committee found in hospitals which applies quality assurance principles to **inpatient care delivery systems**.

quality of life (QoL)

Any measure of the length of a person's life, taking into account physical and psychological suffering caused by disease and its therapy. The quality of life can be assessed at a functional level (e.g. social, physical, emotional and intellectual activities) and at a perceptual level (e.g. the patient's wellbeing and health status). Only by placing a value on life (which is worth more: 5 years of suffering or 1 disease-free year?) can comparisons of different therapies be made, i.e. it is an assessment of the depth as well as the length of life. Quality of life is an important measure in **pharmacoeconomics**.

quantitative structure–activity relationship (QSAR)

Mathematical relationship linking chemical structure and pharmacological activity in a quantitative manner for a series of compounds. Methods which can be used in QSAR include various regression and **pattern recognition** techniques.

See also **structure–activity relationship**.

quantitative variable

One that can be measured (blood pressure, for example).

See also **qualitative variable**.

quarantine

The status of starting or packaging materials, intermediate, bulk, or finished products isolated physically or by other effective means whilst awaiting a decision on their release or refusal.

quasi-experimental study (Clinical Trials)

A study that is similar to a true experimental study except that it lacks random assignments of subjects to treatment groups.

See also **experimental study**.

quiescence

A period during which an infection is present but not active within a host: for example the period between an acute attack of chickenpox (varicella) and a subsequent **recrudescence** of shingles (zoster); not the same as latency.

Compare **latent period**.

R&D
Research and Development.

RADAR (US)
Risk Assessment of Drugs-Analysis and Response.

radioactive drug
Any drug substance that exhibits spontaneous disintegration of unstable nuclei with the emission of nuclear particles or photons. Included is any non-radioactive reagent kit or nuclide generator that is intended to be used in the preparation of a radioactive drug and 'radioactive biological products'. Drugs such as carbon-containing compounds or potassium-containing salts containing trace quantities of naturally occurring radionuclides are not considered radioactive drugs.
Compare **radiopharmaceutical**.

radionuclide
A nuclide of an atom that is radioactive (radioactive isotope).

radionuclide scanning
An imaging technique in which a radioactive substance is introduced into the body and its emitted radiation is detected; specific organs can be studied according to the amount of the radioactive substance that they absorb.

radiopharmaceutical
Drug products (compounds or materials) that may be labelled or tagged with a radioisotope or a preparation containing one or more **radionuclides** (radioactive isotopes). These materials are largely physiological or sub-pharmacological in action, and, in many cases, function much like materials found in the body. It is used in diagnosis, therapy, and research. The principal risk associated with these materials is the consequent radiation exposure to the body or to specific organ systems when they are injected into the body. In the EU, Council **Directive 89/343/EEC** extended the scope of Directives 65/65/EEC and 75/319/EEC to lay down additional provisions for radiopharmaceuticals. It requires labels to be in accordance with the requirements of the Regulations for Safe Transport of Radioactive Materials laid down by the International Atomic Energy Agency.
Compare **radioactive drug**.

radiosensitizing drug
A drug that increases the sensitivity of hypoxic cells (e.g. in ischaemic regions of tumours) to X-rays or γ-rays. Examples of such an agent include vitamin K and some nitro-imidazoles.

RAMA (UK)
A computing system that allows the pharmaceutical industry a controlled access, on subscription basis, to the **MCA**'s major licensing database of **PLUS**.

RAND Corporation (US)
RAND is a US-based non-profit institution that aims to improve public policy through research and analysis. RAND aims to carry out high-quality, objective research addressing problems of domestic policy including health care.

random (Clinical Trials)
Random is the process by which an **outcome** of an experiment or action is determined solely

by a probabilistic mechanism, for example, a coin flip or the roll of a dice. A random **sample** is a group of **subjects** in a **clinical trial** selected by such a mechanism.

random allocation (Clinical Trials)
Assignment of subjects to treatment (or **control**) groups in an unpredictable way. Assignment sequences are concealed, but available for disclosure in the event a subject has a serious adverse experience.

randomization (Clinical Trials)
The process used in research to prevent bias. Trial subjects are assigned by chance rather than systematically (e.g. as dictated by the standard or usual response to their condition, history, or prognosis, or according to demographic characteristics) either to receive the study agent (intervention group) or not (control group). Randomization is often done by a computer.
See also **bias**.

randomization code (Clinical Trials)
A code of treatment allocated to patients in a **controlled clinical trial**. In an emergency (e.g. if a serious **adverse event** has occurred) the **investigator** may need to break the code to uncover which treatment the patient had been receiving. The code for each patient may be contained in a separate envelope or it may be contained in a tear-off strip which was detached from the supplies when they were dispensed to the patient. If the code is broken for any patient then that patient must be withdrawn from the study.

randomized clinical trial (RCT)
Randomized refers to the principle of **random**ness applied to the assignment of **subjects** in a **clinical trial** to avoid study **bias**. This is done using a probabilistic mechanism (crudely, a coin flip) to choose the treatment. Patients with similar traits, such as extent of disease, are chosen or selected by chance to be placed in separate groups and are followed up for the variables/**outcomes** of interest. The **investigator** does not know who is receiving which treatment. Since irrelevant factors or preferences do not influence the distribution of patients, the treatment groups can be considered comparable and results of the different treatments used in different groups can be meaningfully compared. It is the patient's choice to be in a randomized trial or not. Such trial designs offer unbiased distribution of confounders; true blinding and randomization which facilitates statistical analysis. Disadvantages include expense, length of time and possibility of **volunteer bias**, and can be, at times, ethically problematic.
See also **clinical trials**, **randomization**.

randomized, double-blind, placebo-controlled, multicentre trial
A **clinical trial** in which patients have been randomly assigned to receive either the **investigational product** or alternative treatment, in which neither the patient nor the investigator(s) conducting the study know which treatment is being given. The alternative to the study drug is a **placebo**. The study is conducted at several centres.

randomized subject (Clinical Trials)
Any **subject** who has been assigned to either a specific dose regimen or treatment group after signing the **informed consent** and meeting all **inclusion** and **exclusion criteria** of the **protocol**.

random number table (Clinical Trials)
Table of numbers with no apparent pattern used in the selection of random samples for **clinical trials**.

random sample
Members of a **population** selected by a method designed to ensure that each person in the target group has an equal chance of selection.

random screening
Also referred to as 'serendipity'. The biological screening of large databases of chemical compounds from which data on compounds and plant extracts are available to pharmaceutical companies. The chance of discovering a good drug by this approach is estimated to be only 1 in 10 000, i.e. one compound out of 10 000 screened. This process, which used to take several years, has been expedited in recent years with the help of current screening technology and can take only a few months.

rapporteur
A member of the **Committee for Proprietary Medicinal Products** (CPMP) appointed by the committee itself (following preference from the company and bids from Members of CPMP) to coordinate the evaluation of an application for a **marketing authorization**. A rapporteur is selected to act on behalf of the Committee, not their **Member State**. The CPMP will take into account preferences expressed by applicants in selecting rapporteurs, although there is no obligation to follow these preferences.

The rapporteur is responsible for the pre-authorization assessment and continues with post-authorization evaluation (i.e. specific obligations, variations and renewals), **pharmacovigilance** and inspection. With regard to pharmacovigilance in the **centralized procedure**, the rapporteur takes the lead in the pre-authorization phase, unless otherwise decided by the CPMP. The rapporteur is responsible for evaluating and producing assessment reports on pharmacovigilance issues related to centrally authorized product, in accordance with an agreed timetable.

A member will also be appointed as rapporteur in cases of referrals due to differences in national decisions where the interest of the **European Community** is involved or for **arbitration** procedure. The rapporteur is responsible for assessing the grounds for appeal.

See also **co-rapporteur**.

RAPS
Regulatory Affairs Professional Society.

RAST
RadioAllergoSorbent Test.

rate
The number of events happening divided by the length of time over which they happen. A rate of change is the amount of change happening in a interval divided by the length of the interval.
See also **differential equation**.

raw data
The original records or certified copies of original researcher's observations, measurements, and activities (such as laboratory notes, patient charts, evaluations hospital records, X-rays, and attending physician's notes, and data recorded by automated instruments) without conclusions or interpretations. In the US, these records may or may not accompany a **New Drug Application**, but must be kept in the researcher's file. The **Food and Drug Administration** may request their submission or may audit them at the researcher's office.

RAWP (UK)
Resource Allocation Working Party.

RCCS
Read Clinical Classification System, see **Read Codes**.

RCGP (UK)
Royal College of General Practitioners.

RCOG (UK)
Royal College of Obstetrics and Gynaecology.

RCT see **randomized controlled clinical trial**.

RDA
Recommended daily allowance.

RDE
Remote data entry.

rDNA see **recombinant DNA**.

RDRC (US)
Radioactive Drug Research Committee.

Read Codes (UK)
Used widely within the **National Health Service** (NHS) by clinicians and management for both clinical and resource management purposes. The code includes a Drug and Appliance section. The Read Codes are currently used in 75–80% of the computerized general practitioner (GP) practices. This is likely to rise towards 100% as practices purchase new accredited systems. The Requirement for Accreditation (RFA) stipulates that the system should utilize the Read Codes.

Within the secondary health care sector, 150 Trusts have a Read Code presence, 50 of which use Read Codes hospital-wide. There are national licences in place for Scotland and New Zealand and growing international interest in the application of Read Codes within clinical settings, particularly within Northern America.

Read Codes were initially developed by Dr James Read, a GP in Loughborough, as a means of recording a comprehensive summary of a patient's health care on a computer. This coding scheme covered a broad range of data items including disorders, signs and symptoms, procedures, investigations and laboratory results, radiology, administration, preventative care and a full listing of prescribable drugs.

To facilitate implementation of the recommendation, by the Joint Computing Group of the RCGP and the General Medical Services Committee of the **British Medical Association**, the Read Codes were purchased by the Secretary of State for Health and made Crown Copyright in 1990. To ensure that the Read Codes continued to evolve to serve the needs of the Health Service the NHS Centre for Coding and Classification (CCC) was established.

More than 2000 clinicians collaborated with the NHS CCC within three major Terms Projects between 1992 and 1995. The output of these projects has formed the basis for Version 3 of the Read Codes.

Computer Aided Medical Systems Limited (CAMS) is the organization that copies and distributes the Read Codes to end users under Licence from the **Department of Health**. In addition each user is provided with services, either directly or indirectly through the GP System Supplier to include:

- Quarterly updates of the full Read Code set
- Monthly updates of the Drug Dictionary
- Telephone help line for Read Code queries

- A mechanism to request the addition of new Read Codes and Terms
- Supporting documentation etc.

CAMS provides the main channel of communication between end users and the NHS CCC.

It is the intention of the NHS CCC only to provide a Dictionary of medications and appliances etc. Whilst the Read Code Thesaurus may include all of those terms which describe the drug–drug and drug–disease interactions, there are no links between these terms to represent this knowledge.

Similarly, projects such as **PRODIGY**, may use Read Code terms to provide guidelines and decision support, but again these links remain the responsibility of the organization which maintains and supplies the product.

The Read Code hierarchy is utilized to represent the **British National Formulary** (BNF) structure and therefore the chapter headings follow the body systems as laid out in the BNF. Further factual information includes cross-references to the BNF Codes and the **Anatomical Therapeutic Chemical Classification**.

The objective of the Version 3 Drug and Appliance Dictionary is to ensure that all the concepts applying to medical products, appliances, dressings, special foods and reagents are included within the Dictionary, which is part of the Read Thesaurus.

The NHS CCC maintain both Version 2 and Version 3 of the Drug and Appliance Dictionaries. These are updated and released each month. Pharmaceutical companies may notify the NHS CCC of their intention to release new products or change factual information relating to those products in a number of different ways. The NHS CCC will accept notification directly, as long as all the facts and information listed above is accompanied by a **Summary of Product Characteristics** (SPC) and licence number. The NHS CCC undertake to incorporate these new products, if appropriate, but do not provide any form of feedback which confirms the product's inclusion. Members of the NHS CCC also scan current literature to find products not currently listed, so that they may be included and may contact the company directly if necessary, for further details.

After consultation with a number of pharmaceutical companies, CAMS provide a commercially available service in which each licensed pharmaceutical company receives Read Code Request Forms which they fill in for each individual new product. These are then forwarded to CAMS along with the SPC, which is checked for completeness and then forwarded to the NHS CCC within 1 working day of receipt.

Direct feedback is then provided to the pharmaceutical company following inclusion within the Drugs and Appliance Dictionary, including details of the term allocated and the Read Code attached. Should the product not be included, reasons can be ascertained and passed on to the company concerned. In some instances the pharmaceutical company may question the response, in which case CAMS will arbitrate on their behalf with the NHS CCC, until such time as a satisfactory conclusion is reached.

It is CAMS' intention to further automate this process via the Internet, to enable a more responsive service to be provided.

reader bias

Systematic errors of interpretation made during inference by the user or reader of clinical information (papers, test results). Such biases are due to clinical experience, tradition, credentials, prejudice and human nature. The human tendency is to accept information that supports preconceived opinions and to reject or trivialize that which does not support preconceived opinions or that which one does not understand (*JAMA* 247:2533).

See also **bias**.

reagent
Substance used in a chemical reaction.

REB see **Research Ethics Board**.

recall
The act of recalling a product from the market and distributors by the **manufacturer/ marketing authorization** (MA) holder. In the **European Union**, in accordance with Article 28 of **Directive 75/319/EEC**, a system should be designed, by the MA holder, to recall, if necessary, promptly and effectively products known or suspected to be defective from the market. A person should be designated as responsible for execution and coordination of recalls and should be supported by sufficient staff to handle all the aspects of the recalls with the appropriate degree of urgency. This **responsible person** should normally be independent of the sales and marketing organization. If this person is not the '**qualified person**', the latter should be made aware of any recall operation.

There should be established written **procedures** in order to organize any recall activity that should be capable of being initiated promptly and at any time. All **competent authorities** of all countries to which the product may have been distributed should be informed promptly if products are intended to be recalled. Recalled products should be stored separately in a secure way while awaiting a decision on their fate.

recall bias (Clinical Trials)
Systematic error due to the differences in accuracy or completeness of recall to memory of past events or experiences. The recall of exposures or events may differ in cases and controls. Questions may be asked more times and more intensively in cases compared to controls. Patients with the disease are more likely to carefully consider whether or not an exposure occurred.
See also **bias**.

receptor
The macromolecule with which drugs interact to produce their characteristic biological effects. These are specific, functionally important tissue components such as proteins or nucleic acids for which the drug molecule has a high degree of selectivity. A few substances, however, owe their effectiveness to physiochemical mechanisms and because they lack receptor interactions they tend to be less specific.
Compare **affinity, antagonism, blocking agent, intrinsic activity**.

receptor mapping
The technique used to describe the geometric and/or electronic features of a binding site when insufficient structural data for this **receptor** or enzyme are available. Generally the active site cavity is defined by comparing the superposition of active to that of inactive molecules.

rechallenge
The deliberate or inadvertent administration of a further **dose(s)** of the same drug to a person who had previously experienced an **adverse event**, which might be drug-related. The response to rechallenge is a major factor used in the assessment of drug **causality**. A positive rechallenge means that the reaction recurs when the drug is re-administered while a negative rechallenge means the reaction does not recur when the drug is re-administered.

recombinant DNA (rDNA)
DNA artificially constructed by insertion of foreign DNA into the DNA of an appropriate organism (usually bacteria or yeast) so that the foreign DNA is replicated along with the host DNA.

recombinant DNA technology
'The ability to chop up DNA and move the pieces, (which) permits the direct examination of the human genome', and the identification of the genetic components of a wide variety of disorders (Holtzman (1989), p. 1). Recombinant DNA technology is also used to develop diagnostic screens and tests, as well as drugs and biologics for treating diseases with genetic components.

Recommendations (European Union)
As applicable to the **European Union** law, these are legal instruments, which have a persuasive force on those addressed. They are not mandatory to the **Member States**. They do, however, reflect the views of the **European Commission** institutions on a particular question at a particular moment, and are strongly advisory. Many of the early **Guidelines** on various aspects of testing of pharmaceutical products to provide information for a **marketing authorization** application were Council Recommendations. The **Committee for Proprietary Medicinal Products** itself has directly issued Guidelines without involving the **Council of Ministers**.

See also **Communications, Decisions, Directives, Opinions, Regulations**.

reconciliation
A comparison, making allowance for normal variation, between the amount of product or materials theoretically and actually produced or used.

record linkage
Bringing together of data on the same individuals, from different sources, e.g. linking hospital discharge data with patients' general practitioner prescriptions. It is normally a very long-term project but particularly useful when looking for truly long-term adverse reactions from drugs or from other factors such as the occurrence of uterine adenocarcinoma in adolescents whose mothers had received diethylstilbestrol during pregnancy.

recovery
The introduction of all or part of previous batches of the required quality into another batch at a defined stage of **manufacture**.

recrudescence
Reappearance of disease in a host whose infection has been **quiescent**.

recruitment (Clinical Trials)
Process used by sponsor to select **investigators** and/or subjects for a clinical study.

recruitment target (Clinical Trials)
Number of subjects that must be recruited into a study to meet the requirements of the study **protocol**. In multicentre studies, each **investigator** has a recruitment target.

Reference Member State (RMS) (European Union)
The **Member State** (MS), within the **European Union**, chosen by the company for a **mutual recognition procedure** for a new application, **variation**, or **renewal**. Recognition by other MSs is based on the recognition by the RMS.

With regard to **pharmacovigilance**, the responsibilities rest with the **competent authorities** of all the MSs in which authorizations are held. For practical reasons, the MSs agree that the RMS will normally take the lead for products authorized through **mutual recognition procedure** and responsibility for producing and evaluating assessment reports. The RMS takes responsibility for the coordination of communication with the **marketing authorization** holders on such matters.

See also **mutual recognition procedure**.

reference range see **normal range**.

referral
The process of sending a patient from one practitioner to another for health care services. **Health Plans** may require that designated primary care providers authorize a referral for coverage of specialty services.

referral bias (Centripetal Bias)
Physicians and medical centres may attract individuals with specific disorders or exposures.

Referral Center (US)
This is a mechanism established by **health plans** to direct patients to approved hospitals and doctors. Often the referral center serves an underwriting function and certifies or pre-certifies the care. These centres are also used by hospitals to refer patients to certain doctors, reduce use of the emergency room or to provide follow-up patient contact. **Managed Care Organizations** utilize these centres as their central hub of communications with patients and providers at the time of service.

Also called Triage, a Call Center, a 24-Hour Certification or a 1-800.

referrals (European Union)
Referrals to the **Committee for Proprietary Medicinal Products**, by **Member States**, the **European Commission** or **MAH**, where there are concerns on safety, quality or efficacy, under:
Article 10 of **Directive 75/319** – arbitration in **MRP**
Article 11 of **Directive 75/319** – divergent decisions
Article 12 of **Directive 75/319** – community interest
Article 15 of **Directive 75/319** – MRP or ex-concertation products.

Regional Health Authority (RHA) (UK)
Formerly, the intermediate tier between the **Department of Health**, on one hand, and the **District Health Authority** and **Family Health Services Authorities** on the other. RHAs worked as a corporate body and were accountable to the Secretary of State. There were 14 RHAs in England. Each RHA had a chairman, five non-executive members appointed by the Secretary of State, and up to five executive members. Two of the executive members, the General Manager and the Chief Finance Officer, are *ex-officio* members. The remainder are appointed by the chairman and non-executive members together with the general manager. RHAs performed a number of functions in the **National Health Service** (NHS) which were concerned with planning, resource allocation and monitoring of performance. They also had a significant part to play in planning the Government's reforms of the NHS. This includes guiding the introduction of **NHS Trusts**, overseeing implementation of new funding systems for general practitioners and NHS authorities, leading the development of contracting and ensuring that the reforms are introduced timely and in a managed way.

As part of the Health Authorities Act, RHAs were abolished with effect from April 1996 and replaced by eight regional offices of the NHS Executive.

See also **District Health Authority**, **National Health Service**, **Special Health Authorities**.

registration
Authorization given to allow marketing, importing, or manufacturing of a **drug**. It is issued by the **regulatory authority**.

Regulation EEC No. 1768/92
   European Union Council regulation concerning the creation of a supplementary protection certificate for **medicinal products**.

Regulation EEC No. 2309/93
   European Union Council regulation laying down Community procedures for the authorization and supervision of **medicinal products** for human and veterinary use and establishing a European agency for the evaluation of medicinal products.

Regulation EEC No. 297/95
   European Union Council regulation concerning the fees payable to the European agency for the evaluation of medicinal products.

Regulation (EC) No. 540/95
   European Commission regulation laying down the arrangements for reporting suspected unexpected **adverse drug reactions** which are not serious, whether arising in the Community or in a third country, to **medicinal products** for human or veterinary use authorized in accordance with the provisions of Council **Regulation EEC No. 2309/93**.

Regulation (EC) No. 541/95
   European Commission regulation concerning the examination of variations to the terms of a **marketing authorization** granted by a **competent authority** of a **Member State**.

Regulation (EC) 542/95
   European Commission regulation concerning the examination of variations to the terms of a **marketing authorization** falling within the scope of Council **Regulation (EEC) No. 2309/93**.

Regulation (EC) No. 1662/95
   European Commission regulation laying down certain detailed arrangements for implementing the Community decision-making procedures in respect of **marketing authorizations** for products for human or veterinary use.

Regulation (EC) 2141/96
   European Commission regulation concerning the examination of an application for the transfer of a **marketing authorization** for a medicinal product falling within the scope of Council **Regulation (EEC) No. 2309/93**.

Regulations
   As applicable to **European Union** law, these are legal instruments which have general scope, a mandatory, binding effect, and the force of law in the **Member State**s (MS) without the need of transformation into national law. They cannot be overridden by national legislation that happen to be incompatible with it. While **Directives** leave the means of achieving the desired results up to the individual MS, regulations are passed through the **European Parliament** and applied to all MS.
   In the US, a regulation is a written rule or order issued by an executive authority of the government having the force of law. US regulations are derived from laws and provide details that are not included in the laws themselves. They are codified in the **Code of Federal Regulations**, which is published annually by the Government Printing Office.
   See also **Communications**, **Decisions**, **Directives**, **Opinions**, **Recommendations**.

Regulatory Affairs
   A pharmaceutical company's department responsible for obtaining **clinical trials**' approvals

from the regulatory authorities by submitting the drug data. They are also responsible for submitting the clinical trials' data to the authorities to obtain a **marketing authorization** (MA)/**product licence** (PL) for marketing the drug. Other functions of this department include the provision of advice on aspects of the national and international governmental Acts on **medicinal products** (e.g. promotional activities) as well as aspects of business development and licensing.

The profession of '**Regulatory Affairs**' developed because in almost all countries of the world, governments have responded to public concern over public health and product **safety** in a number of areas (such as **pharmaceuticals**, veterinary medicines, **medical devices**, **pesticides** and the like) by placing requirements on **manufacturers** to conform to stringent safety testing procedures and obtain MAs before placing products on the market.

Companies having products subject to such legislation have established specialist departments staffed by regulatory affairs professionals whose job it is to: keep track of the legislation in all the regions in which the company wishes to distribute its products; ensure that the product information submitted to the authorities is as complete as possible and in the correct form; and act as the point of subsequent contacts with the **regulatory authorities**. Such professionals also advise on the legal and scientific restraints and requirements, collect, collate, evaluate scientific data and present registration documents (dossiers) to regulatory agencies, and carry out all the subsequent negotiations necessary to obtain and maintain MAs for the products concerned.

Because MAs are issued for a specified time, and have to be renewed before expiry, a very important part of the Regulatory Affairs function consists of the maintenance and updating of existing authorizations, and in handling the inevitable variations that crop up from time to time. It may take anything up to 15 years to develop and launch a new pharmaceutical product and many problems may arise in the process of scientific development. It is the job of the regulatory affairs professional to help the company avoid deficiencies in their data which may create difficulties in the registration of the product. In most product areas where regulatory requirements are imposed, restrictions are also placed upon the claims which can be made for the product on **labelling** or in advertising. The regulatory affairs department will accordingly take part in the development of the product marketing concepts and is usually required to approve packaging and advertising before it is used commercially.

Regulatory Authority (RA)

A government body, consisting of scientific experts and administrators who have the power to regulate and control the use of medicines and research on new drugs.

In the **International Conference on Harmonization** guideline on **good clinical practice**, the expression 'regulatory authorities' includes the authorities that review submitted clinical data and those that conduct inspections. These bodies are sometimes referred to as **competent authorities**.

In order for a RA to be able to issue a **marketing authorization** (MA)/**product licence**), it must carry out a close scrutiny of all the technical reports generated during the development of the product and review the proposed manufacturing methods, quality control procedures and evidence of pharmacological activity, clinical **safety** and **efficacy**. This activity is known as 'assessment' and there is close contact between the assessors and the regulatory affairs staff involved with a particular application.

In broad terms, the assessor will critically review all the scientific evidence presented by the applicant company to establish that the product's quality, safety and efficacy are acceptable and that this evidence supports packaging and product claims. Product safety legislation is often subject to very rapid change in accordance with the development of scientific methods. Of necessity, the regulations and guidelines are based upon a complex combination of law and technology and call for very specialized training and background to interpret correctly.

regulatory documents (Clinical Trials) (US)
The **Food and Drug Administration** (FDA) requires that companies/sponsors submit regulatory documents for all sites where the trial is conducted, most notably a '**FDA Form 1572**', prior to the start of each study. Usually included are agreement contracts, copies of physicians' licences and all required regulatory forms.

relative risk (RR)
The ratio of the probability of developing, in a specified period of time, an **outcome** among those receiving the treatment of interest or exposed to a **risk factor**, compared with the probability of developing the outcome if the risk factor or intervention is not present.

relative risk reduction (RRR)
The per cent reduction in events in the treated group, **experimental event rate** (EER) compared to the **control event rate** (CER) group, i.e. it is the extent to which a treatment reduces a risk, in comparison with patients not receiving the treatment of interest:

$$RRR = \frac{(CER - EER)}{CER} \times 100$$

In clinical studies it is important to look at both the **absolute risk reduction** (ARR) and the RRR. For example, if disease A occurs in 1 in 100 000 people but taking drug X reduces the incidence to 1 in 10 000 000. The absolute risk of disease is 0.001%. The relative risk is 0.00001/0.001 = 0.1 and the RRR is 1−0.1 = 0.9 or 90%, while the ARR is 0.00001 − 0.001 = −0.00099 or 0.099%, which is probably not apparently significant unless the disease is rapidly fatal and the drug has absolutely no side-effects. In contrast, disease B has a **mortality** rate of 50% and drug Y reduces mortality from 50% to 40%. The absolute risk of death with disease B is 0.5 or 50% and the relative risk is 0.4/0.5 = 0.8 or 80%. The RRR is 1−0.8 = 0.2 or 20%, while the ARR is 0.4−0.5 = 0.1 or 10%. In this case the RRR is 20% (much below the RRR for drug X in disease A) while the ARR is much higher, 10%. Therefore, even though the drug is not very effective, you would still prescribe drug Y in disease B to reduce mortality by 10% unless a more effective drug was available.

See also **absolute risk reduction**.

relevance see **applicability**.

relevant market (European Union)
The **European Commission** (EC) adopted a Notice which gives **guidelines** on its procedures for defining the 'relevant market' when investigating mergers and competition cases under Articles 85 and 86 of the EC Treaty. This Notice sets out the criteria used by competition officials in the Commission for assessing the product and geographic market in which a company or group of companies operate. The purpose of the Notice is to provide guidance as to how the EC applies the concept of relevant market and geographic market in its ongoing enforcement of Community competition law.

The Commission emphasizes that the assessment of the relevant market will vary according to the nature of the competition issue being assessed. For example, in a merger investigation the Commission will look at the prospective effects of the new merged entity on competition in the relevant market. While in competition cases under Article 86 (which prohibits an abuse of a dominant position by a company or group of companies), the Commission is essentially looking at the behaviour of the company in the past to decide whether it has abused its position of market power.

Market definition is used to define the boundaries of competition between firms. It gives the Commission a framework in which to apply the competition rules. Market definition makes it possible to calculate whether a company is in a dominant position (Article 86) and whether its agreements with other companies are restrictive of competition on a particular market (Article 85). It also allows the Commission to calculate how a merger between companies will change the structure of a market (EC Merger Regulation). Market definition consists of identifying the competitive constraints that operate on companies in order to assess whether a company has market power. The Commission Notice identifies three main sources of competitive constraints: demand substitutability, supply substitutability and potential competition. The Commission places the most emphasis on demand substitutability.

reliability see **reproducibility**.

remission

The temporary disappearance of a **disease** or its **symptoms**, either partially or completely; also refers to the time period in which this occurs.

renewal

As applied to pharmaceutical licensing in the **European Union**, it is the restoration of an existing **marketing authorization**. Medicines are authorized for a 5-year period. Thereafter a pharmaceutical company must submit a renewal application for each authorization. This application is evaluated, by the relevant national/European regulatory authority (according to the initial route of authorization), in the context of experience with the medicine over the previous 5 years. Consideration is given to any changes in the state of the art of **manufacture, quality assurance**, or clinical practice. Renewal applications need to be accompanied by a **Periodic Safety Update Report** listing any **adverse drug reactions** recorded since the last renewal.

repeatability see **reproducibility**.

repeat-dose toxicity studies

A term that is interchangeable but preferable to 'sub-acute' and 'chronic' tests. National regulatory authorities differ in their requirements for these tests. It is necessary to examine a range of doses so that any likely effect will be produced and the dose–response relationship and reversibility can be examined. The route of administration used should, as far as possible, be that intended for humans. The species used must include two mammalian species: a rodent and a non-rodent. The concentration of the drug in plasma is assayed so that it is possible to check that animals have been dosed on any given day or whether there is any build-up.

replacement subject (Clinical Trials)

A subject who replaces another previously enrolled into a study and is not reassigned a new patient number or randomized (if randomization was applicable).

reportable adverse reaction

In the **European Union**, a reportable adverse reaction requires the following minimum information:
1. an identifiable **health care professional** – the reporter can be identified by either name, initials, or address or qualifications (e.g. physician, dentist, pharmacist, coroner, nurse)

2. an identifiable **patient** – the patient can be identified by initials or patient number, or date of birth (or age information if date of birth not available) or sex.
3. at least one suspected substance/**medicinal product**.
4. at least one suspected **adverse drug reaction**.

The minimum information is the smallest amount of information required for the submission of a report.

representative see **legally acceptable representative**.

reprocessing
The reworking of all or part of a batch of product of an unacceptable quality from a defined stage of production so that its quality may be rendered acceptable by one or more additional operations.

rescue medication (Clinical Trials)
Medicine offered to a patient in case the **investigational product** (which could be the **placebo**) is not successful in controlling some **symptom** of the patient's illness. The majority of rescue medications are **analgesics**.

research and development phase
The initial phase of **drug product** development. It generally includes laboratory 'bench top' formulation and testing; sometimes it can include **preclinical** studies as well.

research base
An institution or cooperative group that assumes a broad range of responsibilities and functions for the support of **clinical trials** conducted under its name. It supports the **investigator** in developing, organizing, implementing and analysing clinical trials. It assumes responsibility for the quality of the research, both in concept and execution, and has an important role in assuring patient **safety**.

research ethics
This term is used broadly to include many ethically significant issues that arise in research, from fair apportionment of credit among members of a research team, to responsible behaviour in submitting or reviewing grant applications, to responsible treatment of research subjects. In the US, since the government and institutional regulations regarding the treatment of human and animal research subjects pre-dated the increased attention and regulation of matters of research integrity (including fair credit) that began in the 1980s, some sources on the responsible conduct of research address only issues of research integrity and not the treatment of research subjects. Similarly, laboratory safety has long been regulated by the **Occupational Health Safety Administration**, and is not a matter of research integrity. Therefore, it too is often omitted from discussions of responsible behaviour in research. For example, *On Being a Scientist, Responsible Conduct in Research*, put out by the National Academies (NAS, NAE, IOM), in both its first and second edition omits any discussion of the treatment of research subjects, or laboratory safety. The treatment of research subjects and laboratory safety are reasonably classed as matters of research ethics, even if they are not always included under this designation.

Research Ethics Board (REB) (Canada)
Every institution or hospital that conducts research involving human subjects must, under guidelines issued by the **Medical Research Council**, have a REB that initially approves and

periodically reviews the research to protect the rights of the people in the trial. The REB is made up of people from various communities who are not involved in the research being done.
See also **Ethics Committee**, **Institutional Review Board**.

research fraud see fraud.

research hypothesis see hypothesis.

response model
Systems to measure how well a compound binds to the **receptor** (**ligand** binding assays) and to measure the biological effect of a compound in cell-based assays.

responsible person (RP) (European Union)
According to **European Union** law, as stated in **Directive 92/25/EEC**, is a person who is responsible for safeguarding product users against potential hazards arising from poor distribution practices – as a result, for example, of purchasing suspect products, poor storage or failure to establish the bona fides of purchasers. The RP's responsibilities include certifying that the conditions of the **wholesale dealer's licence** are met and the **good design practice** guidelines are followed.

restriction (specification) (Clinical Trials)
Eligibility for entry into an analytic study is restricted to individuals within a certain range of values for a confounding factor, such as age, to reduce the effect of the **confounding factor** when it cannot be controlled by randomization. Restriction limits the external validity (generalizability) to those with the same confounder values.

retrospective study (Clinical Trials)
A study design in which the trialists select patients, who had an outcome event in question and who satisfy the inclusion and **exclusion criteria**, and collate their clinical data from their records after the outcomes have occurred. The data is then analysed in the normal way to establish risk, incidence, treatment efficacy, etc.
See also **case–control study**.

RFDD (US)
Regional Food and Drug Director.

RHA see Regional Health Authority.

ringfencing
The identification of funds to be used for a particular purpose only, e.g. mental illness-specific grant.

risk–benefit ratio
1. The risk of causing side-effects versus the therapeutic benefit from having a medical intervention (drugs, surgical, etc.). The acceptability of the risk depends on the disease in question. For example, side-effects such as nausea may be acceptable for a beneficial cancer chemotherapy but not for a sore throat medicine.
2. (Clinical Trials) The relation between the risks and benefits of a given treatment or procedure. The **Ethics Committee** (or **Investigational Review Board** in the US) located where the study is to take place, determine that the risks in a study are reasonable with respect to the potential benefits. It is also up to patients to decide if it is reasonable for them to take part in a study.

risk factor
1. Patient characteristics or factors associated with an increased probability of developing a condition or disease in the first place. Neither risk nor prognostic factors necessarily imply a cause and effect relationship. Risk factors include anything that raises the chance that a person will get a disease. For example, in non-insulin-dependent diabetes patients have a greater risk of getting the disease if they weigh a lot more (20% or more) than they should.
    Compare **prognostic factors**.
2. (Pharmacoeconomics) Any characteristic, behaviour, or condition which, based on history, utilization, or theory, is thought to directly influence susceptibility to a specific health problem, increase costs or result in increased utilization.

risk ratio
The ratio of risk in the treated group (EER) to the risk in the control group (CER): RR = EER/CER. RR is used in randomized trials and cohort studies.
Where: CER = control event rate, EER = experimental event rate.

RL (US)
Regulatory Letter (**Food and Drug Administration** Post-audit Letter).

RMN
Registered Mental Nurse.

RMO
1. Resident Medical Officer.
2. Responsible Medical Officer.

RMS see **Reference Member State**.

RN
Registered Nurse.

roborant
Former term for a **tonic**.

Royal Pharmaceutical Society of Great Britain (RPSGB) (UK)
Founded in 1841 by a group of leading London chemists and druggists to fend off the threat to their livelihood posed by a Bill before Parliament that sought to reform the law governing the practice of medicine. The Bill would have placed chemists and druggists, as pharmacists were then known, under the control of apothecaries, or general practitioners, and would have effectively prevented them from giving advice on the treatment of minor ailments and recommending **over-the-counter** treatments.
The RPSGB has a membership of 42 000 and performs various roles:
- Acting as the registration and professional body for pharmacists
- Safeguarding the public, and regulating and promoting the profession
- Maintaining the Register of Pharmaceutical Chemists and a register of pharmacy premises
- Management of four Membership groups:
    - Agricultural and Veterinary Pharmacists Group
    - Community Pharmacists Group
    - Hospital Pharmacists Group
    - Industrial Pharmacists Group
- **Joint Formulary Committee of RPSGB and the British Medical Association**

(together with the **Department of Health** for the co-production of the **British National Formulary**)
- Management of two special interest groups:
  - Academic Pharmacy Group
  - **Pharmaceutical Sciences Group**
- Management of other groups:
  - British Pharmaceutical Students Association (BPSA)
  - **Joint Pharmaceutical Analysis Group** (JPAG)
- Publication of:
  - *The Pharmaceutical Journal*
  - *Hospital Pharmacist*
  - *The Pharmacy Assistant*
  - *International Journal of Pharmacy Practice*
  - *Industrial Pharmacist*
  - *Agricultural and Veterinary Pharmacist*
  - *Tomorrow's Pharmacist*
- Overseas activities:
  - Administration of The Commonwealth Pharmaceutical Association (CPA)
  - Representing the profession at the:
    - EU Pharmacy Group
    - EU Advisory Committee on Pharmaceutical Education and Training
    - The WHO Europharm Forum.

Royal Society of Chemistry (RSC) (UK)

A learned and professional society with a worldwide membership of 6000. It has as its main objective the advancement of the science of chemistry and its applications, and the maintenance of high standards of competence and integrity among practising chemists. The Society has been involved with the publication of scientific literature since 1841. Surplus generated from sales funds the promotion of chemistry.

RPSGB see **Royal Pharmaceutical Society of Great Britain**.

RRR see **relative risk reduction**

RSAF
Rating Scale for Affective Flattening.

RSC see **The Royal Society of Chemistry**.

RSM (UK)
Royal Society of Medicine.

RSS (UK)
Royal Statistical Society.

R&TD
Research and Technological Development.

Rules Governing Medicinal Products in the European Community (EC) (EC texts)
Published as a series of volumes by the Office of Official Publications of the European Communities in Luxemburg. The individual volumes are as follows:
Volume I: The rules governing **medicinal products** for human use in the EC.

Volume II: Notice to applicants for **marketing authorization** for medicinal products for human use in the **Member States** of the **European Community**.
Volume IIA: Procedures for marketing authorization.
Volume IIB: Presentation and content of the application dossier.
Volume III: Guidelines on the **quality, safety** and **efficacy** of medicinal products for human use.
Volume IV: Guide to **good manufacturing practice** of medicinal products.
Volume V: The rules governing medicinal products for veterinary use in the **European Community**.
Volume VI: Notice to applicants on veterinary medicinal products.
Volume VII: Guidelines on veterinary medicinal products.
Volume VIII: Maximum residue limits in veterinary medicinal products.
Volume IX: **Pharmacovigilance** on medicinal products for human use and veterinary medicinal products.

Volume I is the text of the directives. It does not include the text of some of the later Directives (e.g. 89/341/EEC, 89/342/EEC).

An addendum to Volume III was published in 1990. This contains the following guidelines (with their date of adoption by the **Committee for Proprietary Medicinal Products** (CPMP) in brackets).

- Analytical validation (July 1989)
- European drug master file procedure for **active ingredients** (July 1990)
- Production and quality control of cytokine products derived by means of biotechnological process (February 1990)
- Production and **quality control** of human monoclonal antibodies (July 1990)
- **Good clinical practice** for trials on medicinal products in the European Community (July 1990)
- Clinical testing of prolonged action forms with special reference to extended release forms (July 1990)
- Evaluation of anticancer medicinal products in man (July 1990)
- Medicinal products for the treatment of epileptic disorders (revision of earlier version of guideline, December 1989)
- **Data sheets** for antibacterial medicinal products (revision, November 1989).

As guidelines often represent a considerable change to existing practices, they are now given a date on which they should be applied. This is normally 6 months from the date of adoption by the CPMP and the issue of the guideline to the European pharmaceutical industry associations.

All of these publications are available from sales points/distributors/bookshops selling the official publications of the European Community. In the USA, these publications are available from:

UNIPUB
4611 F Assembly Drive
Lanham
MD 20706-4391 USA
Tel: + 1(800) 274 4888

In Japan, these publications are available from:

Kinokuniya Company Ltd
17-7 Shinjuku-ku 3-Chome
Shinuku-ku

Tokyo 160-91, Japan
Tel: + 81(03) 354 0131

For other countries (outside the European Community), these publications may be ordered from:

Office des Publications Officielles des Communautés Européennes.
2, rue Mercier
L-2985 Luxembourg
Tel: + 352 49 92 81

run-in period (Clinical Trials)

A period, at the beginning of a **clinical trial**, during which it is necessary to take patients off their existing medication (if any) and sometimes a non-active trial drug is provided, often used to reduce (effects of) previous treatments, or to establish baseline severity of illness/eligibility for the trial. Often, this period (which may be 7 or 14 days) may also be used to confirm the diagnosis over a longer period of time.

Rx

Common abbreviation for 'prescription'.

Rx List (US)

Free, searchable database of more than 4000 **prescription** and **over-the-counter** (US) drug products on the web. Currently contains simple information, such as generic and brand name, and therapeutic category. Contains top 200 prescribed drugs.

S1 guidance documents
International Conference on Harmonization (ICH) guidance documents on 'Carcinogenicity'.
See also **S1A guidance document, S1B guidance document, S1C guidance document, S1C(R) guidance document**.

S1A guidance document
An International Conference on Harmonization (ICH) guidance document on 'Carcinogenicity' entitled 'Guideline on the Need for Carcinogenicity of Pharmaceuticals'.
See also **S1B guidance document, S1C guidance document, S1C(R) guidance document**.

S1B guidance document
An International Conference on Harmonization (ICH) guidance document on 'Carcinogenicity' entitled 'Testing for Carcinogenicity of Pharmaceuticals'.
See also **S1A guidance document, S1C guidance document, S1C(R) guidance document**.

S1C guidance document
An International Conference on Harmonization (ICH) guidance document on 'Carcinogenicity' entitled 'Dose Selection for Carcinogenicity Studies of Pharmaceuticals'.
See also **S1A guidance document, S1B guidance document, S1C(R) guidance document**.

S1C(R) guidance document
An International Conference on Harmonization (ICH) guidance document on 'Carcinogenicity' entitled 'Addendum to the Dose Selection for Carcinogenicity Studies of Pharmaceuticals: Addition of a Dose Limit and Related Notes'.
See also **S1A guidance document, S1B guidance document, S1C guidance document**.

S2 guidance documents
International Conference on Harmonization (ICH) guidance documents on 'Genotoxicity'.
See also **S2A guidance document, S2B guidance document, S3 guidance documents**.

S2A guidance documents
An International Conference on Harmonization (ICH) guidance document on 'Genotoxicity' entitled 'Genotoxicity: Guidance on Specific Aspects of Regulatory Genotoxicity Tests for Pharmaceuticals'.
See also **S2B guidance document, S3 guidance documents**.

S2B guidance document
An International Conference on Harmonization (ICH) guidance document on 'Genotoxicity' entitled 'Genotoxicity: A Standard Battery of Genotoxicity Testing of Pharmaceuticals'.
See also **S2A guidance document, S3 guidance documents**.

S3 guidance documents
International Conference on Harmonization (ICH) guidance documents on 'Kinetics'.
See also **S3A guidance document, S3B guidance document**.

S3A guidance document
An International Conference on Harmonization (ICH) guidance document on 'Kinetics'

entitled 'Note for Guidance on Toxicokinetics: the Assessment of Systemic Exposure in Toxicity Studies'.
See also **S3A guidance document**.

S3B guidance document
An **International Conference on Harmonization** (ICH) guidance document on 'Kinetics' entitled 'Pharmacokinetics: Guidance for Repeated Dose Tissue Distribution Studies'.
See also **S3A guidance document**.

S4 guidance document
An **International Conference on Harmonization** (ICH) guidance document on 'Toxicity' entitled 'Duration of Chronic Toxicity Testing in Animals (Rodent and Non-rodent Toxicity Testing)'.

S5 guidance documents
International Conference on Harmonization (ICH) guidance documents on 'Reprotoxicity'.
See also **S5A guidance document**, **S5B guidance document**.

S5A guidance document
An **International Conference on Harmonization** (ICH) guidance document on 'Reprotoxicity' entitled 'Detection of Toxicity to Reproduction for Medicinal Products'.
See also **S5B guidance document**.

S5B guidance document
An **International Conference on Harmonization** (ICH) guidance document on 'Reprotoxicity' entitled 'An Addendum on Toxicity to Male Fertility'.
See also **S5A guidance document**.

S6 guidance document
An **International Conference on Harmonization** (ICH) guidance document on 'Biotechnological Safety' entitled 'Preclinical Safety Evaluation of Biotechnology-derived Pharmaceuticals'.

SAC
1. Standardized Assessment of Causality.
2. Safety Assessment Candidate.

SAC-PM see **Specialist Advisory Committee on Pharmaceutical Medicine**.

safety
Relative freedom from harm; in **clinical trials**, this refers to an absence of harmful **side effects** resulting from use of the product and may be assessed by laboratory testing of biological samples, special tests and procedures, psychiatric evaluation, and/or physical examination of subjects. A **drug product** is considered safe if it does not pose a risk to public health when used in accordance with its **labelling**.

Safety and Efficacy Register of New Interventional Procedures (SERNIP) (UK)
Set up under the auspices of the Academy of Medical Royal Colleges in May 1996, with a remit to proscribe unsafe procedures, limit dissemination of unproven techniques and promote primary research into **safety** and **efficacy**.

SERNIP investigates new procedures as they are notified to the secretariat. Advice is sought from the clinicians involved, their specialty associations, experts in the field, device suppliers and the **Medical Devices Agency** (MDA). Systematic literature searches are then undertaken and various **health technology assessment** organizations contacted. A synthesis of the data relating to safety and efficacy is then circulated to members of the SERNIP Advisory Committee, which meets quarterly to discuss these data.

A simple system of grading the safety and efficacy of new procedures has evolved over the 3 years:

A Safety and efficacy established: procedure may be used
B Efficacy established: further evaluation required to confirm safety: procedure can be used as part of a surveillance programme registered with SERNIP
C Safety and efficacy not proven: procedure should be used only as part of a primary research programme, using appropriate methodology and registered with SERNIP
D Safety and/or efficacy shown to be unsatisfactory: procedure should not be used.

From its inception, SERNIP has had close links with the Standing Group on Health Technology (SGHT), **Medicines Research Council** and MDA. Recently, liaison with the surgical community has been strengthened by appointing the President of the Federation of Surgical Specialty Associations (FSSA) to the Advisory Committee. SERNIP have also established a formal link with the **ABHI** and are considering co-opting a consumer representative.

Safety Assessment of Marketed Medicine (SAMM) Study (UK)

A formal investigation conducted for the purpose of assessing the clinical **safety** of marketed medicine(s) in clinical practice. It was developed by collaboration between several organizations and guidelines were published in 1993. They took the place of previous guidelines on post-marketing surveillance which were published in 1988. SAMM studies may be undertaken to identify previously unrecognized safety issues or to investigate likely risks and must not be conducted for the purposes of promotion. Various study designs may be appropriate for a SAMM study including **case–control** and **cohort** observational studies. **Clinical trials**, involving systematic allocation of treatment, may also be used to evaluate the safety of marketed products. These studies must also comply with the guidelines for phase IV trials.

Safety, Efficacy and Adverse Reactions Subcommittee (SEARS) (UK)

A subcommittee of the **Committee on Safety of Medicines**, now disbanded, that was involved with drug **safety** surveillance and evaluation of new drugs. It was one of three advisory committees available to the **Medicines Control Agency**.

safety margin see **standardized safety margin and therapeutic index**.

safety profile

History of a drug safety record.

Safety Update Report (US)

Reports that a **New Drug Application sponsor** must submit to the **Food and Drug Administration** (FDA) about any new **safety** information that may affect the use for which the drug will be approved, or draft **labelling** statements about contraindications, warnings, precautions and adverse reactions. Safety Update Reports are required 4 months after the application is submitted, after the applicant receives an approvable letter, and at other times upon FDA request.

Compare **Periodic Safety Update Report**.

Sales Representative see **Medical Representative**.

salivary excretion

This is not really a method of drug excretion as the drug will usually be swallowed and reabsorbed, thus a form of 'salivary recycling'. Drug excretion into saliva appears to be dependent on **pH partition** and protein binding. This mechanism appears attractive in terms of drug monitoring, i.e. determining drug concentration to assist in drug dosage adjustment. For some drugs, the saliva/free plasma ratio is fairly constant. Therefore drug concentrations in saliva could be a good indication of drug concentration in plasma. For some drugs, localized **side-effects** may be due to salivary excretion of the drug.

SAMM see **Safety Assessment of Marketed Medicines**.

sample (Clinical Trials)
A sub-group or subset of a patient **population** that is used for study in a **clinical trial**. Every attempt should be made to ensure that the sample is representative of the population, including the use of **random** mechanisms.

sample size (n) (Clinical Trials)
The number of **subjects** in a study's **sample**. The larger the sample size, the greater the precision and thus **power** for a given study design to detect an effect of a given size. For statisticians, an $n > 30$ is usually sufficient for the Central Limit Theorem to hold so that normal theory approximations can be used for measures such as the **standard error of the mean**. However, this sample size ($n = 30$) is unrelated to the clinicians' objective of detecting biologically significant effects, which determines the specific sample size needed for a specific study. **Type I** and **type II** errors, the desired **power**, the **signal-to-noise** ratio, and the design of the study are all affected by the sample size.

sampling biases (Clinical Trials)
Systematic error that occurs when there are design and execution errors in sampling, selection, or allocation methods, or when the study comparisons are between groups that differ with respect to the outcome of interest for reasons other than those under study.
Also called **selection biases**.

SAPO (UK)
Specified Animal Pathogens Order 1993.

SAR see **structure–activity relationship**.

SAS (Statistics)
Statistical Analysis System.

SBA (US)
Summary Basis of Approval.

s-c
Sugar-coated drug product.

scabicide
An insecticide suitable for the eradication of mite infestations in humans (scabies).

scale up
The expansion of the manufacturing process of a new drug from research-sized batches to commercial production.

ScHARR see **School of Health and Related Research**.

schistosomicide
An agent that destroys schistosomes, i.e. flukes of the genus *Schistosoma*, causative organism of schistosomiasis.

School of Health and Related Research (ScHARR) (UK)

One of the four schools in the Faculty of Medicine at the University of Sheffield, ScHARR is a university-based concentration of health related resources in Trent and one of the most important in the UK.

ScHARR brings together a wide range of health related skills including *inter alia*: **health economics**, operational research, management sciences, **epidemiology**, medical **statistics** and information science. There are also clinical skills in general practice and **primary care**, psychiatry, rehabilitation and public health. It includes the Medical Care Research Unit, the Institute of General Practice and Primary Care, and the Sections of Public Health, Health Policy and Management, Psychiatry (including Forensic Psychiatry), Health Economics, Operational Research and Information Resources.

SCI

Science Citation Index.

Science Reference and Information Service (SRIS) (UK)

A division within the British Library (BL) that provides access to the BL reference collection in the life sciences, earth sciences and mathematics. Life sciences include biotechnology and medicine but exclude nursing and health service administration. SRIS is freely available for reference use; telephone and written enquiries are accepted.

scientific fraud see fraud.

scientific hypothesis see hypothesis.

scientific knowledge

The current set of peer-evaluated consensus models about how natural phenomena work, which often differ between groups of researchers at the research frontier. These models are established by evidence obtained from critical scientific inquiry that has been subjected to peer evaluation and replication. All scientific knowledge contains varying degrees of uncertainty and is constantly at varying risk of being modified or dismissed as the result of evidence from further inquiry. Models are disproved by multiple findings of discrepant evidence, which is often the result of improvements in measurement technology.

scientific method

The basic approach to conducting any scientific experiment, including a **clinical trial**, that involves stating a **hypothesis**, designing a study to answer the **hypothesis**, gathering data, interpreting the results, and drawing conclusions. It is the conceptual process of organizing empirical facts and their inter-relationships in a structure of theories and inferences. Scientific methods are the philosophical ideals of how scientists advance scientific knowledge by methodically and systematically applying procedures that reduce the likelihood of alternative explanations for their observations. The underlying principles are scepticism (an attitude of doubt), determinism (the principle that all natural phenomena are caused by previous events linked by fundamental physical laws that are the same everywhere in the universe) and empiricism (the practice of relying on observation and experiment for developing an understanding (theory) of natural phenomena).

scientific paradigm

The model shared by most but not all members of a scientific community, designed to describe and interpret observed or inferred phenomena, past or present, and aimed at building a testable body of knowledge open to rejection or confirmation. (Shermer, M. Why People Believe Weird Things [WH Freeman and Co, 1997]).

scientific research

The systematic, controlled, empirical and critical investigation of hypothetical propositions about the presumed relations among natural phenomena (Kerlinger, F. Foundations of behavioural research [Holt, Rinehart and Winston Inc., 1964]). It is the objective inquiry into natural phenomena using currently accepted investigation procedures, the immediate product of which is evidence, with the objective of discovering how that aspect of the physical world works. Scientific research also represents an empirical, conceptual system of learning about the physical world that organizes publicly observable facts and reasoning within a structure of theories and inferences. The methods of inquiry are constructed to minimize the effects of natural human biases in observation and interpretation. By convention, the evidence, the procedures used to acquire it, and subsequent interpretation is subjected to peer evaluation as a prelude to publication in the **primary source** literature where it is publicly available for further scrutiny and use.

Scientific Steering Committee (SSC) – DG XXIV (European Union)

Set up by the **European Commission** to coordinate the work of the scientific committees. Membership comprises eight scientific experts not involved in other scientific committees and the chairpersons of the eight scientific committees. The chairman of the SSC is elected from amongst the membership.

scientific theory

The articulate, interrelated structure of scientific propositions and principles derived over time from scientific evidence that explains a class of observed phenomena or facts. Theories enable us to make sense of what we see and to make predictions. A scientific theory must have predictive power (predict phenomena that can be observed) and must be testable and falsifiable (the theory is false if the predicted phenomena are not observed in the appropriate experiment). A scientific theory must be consistent both internally and with broader, more fundamental theories related to other aspects of the phenomena. For example, a theory of disease treatment cannot be inconsistent with most of the more fundamental theories of chemistry. Although a theory that is consistent with a diversity of evidence generally is stronger (more certain) than one that is not, a theory cannot be proven as an absolute certainty (absolute truth) and is always at some risk of modification if not replacement. To replace a previously held theory, the new theory must explain those phenomena explained by the previous theory as well as those it did not adequately explain. Note that in non-scientific contexts the word theory is often used to mean a mere hypothesis or speculation, a much less reliable proposition than is a scientific theory.

sclerosing agent

An irritant suitable for injection into varicose veins to induce their fibrosis and obliteration.

SCM

Specialist in Community Medicine.

SCOP (UK)

Subcommittee on Pharmacovigilance, see **Committee on Safety of Medicines**.

SCOPME (UK)

Standing Committee On Postgraduate Medical Education.

Scottish Intercollegiate Guidelines Network (SIGN) (UK)

Established in 1993 by the Academy of Royal Colleges and their Faculties in Scotland to develop evidence-based clinical guidelines for the **National Health Service** (NHS) in Scotland. Membership of SIGN includes representatives of the Scottish and UK Royal Medical Colleges, dentistry, nursing, pharmacy, other professions allied to medicine, and patients. Pharmacy is represented by the **Royal Pharmaceutical Society of Great Britain** (Scottish Department).

SIGN supports over 50 working groups developing guidelines for a wide range of clinical conditions and is responsible for publishing and distributing these guidelines throughout the NHS in Scotland. The SIGN programme is coordinated by a small secretariat based at the Royal College of Physicians of Edinburgh. Funding for the SIGN initiative is provided by the Clinical Resource and Audit Group (CRAG) of the Scottish Executive **Department of Health**. SIGN guidelines are distributed free of charge within the NHS in Scotland.

screening
1. The testing of an otherwise healthy person in order to diagnose disorders at an early stage.
2. (Clinical Trials) The process of determining which patients are good candidates for a study, done by asking questions and conducting medical tests. Preliminary screening is done by phone, and the medical tests are done on the patient's first visit. Screening and the inclusion/**exclusion criteria** for studies are done to protect the patient's **safety**.
3. The use of automated or half-automated *in vitro* biochemical assays, such as **ligand** binding assays, or cell-based assays to detect a large number of compounds which modulate the activity of a target (e.g. enzyme inhibitors, **receptor agonists** or **antagonists**).

screening bias
The **bias** that occurs when the presence of a disease is detected earlier during its **latent period** by screening tests but the course of the disease is not changed by earlier intervention. Because the survival after screening detection is longer than survival after detection of clinical **signs**, ineffective interventions appear to be effective unless they are compared appropriately in **clinical trials**.

SCT (US)
Society for Clinical Trials.

SD see **standard deviation**.

SDI
Selective Dissemination of Information.

SDV see **source data verification**.

SEA
Single European Act of 1987.

SEARS see **Safety, Efficacy and Adverse Reactions Subcommittee**.

secondary containment
A system of containment which prevents the escape of a biological agent into the external environment or into other working areas. It involves the use of rooms with specially designed air handling, the existence of airlocks and/or sterilizers for the exit of materials and secure operating procedures. In many cases it may add to the effectiveness of primary containment.
See also **clean/contained area, contained area, containment**.

secondary source
An information source that does not have as a major component the description of formal

observations or experiments but rather is synthesized from some combination of primary sources, experience, or authoritative belief (dogma). The primary literature used may have been selected in a biased or incomplete fashion and may have been used without comprehensive critical appraisal to establish the relative strength of evidence in each source. Examples of secondary sources are review articles, journals specializing in practitioner-oriented reviews, most practitioner-oriented conference proceedings, trade publications, most e-mail conversations, and authorities presenting information without supporting evidence in whatever format (lectures, CE meetings, e-mail forums).

See also **integrative source**, **primary source**, **tertiary source**.

second messenger
An intracellular **metabolite** or ion increasing or decreasing as a response to the stimulation of **receptors** by **agonists** (considered as the 'first messenger'). This generic term usually does not prejudge the rank order of intracellular biochemical events.

seeding trial (Clinical Trials)
Trials carried out with the aim of improving the marketing profile of the **drug product**. Unlike true post-marketing, phase IV, studies, seeding trials tend to lack **compliance** with **good clinical practice** and are **open** in design.

SEER (US)
Surveillance, **Epidemiology** and End Results.

selection bias (Statistics)
A **bias** in assignment or a **confounding factor** that arises from study design rather than by chance. These can occur when the study and **control** groups are chosen so that they differ from each other by one or more factors that may affect the **outcome** of the study.

SEM see standard error of the mean.

SEN
State Enrolled Nurse.

Senior House Officer (SHO)
Hospital practitioner grade after registration.

Sen. Reg.
Senior Registrar.

sensitivity
The proportion of truly diseased persons, as measured by the gold standard, who are identified as diseased by the test under study. It represents the ability of a test to work on people who have infection. More precisely TP/(TP+FN), where TP is the number of true positives and FN is the number of false negatives.

sequential trials (Clinical Trials)
A trial design that allows two treatments to be compared using a small number of patients. Using a cross-over technique ensures such possibility.

serious adverse event (AE)/serious adverse drug reaction (ADR)
According to **International Conference on Harmonization**, an AE/ADR is defined as 'serious' if it is at least one of the following:
- Fatal
- **Life-threatening**

- Requires **inpatient** hospitalization or prolongs hospitalization
- Results in persistent or significant disability/incapacity
- Requires medical intervention to prevent permanent impairment or damage
- Causes a **congenital** anomaly/birth defect
- An event which may jeopardize the patient or may require intervention to prevent any of the above.

Expedited reporting is a legal requirement in these cases. Medical and scientific judgement should be exercised in deciding whether expedited reporting is appropriate in other situations, such as important medical events that may not be immediately life-threatening or result in death or hospitalization but may jeopardize the patient or may require intervention to prevent one of the other outcomes listed in the definition above.

See also **adverse drug reaction, adverse event**.

SERNIP see Safety and Efficacy Register of New Interventional Procedures.

seroprevalence
The proportion of a **population** who are seropositive.

service agreement (UK)
Alternative term for '**contract**' used in the **National Health Service**. It reflects that a contract is 'an agreement enforceable by law' whilst a service agreement is not. Favoured by the Labour Government and used in the 1998/9 planning guidance.

SHA
1. See **Special Health Authorities**.
2. Specialist Health Association.

Sherley Amendment (US)
An amendment to the 1906 food and drug law that made false and fraudulent therapeutic drug claims by a manufacturer illegal.

SHO see Senior House Officer.

SI
1. Statutory Instrument.
2. *Systéme Internationale*, International System.

sialagogue
An agent that promotes the flow of saliva.

side-effect
A non-specific term used to describe an unwanted effect of a drug or other form of therapy but not discriminating between an **adverse event** (AE) and an **adverse drug reaction** (ADR). Note that the term is sometimes used to imply an ADR predictable on pharmacological grounds (i.e. a **type A reaction**).

It usually, but not necessarily, connotes an undesirable effect. For instance, in the treatment of peptic ulcer with atropine, dryness of the mouth is a side-effect and decreased gastric secretion is the desired drug effect. If the same drug was being used to inhibit salivation, dryness of the mouth would be the therapeutic effect and decreased gastric secretion would be a side-effect.

Pharmacological side-effects are true drug effects. With increasing doses of a drug, the intensity of pharmacological side-effects in individuals, and/or the frequency with which a pharmacological side-effect is observed in a population is increased.

The term 'side-effect' is an old, and evidently vague, term. It is recommended that this term no longer be used and particularly should not be regarded as synonymous with an AE or ADR.

Compare **allergic response, dose–response curve, idiosyncratic response.**

SIGAR see **Special Interest Group on Adverse Reactions and pharmacovigilance.**

sign
A mark or indication of a particular disorder that is noticed by the doctor examining a patient but not by the patient himself.
Compare **symptom**.

SIGN see **Scottish Intercollegiate Guidelines Network.**

signal-to-noise ratio
The ratio of the supposed effect of a new intervention on a particular study **outcome** (signal) to the variation (**noise**) in the outcome. A hypothesized value of this ratio is required in order to calculate **sample size**.

significance level (Statistics)
The probability of rejecting a true **null hypothesis** in a statistical test or the probability of a **type I (alpha) error**. Although significance level is relative and dependent on the interpreted clinical significance, it is usually set at the 5% level.

significance tests (Statistics)
Tests applied to a set of data, which seek to establish whether the results could have occurred by chance, and therefore their 'significance'.

significant risk device
An investigational **medical device** that presents a potential for serious risk to the health, **safety**, or welfare of the subject.

SII
Science Index Impact.

simple randomization (Clinical Trials)
A procedure that uses a code to assign all subjects to receive different **investigational products** or treatments at the start of the **clinical trial**.
See also **randomization**.

single-blind clinical trial
Typically, a study design in which the **investigator**/assessor, but not the subject, knows the identity of the treatment assignment. Occasionally the subject, but not the investigator, knows the assignment. Sometimes called 'single-blind design'.

single fault condition (UK)
Condition in which a single means for protection against hazards is defective or a single external abnormal hazardous condition is present in a **medical device**.

single-masked design see **single-blind clinical trial.**

site (Clinical Trials) see **trial site.**

site audit (Clinical Trials)
The audit conducted at the study site. It may be internal (conducted by the company, **sponsor**

or **contract research organization**) or it may be external (from the regulatory authorities, such as the **Food and Drug Administration, Medicines Control Agency,** etc.).

site-specific delivery
An approach to target a **drug** to a specific tissue, using **prodrugs** or antibody recognition systems.

site visit (Clinical Trials)
A visit by the **regulatory authority** officials, representatives, or consultants to the location of a research activity to assess the ethical adequacy (**Investigational Review Board,** or **Ethics Committee**) of protection of human subjects or the capability of personnel to conduct the research.

skew (Statistics)
Non-symmetrical data set. This can be right-skew where the larger data are spread out while the small data are close together or it can be a left-skew where the larger data are close together while the small data are spread out.

skin patch
A sticky patch attached to the surface of the skin that releases drugs into the bloodstream.

slow release see **sustained release**.

SM
Single market.

SMART
1. (US) Submission Management and Review Tracking (**Food and Drug Administration**).
2. **S**pecific, **M**easurable, **A**ttainable, **R**elevant and **T**imed. A notation describing a good objective.

SMDA (US)
Safe Medical Devices Act (1990).

SME
Significant medical event.

SMO (Clinical Trials)
Site Management Organization.

SmPC see **Summary of Product Characteristics**.

SMR see **standardized mortality rate**.

SMT see **specialist medical training**.

SNDA see **Supplemental NDA**.

SNIF
Summary Notification Information Format.

SNIP
1. see **Strength, New, Importance and Potential for prevention**.
2. (France) *Syndicat National De L'Industrie Pharmaceutique*. French pharmaceutical industry association.

SnNout
When a sign/test has a high **sen**sitivity, a **n**egative result rules **out** the diagnosis, e.g. the sensitivity of a history of ankle swelling for diagnosing ascites is 92%, therefore if a person does not have a history of ankle swelling, it is highly unlikely that the person has ascites.

See also **SpPin**.

SNOMED
Systematized nomenclature of medicine.

SOC
System/Organ Class (or Classification). The classification of **adverse events** or listing of drugs (e.g. in formularies) by body systems (e.g. gastrointestinal).

Society of Pharmaceutical Medicine (SPM) (UK)
The Society was founded in 1987 with a specific remit to be a multidisciplinary organization covering all facts of drugs discovery and development – both within the pharmaceutical industry and also outside.

The SPM aims to:
- promote the acquisition and dissemination of knowledge concerning the action and development of **medicinal products** as well as their application in therapeutics
- arrange meetings as appropriate between those engaged in aspects of **pharmaceutical medicine**
- promote a closer relationship between physicians and scientists in the fields of **pharmacology**, **toxicology**, drug **metabolism**, clinical research, clinical pharmacology, therapeutics and drug development
- ensure that the Society activities are in the overall interests of persons suffering from, or at risk from illness and disease.

The Society has successfully linked up with other groups to hold joint meetings with added value, e.g. the International League Against Epilepsy, the Society for Drug Research, The Association of Cancer Physicians and the **ACRIPI**. The Society's meetings have also progressed into more general areas of interest, e.g. **pharmacoeconomics**, implications of **National Health Service** changes for the conduct of clinical research, patient-generated data, etc.

sociodemographic trends
Broad industry trends which impact the market. Comprehension of these trends is essential in order to develop an effective marketing strategy for a health care product. Each country has its own sociodemographic trends. In the US, for example, there are currently two important sociodemographic trends affecting the health care industry:
1. An ageing population, which is causing an increased demand for health care products and services.
2. A growing number of un- and underinsured Americans.

SoCRA (US)
Society of **Clinical Research Associates**.

Soft drug
A compound that is degraded *in vivo* to predictable non-toxic and inactive **metabolites**, after having achieved its therapeutic role.

Compare **hard drug**.

SOHHD
Scottish Office Home and Health Department.

solution
1. The homogenous molecular mixture formed by one or more substances whether solid, liquid or gaseous with another substance usually a liquid but sometimes also a solid.
2. (Formulation) Drugs are commonly given in solution in cough/cold remedies and in medication for the young and elderly. In most cases absorption from an oral solution is rapid and complete, compared with administration in any other oral dosage form. The rate-limiting step is often the rate of gastric emptying. When an acidic drug is given in the form of a salt, it may precipitate in the stomach. However, this precipitate is usually finely divided and is readily redissolved and thus causes no absorption problems. There is the possibility with a poorly water-soluble drug such as phenytoin that a well formulated suspension, of finely divided powder, may have a better bioavailability.

Some drugs which are poorly soluble in water may be dissolved in mixed water/alcohol or glycerol solvents. This is particularly useful for compounds with tight crystal structure, higher melting points that are not ionic. The crystal structure is broken by solution in the mixed solvent. An oily emulsion or soft gelatine capsules have been used for some compounds to produce improved **bioavailability**.

solvate
A compound of a solute with its solvent.

SOP see **standard operating procedure(s)**.

sorbefacient
A medicine or substance that produces absorption.

sorption
The process of taking up by absorption and/or adsorption.

source data (Clinical Trials)
All information in original records and certified copies of original records of clinical findings, observations, or other activities in a **clinical trial** necessary for the reconstruction and evaluation of the trial. They include hospital records, clinical and office charts, laboratory notes, memoranda, subject's diaries or evaluation checklists, pharmacy dispensing records, recorded data from automated instruments, tracings (ECG, EEG etc.), copies of transcriptions certified after verification as being accurate copies, microfiches, photographic negatives, microfilm or magnetic media, X-rays, subject files, and records kept at the pharmacy, at the laboratories and at medico-technical departments involved in the clinical trial.

Also called source documents.

source data verification (Clinical Trials)
Validation of the collected data (**source data**) against that on the **case record forms** to comply with **good clinical practice**. Unlike in the UK, US companies have the right to inspect patients' records.

South Africa Foundation for Research and Development (FRD)
Government-funded organization, pursuing alliances with local and internal industry; it helps develop people in South Africa with research and other expertise in the medical and pharmaceutical sciences.

SPA (UK)
Scottish Prescribing Analysis.

spasmolytic see **antispasmodic**.

SPC
1. see **structure–property correlations**.
2. see **Summary of Product Characteristics**.

Special Health Authorities (SHA) (UK)
Health authorities that administer some **National Health Service** (NHS) services and are responsible for specific areas of activity. Examples include the eight authorities covering London's post-graduate teaching hospitals, the Health Education Authority, the Mental Health Act Commission and Special Hospitals Services Authorities. SHAs are not part of the NHS structure but are directly accountable to the Secretary of State.
See also **District Health Authority**, **GP Fundholder**, **National Health Service**, **Regional Health Authority**.

Special Interest Group on Adverse Reactions and pharmacovigilance (SIGAR) (UK)
The **AIOPI** special interest group for **adverse drug reactions** and **pharmacovigilance**. SIGAR organizes meetings, promotes awareness and best practice, and identifies sources of information in the subject areas of drug **safety** information and pharmacovigilance. SIGAR has a regular section in the AIOPI newsletter. Any AIOPI member may become a member of SIGAR.
See also **Association of Information Officers in the Pharmaceutical Industry**.

specialist medical training (SMT)
Training in pharmaceutical medicine with the purpose of enabling **pharmaceutical physicians** to be certified as specialists by acquisition of the Certificate of Completion of Specialist Training (CCST-UK). SMT consists of two parts, Basic Training and Advanced Training.

Specialist Training Authority of the Medical Royal Colleges (STA) (UK)
The **competent authority** in the UK responsible for setting and maintaining standards of the **specialist medical training** in the UK and ensuring that training programmes comply with the minimum requirements stipulated in the **European Commission** Directive (93/16/EEC).

speciality
A description of a branch of medicine such as gastroenterology.

speciality costing
The allocation of expenditure to clinical areas. It can be useful for inter-unit comparisons, comparisons over time, and between contracts.

specifications
The detailed requirements with which a product or material, used or obtained during manufacture, have to conform. They serve as a basis for quality evaluation.

specificity
The accuracy of a diagnostic test.

SPID
Sum of Pain Intensity Score.

SPM see **Society of Pharmaceutical Medicine**.

sponsor (Clinical Trial)
An individual, company, institution, or organization which takes responsibility for the initiation, management, and/or financing of a **clinical trial**, usually the drug **manufacturer** or research

institution that developed the drug. The sponsor does not actually conduct the investigation, but rather distributes the new drug to **investigators** and physicians for clinical trials. The drug is administered to subjects under the immediate direction of an investigator who is not normally a sponsor. A clinical investigator may, however, independently initiate and take full responsibility for a trial which may subsequently become a part of an application for a **marketing authorization**, the investigator then assumes the role of the **sponsor** as well and serves as a **sponsor-investigator**. The sponsor assumes responsibility for investigating the new drug, including responsibility for **compliance** with applicable laws and **regulations**.

All **clinical trials** conducted in the US must have a **Food and Drug Administration** (FDA) approved sponsor. The sponsor is responsible for all aspects of the trial, from design to implementation. New **drug products** and **medical devices** are typically sponsored by their **manufacturer** during the **clinical phase** of study. The sponsor, for example, is responsible for obtaining FDA **approval** to conduct a trial and for reporting the results of the trial to the FDA.

sponsored journal

A journal that publishes articles paid for by a sponsor but it is subject to acceptance and approval by the editorial personnel.

sponsor-investigator

An individual who both initiates and conducts, alone or with others, a **clinical trial**, and under whose immediate direction the investigational product is administered to, dispensed to, or used by a subject. The term does not include any person other than an individual (e.g. it does not include a corporation or an agency). In the US, the obligations of a sponsor-investigator include both those of a sponsor and those of an investigator. Under 21 **Code of Federal Regulations** 50.3, the term is used only for an individual person; it does not apply to corporations or agencies.

spontaneous notification see spontaneous reporting.

spontaneous reporting (SR)

A voluntary communication to a company, **regulatory authority**, a journal or other organization from health professionals, consumers (in some countries e.g. US), lawyers, etc. that describes an **adverse event (AE) adverse drug reaction** (ADR) in a patient given one or more **medicinal products** and which does not derive from a study. The **Yellow Card Scheme** in the UK is one of the best examples of such reporting. SR benefits include:
- Characterization of ADRs
- Possibility of identification of **risk factors**
- Relatively inexpensive and simple
- Can be applied to all drugs
- It provides 'early warnings' of previously unsuspected ADRs, i.e. new signals.
- It can be used to elicit factors that predispose to particular ADRs
- It permits continued safety monitoring throughout the duration of a product's use as a marketed medicine
- It can compare ADR profiles between medicines within therapeutic classes
- Can cover the whole population including subgroups.

SR, however:
- Cannot be used to calculate **incidence** as it does not have a denominator and it does not, usually, confirm a **hypothesis**
- Suffers from under-reporting by doctors whose reporting trends tend to be high soon after launch but diminish afterwards

- The reports are observations of suspected association and there is no control group
- Reporting rates may be raised by publicity about a problem with a particular drug
- There are problems analysing prescribing rates (repeat prescription, prescriptions, differences in quantities, doses prescribed)
- Similar drugs may be used in different types of patients, making comparison of ADR rates difficult to comprehend.

Note that in the US, spontaneous ADR reports are accepted from the consumer (i.e. the patient or the patient's guardian) whereas in the **European Union**, if the information is received directly from a patient (or a relative) suggesting a serious ADR may have occurred, the **marketing authorization** holder should attempt to obtain relevant information from the **health care professional** involved in the patient's care. On receipt of such information, the case can be considered reportable.

See also **adverse drug reaction, reportable adverse reaction**, **Yellow Card Scheme**.

SPP see **strategic publication plan**.

SpPin

When a sign/test has a high **Sp**ecificity, a **P**ositive result rules **in** the diagnosis; e.g. the specificity of fluid wave for diagnosing ascites is 92%. Therefore, if a person has a fluid wave, it is highly likely that the person has ascites.

See also **SnNout**.

spray

A suspension of minute drops of liquid in air or other gas used, e.g. for the medication of the throat and nasal passages.

See also **aerosol**.

sprue

A digestive disorder in which nutrients cannot be properly absorbed from food (or **medicinal products**), causing weakness and loss of weight (or ineffective treatment).

Compare **celiac disease**.

SPSS

Statistical Package for the Social Sciences.

SPUR (UK)

Support for Products Under Research.

Sr

Sister.

SR

1. see **sustained release**.
2. Senior Registrar.
3. significant risk.
4. see **spontaneous reporting**.

SRN

Senior Registered Nurse.

SRS

Spontaneous Reporting System.

SSCT (Sweden)
Swedish Society for Clinical Trials.

SSFA (Italy)
Società di Scienze Farmacologiche Applicate (Italian association of pharmaceutical physicians).

stability
Refers to a product's ability to remain physically unchanged during storage and to resist decomposition either spontaneously or in the face of conditions tending to bring it about. Stability testing is performed on drugs to determine appropriate storage conditions. Typically, this involves placing samples into storage at different temperatures, then testing the samples at previously specified intervals, such as 30 days, 3 months, 6 months, 1 year, 2 years, or more.

stabilizer
In a chemical action it is any substance employed to maintain an equilibrium or moderate the velocity, also any compound which improves the stability of another compound.

stable endemicity
Where the **incidence** of infection or disease shows no global trend for increase or decrease.
See also **endemic**, **endemic fadeout**.

staging
Methods used to establish the extent of a patient's disease.

standard deviation (SD) (Statistics)
It is the square root of the **variance** representing a measure of **variability**. The standard deviation quantifies how much the values vary from each other. A measure of the spread of individual observations around the **mean** value of the sample. A normal, unskewed curve will have 34% of the cases between the mean and 1 SD above or below the mean, 68% of cases between 1 SD above and 1 below the mean. 95.5% of cases will be within two standard deviations of the mean.

standard drug see **bioassay, positive control drug**.

standard error of the mean (SEM) (Statistics)
A measure of **variability**. The extent to which **means** of several different samples would vary if they were taken repeatedly from the same **population**. It is a measure of the accuracy with which a population **mean** is estimated. SEM is calculated by dividing the **standard deviation** by the square root of the number of subjects. Differences from the means are said to have **statistical significance** when they are greater than twice the standard error of those means, since the probability of this difference or a larger one occurring by chance is less than 5%. The larger the **sample size** the smaller the standard error of the mean. Used in computing **confidence intervals**. In a **clinical trial**, the larger the sample size the tighter the 95% confidence interval is around the point estimate of the study.
See also **significance level**.

standardized mortality rate (SMR)
Mortality rate adjusted for a confounding variable such as age. It represents the number of deaths in a given area compared with those expected. The expected number is a standard sex/age mortality of a reference period.
Also called standardized mortality ratio.
See also **confounding factor**.

standard operating procedure (SOP)
Detailed written instructions stating who does what, when and how to achieve uniformity of the performance of a specific function. Every activity related to **good clinical practice** must be covered by a SOP. SOPs must take into account:
- The Department/Division within the company
- Corporate requirements
- National/International regulatory/ethical/legal requirements.

SOPs must be reviewed and updated regularly.

As applied to **clinical trials**, SOPs are the **sponsor**'s standard; detailed, written instructions for the management of the trials. They provide a general framework enabling the efficient implementation and performance of all the functions and activities for a particular trial as described in this document.

standard treatment
A treatment or other intervention currently being used and considered to be of proven effectiveness on the basis of past studies. Not to be confused with **standard drug**.

Standing Committee of European Doctors (or CP for *Comité Permanent*)
An international organization that consists of the national medical organizations in 17 countries of the **European Union** (EU)/European Economic Area and **EFTA**. The CP was created in Amsterdam in October 1959, two years after the signing of the **Treaty of Rome** establishing the Common Market. Its original members were the medical organizations of the six countries which formed the **European Commission** (EC) at that time: Belgium, France, Federal Republic of Germany, Italy, Luxembourg, and The Netherlands. The CP was meant to act as a permanent liaison committee with European bodies.

From 1 January 1973, the medical organizations of Denmark, Ireland and the UK were incorporated. In 1980 Greece joined and on 1 January 1986 Spain and Portugal joined. On 1 January 1994 the medical organizations of Austria, Finland, Norway, Iceland and Sweden were accepted as CP members, after the decision of the plenary Assembly to open the possibility of membership to national medical organizations of the **European Free Trade Association** countries. Since 1 January 1998 the CP has the legal status as a non-profit organization under the Belgian law. In 2000, the CP represented 1.3 million doctors.

Over the years, the CP has worked to keep its policy responsive to developments in Europe as well as to take the lead in matters of importance and urgency for the profession. While it has devoted great attention to the practice of the profession, it has also considered major aspects of medical ethics (doctors and torture, aid to the dying, AIDS, artificial procreation, living wills, medical confidentiality, the human genome, and other topics). The CP has long been the main interlocutor of the EU to discuss, advise and work towards the free movement of doctors and the mutual recognition of diplomas, certificates and other evidence of formal qualifications within the EU, resulting in several directives, which are binding for **Member States**.

The limitation of health costs is also an area about which the CP is very much committed and its declarations on this issue have been warmly greeted. The relation with the pharmaceutical industry and the pharmacists, substitution on medical products, alternative medicine and the comparison of health systems are other issues which have been dealt with.

In the field of preventive medicine, its recommendations and declarations (about primary and secondary prevention, the ageing problem, occupational health etc.) have been well received as well as its remarks about the relation between health and the environment. The CP has been the first doctors' association to declare medication should not destroy the ozone layer. The CP has strongly supported major effects made by the European bodies to fight and eradicate major health scourges.

starting material
Any substance used in the production of a medicinal product but excluding packaging materials.

Statement of Investigator see **FDA Form 1572**.

statistic
A numerical value calculated to summarize the values in a sample and that provides an estimate of that characteristic in the **population**.

statistical significance
The state achieved after a statistical analysis of study **data** at which an **investigator** can conclude that observed differences (results) are considered to be representative of a meaningful treatment effect and not just a **chance** occurrence. Significance is usually assessed in terms of a probability or ***P*-value** that by convention is supposed to be less than 5% (i.e. a 5% [1 chance in 20] probability of the result occurring by chance. Also called significance at the 0.05 level).
See also **clinical significance**.

statistics
The branch of mathematics that deals with the methods used to evaluate and interpret **data** collected from **sample**s in order to draw conclusions or inferences about a **population** and to evaluate the effects of **chance**. They are the methods to quantify and evaluate information containing uncertainty of random origin (noise) in results from groups of individuals, each with inherent biological differences and thus biological **variability**, when these individuals represent a sample drawn from a population that could not be evaluated in its entirety (e.g. all the individuals on which the test could have been done, to which the treatment could have been applied, could have been treated with the product). Statistics are valid only to the degree that the opportunity for bias is minimized in the design and execution of the study.

sterile
Free from all living organisms.

sterility
The absence of living organisms. The conditions of the sterility test are given in the **European Pharmacopoeia**.

sterilization
The process of killing microorganisms, including spores, on objects such as surgical instruments.

StN
Student Nurse.

stochastic (Statistics)
Involving a **random** variable; involving chance or probability.

stochastic model (Statistics)
A mathematical model which takes into consideration the presence of some randomness in one or more of its parameters or variables. The predictions of the model therefore do not give a single point estimate but a probability distribution of possible estimates.
We might distinguish demographic stochasticity which arises from the discreteness of

individuals and individual events such as birth, and environmental stochasticity arising from more-or-less unpredictable interactions with the outside world.
Compare **deterministic model**.

stomachic
A drug that is used to stimulate the appetite and gastric secretion.
See also **tonic**.

strategic plan
A company's strategic plan is a broad plan for meeting the goals of its **mission statement**. It is used to outline more specific business goals and the general strategy for meeting them.

strategic publication plan (SPP)
A plan developed by the drug **company** or on behalf of the company by a **medical education agency** with the objective of ensuring that **clinical trials** data reaches target audiences at the right time and to a maximum effect. Both **peer-reviewed** journals and congresses are targets for SPP.

stratification (Clinical Trials)
Division into groups. The procedure of assigning patients to an **investigational product** or treatment in a **clinical trial** based on their age, weight, race, severity of disease, or any other relevant factor that is expected to have an important influence on the **outcome** of the trial. A process to control differences in **confounding factors**, by making separate estimates for groups of individuals who have the same values for the confounding factors.

strength
The concentration of the drug substance in the **drug product**.

Strength, New, Importance and Potential for prevention (SNIP)
Criteria used at each stage of the review process that facilitate the consistent and effective evaluation of drug **safety** signals, producing a standard approach that allows rapid decisions to be made as to whether potential signals are worthy of further attention. Different elements of SNIP have different weights, depending on the signal being reviewed. However, not all elements need to be met for a given signal before a decision is made to investigate further.

strength of inference (Statistics)
The likelihood that an observed difference between groups within a study represents a real difference rather than mere **chance** or the influence of **confounding factors**, based on both *P*-values and **confidence intervals**. Strength of inference is weakened by various forms of bias and by small **sample sizes**.

strict liability (UK)
An aspect of a UK law which makes the **manufacturer** liable if a medicine is defective, i.e. it causes an **adverse drug reaction** that was not identified and notified to the prescriber prior to the time of prescribing. Negligence does not have to be proven, only that injury has taken place.

structure–activity relationship (SAR)
The relationship between chemical structure and pharmacological activity for a series of compounds.
See also **quantitative structure–activity relationship**.

structure-based design see **structure-based drug design**.

structure-based drug design
Design of novel compounds based on the three-dimensional (3D) structure of a validated target, for example, a **receptor** protein determined by physical methods (**X-ray crystallography**, nuclear magnetic resonance or **computational chemistry** techniques) to direct chemical synthesis of the **drug candidates**.

structured abstract
An abstract format, adopted by many clinical journals, that generally contains the key components of study **population** and source, study subject, study design, main findings and clinical implication in a concise outline format. This format was developed because unstructured abstracts are of varying quality, often omitting key components, and many clinicians, particularly those using the derivative sources, read only the abstracts because of time constraints.

structure–property correlations (SPC) (Statistics
All statistical mathematical methods used to correlate any structural property to any other property (intrinsic, chemical or biological), using statistical regression and **pattern recognition** techniques.

study agent see **investigational product**.

study arm
One of the groups in a **clinical trial** (the other is normally the **control** arm). Typically, patients in clinical trials are assigned to one part or segment of a study – a study 'arm'. One arm receives a different treatment from the other.

study coordinator see **clinical trials coordinator**.

study medication see **investigational product**.

Study Report see **Final Report**.

Styptic
An agent which has **astringent** properties and arrests bleeding.

sub-clinical infection
An infection in which **symptom**s are sufficiently mild or unapparent to escape diagnosis other than by positive confirmation of the ability to transmit the infection or serologically.

subcutaneous (SC) injection
Administering a fluid into the tissue beneath the skin with a needle and syringe. Subcutaneous tissue is loose connective tissue, often fatty, situated under the dermis.
See also **intramuscular injection, intravenous injection**.

sub-investigator (Clinical Trial)
Any individual member of the **clinical trial team** designated and supervised by the **investigator** at a **trial site** to perform critical trial-related procedures and/or to make important trial-related decisions (e.g. associates, residents, research fellows).
See also **investigator**.

subject see **human subject**.

subject discontinuation see **subject withdrawal**.

Subject Identification Code (Clinical Trials)
A unique identifier assigned to each trial subject to protect the subject's identity and used *in lieu* of the subject's name when the **investigator** reports **adverse event**s and/or other trial-related data.

subject withdrawal (Clinical Trials)
The situation where a subject/patient withdraws or discontinues from a trial prior to completion of all evaluations, as per the **protocol**. Withdrawal from the trial may be due to the following:
1. **informed consent** revoked
2. medical reason
3. **adverse event**
4. other reason.

submission (US)
A collection of information sent to the **Food and Drug Administration** in response to a particular regulatory requirement. This term is often used to refer to a market **approval** application, such as an **New Drug Application, Product Licence Application**, or **Pre-market Approval Application**.

subpopulation (Clinical Trials)
A particular segment of a study **population** for which the effect of the study treatments may be different, usually better, than for other members of the population.

subsidy (New Zealand)
Defined at the level of the **manufacturer**'s price. The actual payment to the pharmacy is the subsidy plus any wholesale mark-up, a retail mark-up and dispensing fee(s), less the Government prescription charge. Manufacturer's price is based on the latest information notified to **PHARMAC** and may change at the manufacturer's discretion, without notice to PHARMAC.
Also referred to as price ex-supplier, or price to wholesaler.
Pharmacy price is manufacturer's price plus mark ups and fees. The mark ups and fees are also referred to as the pharmacy margin.

SUD
Sudden unexpected death.

sudorific see **diaphoretic**.

sugar-free
Oral liquid **medicinal products** that do not contain fructose, glucose, or sucrose are normally described as 'sugar-free'. The term is also used to describe those oral medicines that contain hydrogenated glucose syrup, mannitol, or sorbitol since there is evidence that they do not cause dental problems.

Summary Basis of Approval (Clinical Trials) (US)
A document that contains a summary of the **safety** and effectiveness data and information evaluated by the **Food and Drug Administration** (FDA) during the **approval** process. A draft may be prepared and submitted by the **New Drug Application** (or **Abbreviated NDA**) applicant, usually the **sponsor**, for review and revision by FDA or the summary basis of approval may be prepared by the FDA.

Summary of Product Characteristics (SPC, SmPC)
Formerly used term 'Data Sheet'. A key company document which contains basic information,

for prescribers. The SPC is necessary for **marketing authorization** (MA) within the **European Union**. In accordance with Article 4a of **Directive 65/65/EEC**, as amended by **Directive 83/570/EEC** the applicant is required to produce a draft SPC as part of the application documentations. The **regulatory authorities** then review this, and the applicant is given the revised and accepted version when the MA is revised. The MA holder, in any subsequent advertising and promotion of product, then uses the wording of the SPC. The SPC also, once an MA has been gained, controls the claims that can be made for the product. The advertising material and the information provided to practitioners has to be in line with the information in the approved SPC. Within the **Committee for Proprietary Medicinal Products**, there is an increasing desire to arrive at a common SPC (Euro-SPC) throughout the **European Commission** for any given product. 'The SPC, therefore, sets out the agreed position of the **medicinal product**, as distilled during the course of the assessment process. It is the definitive statement between the competent authority and the MA holder, and it is the common basis of communication between the **competent authorities** of all **Member States**. As such the content cannot be changed except with the approval of the originating competent authority.' Notice to applicants for MAs for medicinal products for human use in the European Union. Volume IIA. The SPC contains the following sections:

1. Trade name of the medicinal product
2. Qualitative and quantitative composition (active ingredients, excipients)
3. Pharmaceutical form, type and contents of the container
4. Clinical particulars
   4.1. Therapeutic indications
   4.2. **Posology** and method of administration
   4.3. **Contraindications**
   4.4. Special warnings and special precautions for use
   4.5. Interaction with other medicaments and other forms of interaction
   4.6. **Pregnancy** and lactation
   4.7. Effects on ability to drive and use machines
   4.8. Undesirable effects
   4.9. Overdose
5. Pharmaceutical properties
   5.1. **Pharmacodynamic** properties
   5.2. **Pharmacokinetic** properties
   5.3 Preclinical **safety** data
6. Pharmaceutical particulars
   6.1. List of **excipients**
   6.2. Incompatibilities
   6.3. Shelf life
   6.4. Special precautions for storage
   6.5. Nature and contents of container
   6.6. Instructions for use/handling
7. Marketing authorization holder; name or style and permanent address or registered place of business of the holder of marketing authorization
8. Marketing authorization number
9. Date of first authorization/renewal of authorization
10. Date of (partial) revision of the text.

See also **Patient Information Leaflet**.

Supervisory Committee (Clinical Trials)
A committee of appointed personnel who are not actively conducting the trial. They could have access to data during the trial and could perform planned **interim analyses** and make necessary recommendations, based on the analyses' outcome, to the Steering Committee.

supplement see **Supplemental New Drug Application**.

Supplemental New Drug Application (SNDA) (US)
The documentation, for marketing application, submitted to the **Food and Drug Administration** (FDA) for changes on a drug substance or **drug product** that is already the subject of an approved NDA. FDA must approve all important NDA changes (in **packaging** or ingredients, for instance) to ensure that the conditions originally set for the product are not adversely affected. SNDA may be submitted for a variety of reasons such as **labelling** changes, a new or expanded clinical indication, or new dosage form. For example, for labelling changes, the **sponsor** may want to add a new specification or test method or changes in the methods, facility, or controls to provide increased assurance that the drug will have the characteristics of identity, strength, quality, and purity that it purports to possess.
See also **New Drug Application**.

suppository
A solid cone or bullet-shaped medicated object made up of a chemically inactive base of fatty substance (e.g. cocoa butter or gelatine) that is inserted into the rectum or vagina; and intended for the treatment of local conditions or as a means of delivering a drug to the body. Suppository bases are solid at room temperature but melt or dissolve at body temperture.

surfactant
1. A mixture of substances secreted by the air sacs of the lungs that prevents the air sacs from collapsing during exhalation.
2. A surface active agent that decreases the surface tension between two miscible liquids or between solid and liquid used, to prepare emulsions, suspensions and act as cleansing agent.

surrogate see **surrogate marker**.

surrogate endpoint see **surrogate marker**.

surrogate marker
A type of measurement (laboratory finding or physical sign) that may not, in itself, be a direct measurement of how a patient feels, functions or survives but nevertheless is used in studies of chronic diseases which in the short-term helps to predict the long-term therapeutic benefit/effect of treatment. For example, the measurement of CD-4 counts is a surrogate used to measure the strength of the immune system for **mortality** in AIDS patients.

surveys
Studies designed to obtain information from a large number of respondents through written questionnaires, telephone interviews, door-to-door canvassing, or similar procedures.

survival analysis (Statistics)
Statistical procedures for estimating survival (prognosis) in a population under study.

survival curve (Statistics)
A graph of the number of events occurring over time or the **chance** of being free of these events over time. The events must be discrete and the time at which they occur must be precisely known.

In most clinical situations, the chance of an **outcome** changes with time. In most survival curves the earlier follow-up periods usually include results from more patients than the later periods and are therefore more precise.

suspension
A system consisting of a solid dispersed in a liquid medium in which the size of the solid particles is greater than 1 µm, i.e. larger than colloidal systems; may also be a solid in a gas or liquid in a gas. A well formulated suspension is second only to a solution in terms of superior **bioavailability**. **Absorption** may well be dissolution limited, however a suspension of a finely ground powder will maximize the potential for rapid dissolution. A good correlation can be seen for particle size and absorption rate. With very fine particle sizes, the dispersibility of the powder becomes important. The addition of a surface active agent will improve dispersion of a suspension and may improve the absorption of very fine particle size suspensions otherwise caking may be a problem.

sustained release (SR)
The property of prolonged release dosage forms (**drug product**) that are formulated in such a way so as the liberation rate of the **active ingredient**(s) is lower than its absorption.

Also called slow release.

sustained release tablets
Tablets which have been formulated with a **sustained release** (SR) mechanism.
Benefits:
- For short half-life drugs, SR can mean less frequent dosing and thus better **compliance**.
- Reduce variations in plasma/blood levels for more consistent result.

Problems:
- More complicated **formulation** may be more erratic in result. A SR product may contain a larger dose, i.e. the **dose** for two or three (or more) 'normal' dosing intervals. A failure of the controlled release mechanism may result in release of a large toxic dose.
- More expensive technology.

Types of products:
- Erosion tablets
- Waxy matrix
- Matrix erodes or drug leaches from matrix
- Coated pellets
- Different pellets (colours) have different release properties
- Coated ion exchange
- Osmotic pump
- Insoluble coat with small hole. Osmotic pressure pushes the drug out at a controlled rate.

SWOT Analysis – Strengths/Weaknesses/Opportunities/Threats
A tool used to assess, amongst other areas, marketing strategies. It consists of two parts: (1) **internal assessment**: an examination of the internal **S**trengths and **W**eaknesses of a company and its products, (2) **external assessment**: an examination of any external **O**pportunities and **T**hreats. This tool is used to help develop strategic and tactical marketing plans.

symmetry principle (Clinical Trials)
In a study, the principle of keeping all things between groups similar except for the treatment of interest. This means that the same instrument is used to measure each individual in each group, the observers know the same things about all individuals in all groups, randomization

is used to obtain a similar allocation of individuals to each group, the groups are followed at the same time.

sympathicotonic
Sympathomimetic.

symptom
A condition of the body reported by an individual when suffering from a disease; it is different from a sign (which is noticed by the doctor but not necessarily by the patient).

See also **sign**.

syndrome
A group of signs and/or symptoms or a series of events that indicate a certain disorder, make up a disease or health problem when they occur together.

synergist
A drug which supplements the action of another often to such an extent that the combined effect is greater than the sum of the two drugs administered independently.

syringe driver
A portable device used to continuously administer a drug, mainly strong analgesics, by subcutaneous route. It is used when parenteral administration is necessary as an alternative to repeated intramuscular injections (particularly to a cachectic patients). It is commonly used in **palliative** care.

syrup
A liquid medicament for oral administration containing a large percentage of sugar either for the purpose of flavouring or as a preservative or both.

systematic availability
The **bioavailability** of a drug following any route of administration: e.g. oral, topical, intravenous, intramuscular, etc.

systemic
A word used to describe conditions that affect the entire body. Diabetes is a systemic disease because it involves many parts of the body such as the pancreas, eyes, kidneys, heart and nerves.

systemic effects
The effect obtained when the drug released from the drug product enters the blood and/or a lymphatic stream and is distributed within the body regardless of the site and the route of administration.

$t_{1/2}$ see **half-life**.

tablet

A solid disk containing one or more medicaments prepared by compressing a granulated powder in the die of a machine. The tablet is the most commonly used oral dosage form. It is also quite complex in nature. The biggest problem is overcoming the reduction in effective surface area produced during the compression process. One may start with the drug in a very fine powder, but then proceed to compress it into a single dosage unit. Tablet ingredients include materials to break up the tablet formulation.

- Drug – may be poorly soluble, hydrophobic
- Lubricant – usually quite hydrophobic
- Granulating agent – tends to stick the ingredients together
- Filler – may interact with the drug, etc., should be water soluble
- Wetting agent – helps the penetration of water into the tablet
- Disintegration agent – helps to break the tablet apart.

Coated tablets are used to mask an unpleasant taste, to protect the tablet ingredients during storage, or to improve the tablet appearance. Another barrier is placed between the solid drug and drug in solution. This barrier must break down quickly or it may hinder a drug's **bioavailability**.

See also **capsule**.

tachyphylaxis see **tolerance**.

taenifuge

An agent that expels tapeworms from the body.

Taft, William Howard

President of the US who, along with Congress, enacted the **Sherley Amendments** to the 1906 food and drug law.

target allocation

A **National Health Service** term used to describe the health authority share of the national allocation. It is calculated by reference to a **weighted capitation** formula including age, sex, **mortality**, service costs, etc.

target validation

The association of a gene and/or its gene product as a molecular target for drug intervention in a particular pathology.

TDM see **therapeutic drug monitoring**.

tds

Three times daily dose regimen (also TDS).

teaching hospital

A hospital that is attached to a medical school.

teratogen

Anything that causes abnormalities/malformation in a developing embryo or fetus, such as a drug or virus.

teratology

The study of developmental abnormalities and their cause.

TERT see **Trust for Education and Research in Therapeutics**.

tertiary source
A compilation of information for application across a broad spectrum typically represented by class notes and textbooks intended for use in core courses. The information is often presented in a dogmatic, authoritative fashion as a sequence of facts and interpretations of their meaning that the reader is to believe without reservation or evaluation. Much of the evidence-based information contained in textbooks is filtered sufficiently that it is accepted by most or all of the experts in the field, much of it is unlikely to change in the future, and most or all of the changes will be minor. The strength of the underlying evidence is not indicated and any current controversy between researchers in the area is not addressed. The bibliography is usually predominately secondary literature and is usually intended to provide the interested reader with entry points to the underlying primary literature. However, depending on the field, textbooks contain a varying amount of dogma and interpretations of facts that will change with the progress of research in the area, sometimes significantly. Because clinical experience is often not examined critically, clinical textbooks tend to contain a larger proportion of dogma than do basic science textbooks. Class notes usually contain much more limited information than do textbooks and do not undergo the auditing process as part of publication as textbooks do.

test article
This term has been used interchangeably with 'investigational product', which is the usual term in Europe. According to the US version of **good clinical practice**, however, it is defined as 'Any drug (including a biological product for human use), **medical device** for human use, human food additive, electronic product, or any Public Health Service Act (42 U.S.C. 262 and 263b–263n).'

See also **investigational product**.

TFR see **total fertility rate**.

TGA (Australia) see **Therapeutic Goods Administration**.

thalidomide
A **sedative** and hypnotic drug that, in 1961, caused severe deformities in infants born to mothers using it during **pregnancy**. It is still considered safe for particular indications and is used in many countries throughout the world. It was first marketed by a German company as part of a combination product called Grippex indicated for respiratory infections. It was not until May 1960 when it was first shown to cause deformation in infants (phocomelia or sealed limbs) and not until November 1961 before it was withdrawn from the German and British markets.

The tragedy forced the passage of the **Kefauver–Harris Amendments** to the **Food, Drug and Cosmetic Act** in the US in October 1962. This was the first time in the US where a new law required evidence of **efficacy** in the proposed indications. The **Food and Drug Administration** (FDA) then introduced the **Investigational New Drug** application as well as the requirement to notify **adverse drug reactions** to the FDA.

In the UK, the catastrophe led to the creation of the **Committee on Safety of Drugs (CSD)**.

therapeutic alternates
Drug products belonging to same pharmacological or therapeutic class that are expected to have similar therapeutic effects when administered in therapeutically equivalent doses (i.e. prednisone and prednisolone).

therapeutic drug monitoring (TDM)

TDM becomes important when:
1. the drug has a narrow therapeutic-toxic range
2. there is a large variability in **pharmacokinetic** parameter values between patients
3. the therapeutic effect is not readily assessed (e.g. antibiotics) or clinical symptoms are to be avoided (e.g. seizure). Not as useful for blood pressure (BP) lowering (can measure BP directly) or anticoagulants (can measure clotting time directly)
4. there is a direct relationship between plasma concentration or concentration in other biological sample (e.g. saliva) and pharmacological effect
5. an appropriate (accurate, short turn around, inexpensive) analytical method is available for the drug
6. the expected or desired therapeutic effect is not observed (may be absorption or compliance problem)
7. a drug with high first pass effect is involved
8. a patient has altered and/or variable renal state and the drug is eliminated mostly as unchanged drug in urine.

Typical drugs for which TDM is done include:

Drug	Therapeutic concentration range
Aminoglycoside (gentamicin, tobramycin)	0.5 <–> 8 mg/L
Digoxin	0.5 <–> 8 2.0 ug/L
Phenytoin	10 <–> 8 20 mg/L
Theophylline	10 <–> 8 20 mg/L

Assay methods for TDM are usually under the direction of the pathology or clinical chemistry laboratory. GLC, **HPLC**, RIA, EMIT, fluoroimmunoassay, luminescence.

therapeutic equivalence

The pharmaceutical equivalents which provide the same therapeutic effect (control of a **symptom** or disease or other measures) are said to be therapeutically equivalent.

Therapeutic Goods Act 1989 (Australia)

The Act provides the basis for a national regulatory system for therapeutic goods supplied in Australia. Therapeutic goods, defined broadly, include chemically-made products and products obtained from biological sources (such as vaccines and antibiotics) and devices such as intra-ocular lenses, intra-uterine contraceptive devices, pacemakers, heart valves and defibrillators, along with a wide range of herbal products, vitamin and mineral supplements, the more concentrated homoeopathic products, and sunscreens. Cosmetics and food are generally exempt but if therapeutic claims are made then they are regarded as therapeutic goods.

Therapeutic Goods Administration (TGA) (Australia)

A Division of the Federal Department of Health and Aged Care, responsible for administering the provisions of the Therapeutic Goods Act. The TGA carries out a range of assessment and monitoring activities to ensure therapeutic goods available in Australia are of an acceptable standard. At the same time the TGA aims to ensure that the Australian community has access, within a reasonable time, to therapeutic advances. Overall control of the supply of therapeutic goods is exercised through three main processes:
- pre-market assessment

- licensing of manufacturers
- post-market vigilance.

Pre-market assessment
Products assessed as having a higher level of risk (prescription medicines, some non-prescription medicines and **medical devices**) are evaluated for **quality, safety** and **efficacy**. Once approved for marketing in Australia these products are included in the **ARTG** as 'registered' products and are identified by an AUST R number.

Products assessed as being lower risk (many non-prescription medicines including most complementary medicines and low-risk medical devices) are assessed for quality and safety. Once approved for marketing in Australia, these products are included in the ARTG as 'listed' products and are identified by an AUST L number.

In assessing the level of risk, factors such as the strength of a product, **side-effects**, potential harm through prolonged use, **toxicity** and the seriousness of the medical condition for which the product is intended to be used, are all taken into account.

Licensing of manufacturers
Australian manufacturers of therapeutic goods must be licensed. Their manufacturing processes must comply with principles of **good manufacturing practice**. The aim of licensing and standards is to protect public health by ensuring that medicines and medical devices meet definable standards of **quality assurance** and are manufactured in conditions that are clean and free of contaminants.

Post-marketing vigilance
Post-marketing activities include investigating reports of problems, laboratory testing of products on the market and monitoring to ensure compliance with the legislation.

therapeutic index
The difference between the minimal effective dose and the **maximum tolerated dose** to increase the risk to a subject beyond an acceptable level or threshold. It is a measure of the approximate margin of **safety**, 'safety factor' for a drug; a drug with a high index can presumably be administered with greater safety than one with a low index.

therapeutic intent (Clinical Trials)
The research physician's intent to provide some benefit to improving a subject's condition (e.g. prolongation of life, shrinkage of tumour, or improved **quality of life**, even though cure or dramatic improvement cannot necessarily be effected). This term is sometimes associated with phase I drug studies in which potentially toxic drugs are given to an individual with the hope of inducing some improvement in the patient's condition as well as assessing the **safety** and **pharmacology** of a drug.

therapeutic personality bias
Occurs when the observer is not blinded. The observer's beliefs about therapeutic effectiveness may influence outcomes and their measurements.

therapeutic range
The range of doses of a **drug** that will produce beneficial results without **side-effects**.

therapeutic ratio see therapeutic index.

therapeutic substitution
The practice whereby a pharmacist, with the prescribing physician's knowledge and approval, dispenses a chemical entity different from the one prescribed but in the same therapeutic class.

In the US, therapeutic substitution is common in **Health Maintenance Organizations**, hospitals and other institutions under guidelines agreed to by the institution.

Compare **generic substitution**.

therapeutic window see **therapeutic index.**

third party administration (TPA)
The administration of a **group insurance** plan by some person or firm other than the insurer or the policyholder.

Third-Party Prescription Drug Programs (US)
A method of health care delivery that includes reimbursement to pharmacies for drugs dispensed. The programmes can be either governmental or private. The primary government programme is **Medicaid**. Several States also have prescription programmes to assist the low-income elderly who do not qualify for Medicaid. In private third-party programmes the ultimate **payers**, for the most part, are companies – that is, employers – which often buy **coverage** from an **insurer** by paying a **premium**.

three-dimensional quantitative structure–activity relationship (3D-QSAR)
The analysis of the quantitative relationship between the biological activity of a set of compounds and their spatial properties using statistical methods.

thrombogenic
Causing thrombosis or coagulation of the blood.

thromboprophylaxis
Prevention of thrombosis.

TIA
Transient ischaemic attack.

TICTAC (UK)
A British computer-aided tablet and capsule identification system that is available to authorized users including Regional Drug Information Centres and Poisons Information Centres.

TID
Tres In Die; Three times daily dose regimen (also TDS and tid).

tincture
An alcoholic extract of an animal or vegetable drug prepared usually by percolation or **maceration** process.

TIND (US)
Treatment Investigational New Drug.

tissue-profiling
A systematic testing of compounds for their effect in cell assays derived from different organs of relevance for the indication in question. Tissue profiling facilitates the identification of compounds with tissue selective activity and minimizes the need for animal studies at this stage of the drug development.

TMF see **Clinical Trial Master File.**

TMO
Trial Management Organization, see **Clinical Research Organization.**

tolerance

A condition produced by a drug in which there is a decreased sensitivity (or producing progressively smaller effects) of the body to a certain drug following repeat doses. The apparent loss of potency of a drug observed during the course of successive administrations is usually either because the liver becomes more efficient at breaking down the drug or the body's tissues become less sensitive to it. The condition is characterized by the necessity to increase successive drug doses in order for them to produce identical effects.

Tachyphylaxis is tolerance that develops over a short interval (usually measured in minutes or hours rather than days or weeks). 'Tolerance' should not be used to mean 'lack of sensitivity' manifested toward a dose of drug. A non-addicted morphine abuser who is unaffected by several doses of morphine in rapid succession is probably insensitive to morphine rather than tolerant to its effects.

Compare **addiction, dependence, habituation, sensitivity**.

tonic

An agent used to stimulate the functions of the body or more generally to increase the patient's feeling of **well-being** and to stimulate appetite.

See also **stomachic**.

topical anaesthetic

An agent that causes loss of sensation from the skin or external mucous membranes when applied directly to the area to be anaesthetized.

Topliss tree

An operational scheme for **analogue** design.

total fertility rate (TFR)

The number of children an average woman would have assuming that she lives her full reproductive lifetime.

Total Purchasing Group (UK)

A group of general practitioner practices that have joined together to hold a fund to negotiate contracts and purchase the entire health care for their patients.

Toxbase (UK)

A British on-line database which provides information about routine diagnosis, treatment and management of patients exposed to drugs, household products, and industrial and agricultural chemicals. It is available via a Viewdata system to authorized users such as an Accident and Emergency Department.

toxicity

The relative extent to which a substance is poisonous or toxic. It is one of the factors of a new drug or **biological** that **preclinical** and **clinical trials** attempt to measure.

toxicity studies

This term refers to the animal toxicity studies. They consist of a series of studies that are conducted over several years with the objective of evaluating the toxicity of the investigational compound and identifying the target organ for the compound's toxicity. The content of this series of studies varies according to the intended indication of the drug. In general, the series include the following five types of studies:

1. Acute-single dose such as the LD_{50} study identifying the single dose that results in fatality of 50% of animals treated over a 7-day duration.
2. Sub-acute, sub-chronic multiple-dose studies which are designed according to the

intended duration of treatment in humans (e.g. animal's exposure of 14 days would allow a human exposure 1–3 doses, and 28 days (animal exposure) corresponds to 10 days in humans respectively).
3. Fertility, teratogenicity and other reproductive studies. Fertility studies involve both sexes being dosed 60 and 14 days pre-coitus. Administration of drugs to women of child-bearing age is not permitted, by the **regulatory authorities** (RAs), until animal teratology studies (on mice, rats and a non-rodent (normally rabbits)) at certain gestational stages have been conducted.
4. Carcinogenicity studies. These are necessary and required by RAs if the drug is:
   - intended for chronic use (normally defined as more than a year)
   - repeated dosing over long periods
   - suspected of being carcinogenic due to structural characteristics common with known carcinogens
   - previous mutagenicity studies have raised certain concerns.
5. Other specialized studies. These are intended to be organ specific should there have been a signal generated by previous studies.

toxicologist

A scientist who investigates such diverse problems as the effects of overdoses of pharmacotherapeutic agents; the diagnosis, treatment, and prevention of lead poisoning in the paint manufacturing industry; the possibility that criminal poisoning was the cause of an otherwise inexplicable death, etc.

See also **toxicology**.

toxicology

The study of the effects and detection of poisons in living organisms. Also, substances that are otherwise harmless but prove toxic under particular conditions. The basic assumption of toxicology is that there is a relationship between the dose (amount), the concentration at the affected site, and the resulting effects.

Compare **hazard**, **pharmacology**, **toxicologist**.

Toxicology Methods

A journal that publishes, quarterly, peer-reviewed forum for toxicologists to share and critically evaluate all aspects of the development, validation, and application of new and existing methods, techniques and equipment, including:
- *in vivo* studies with standard and alternative species
- *in vitro* studies and alternative methodologies
- molecular, biochemical, and cellular techniques
- **pharmacokinetics** and **pharmacodynamics**
- mathematical modelling
- computer programs
- forensic analyses
- risk assessment
- data collection and analysis.

toxin

A poisonous substance.

toxoid

A bacterial exotoxin which has been modified so that it is not toxic but retains its antigenic properties.

trademark
An officially registered and legally restricted name, symbol or representation, the use of which is restricted to its owner. A trademark identifies a product and distinguishes it from others so as to identify the source of the product. Trademarks are property rights belonging to trademark owners that serve to protect the public so consumers can identify the makers or providers of goods or services.

trade secret
Almost anything that is not generally known and that gives its owner a competitive business advantage. Trade secrets can be patentable inventions, or they can be other intangibles such as manufacturing techniques, business methods, sources of supply, customer lists and other industrial or commercial ideas. In order to qualify as a trade secret, the owner must take precautions to ensure that the trade secret remains secret. The owner of a trade secret has the right to prevent use or dissemination of that trade secret by anyone who learned or derived it from the owner. The owner has no trade secret rights against anyone who independently discovers the trade secret. Each form of intellectual property has its place within an organization. Copyrights protect the form of expression of ideas, trademarks protect the identification of the source of ideas, and patents and trade secrets protect the application of ideas.

transcutaneous
Through the skin.

transdermal
Entering through the dermis or skin, as in administration of a drug applied to the skin in ointment or patch form.

transferability see **applicability**.

transfer prices
Charges for products, ingredients or other services made by an overseas affiliate to a nationally-based company.

transgenic
Pertaining to the insertion by biotechnical means of a foreign gene or genes into the genetic makeup of an organism.

transition-state analogue
A compound that mimics the transition state of a substrate bound to an **enzyme**.

Treatment Investigational New Drug (US)
A mechanism that allows promising **investigational drugs** to be used in 'expanded access' protocols – relatively unrestricted studies in which the intent is both to learn more about the drugs, especially their **safety**, and to provide treatment for people with immediately **life-threatening** or otherwise serious diseases for which there is no real alternative. But these expanded access protocols also require researchers to formally investigate the drugs in well-controlled studies and to supply some evidence that the drugs are likely to be helpful. The drugs cannot expose patients to unreasonable risk.

Treaty of Rome
The European Pact that was agreed and signed on 25 March 1957 following the foundation of the European Economic Community by six countries: Federal Republic of Germany, Luxembourg, Italy, France, Belgium and the Netherlands.
See also **European Union**.

treponemicide see **antitreponemal agent**.

triage
A system used to classify sick or injured people according to the severity of their conditions.

trial audit see **audit**.

trial coordinator see **clinical trial coordinator**.

trial drug see **investigational medicinal product**.

trialist see **investigator**

Trial Master File see **Clinical Trial Master File**.

trial site (Clinical Trials)
The place (clinic, hospital, etc.) where a **clinical trial** is conducted. In the case of multicentre trials, it is one of many places where the same trial is being conducted. The site may be private or public.

trial subject see **human subject**.

trial termination (Clinical Trials)
The closing of a trial by either the **sponsor**, **investigator**, **Ethics Committee**, or **Institutional Review Board**. Anyone terminating a trial must provide an appropriate explanation.

TRIP see **Turning Research Into Practice (TRIP) database**.

triple-blind clinical trial
A study design in which knowledge of the treatment is concealed from the people who organize and analyse the data of a study as well as from both the subjects/patients and **investigators**.

TRIPS (UK)
Trade Related Intellectual Property Rights, see **Association of the British Pharmaceutical Industry**.

Trust for Education and Research in Therapeutics (TERT) (UK)
A trust, set up by **AMAPI**, in 1965 as a charity. AMAPI conducted various symposia through TERT. TERT also organized regular courses in **clinical trials** methodology.

TSCA (US)
Toxic Substance Control Act.

tropical sprue see **sprue**

t-test (Student's test) (Statistics)
A statistical test used to analyse two paired or matched samples of data to compare the means; analyse two un-paired, unmatched samples to compare the means of their corresponding **populations**; or to analyse one data sample to compare a population mean with a particular value.

trypanocide see **antitrypanosomal agent**.

Turning Research Into Practice (TRIP) database (UK)
This resource, hosted by the Centre for Research Support in Wales, aims to support those

working in primary care. The database has 8000 links covering resources at 28 different centres and allows both Boolean searching (AND, OR, NOT) and truncation.
> Website: http://www.ceres.uwcm.ac.uk/frameset.cfm?section = trip

Tx
Common abbreviation for 'treatment'.

type I error (Statistics)
The same as **alpha error, consumer risk** and **false positive**. Mistakenly rejecting the **null hypothesis** when it is actually true. It refers to the potential statistical error that can be made in a hypothesis when deciding a treatment has a **statistically significant** effect when in fact it is no better (or perhaps, worse) than the **control**. It is determined before the study begins. Studies commonly set it to 1 in 20 (= 0.05).

type II error (Statistics)
The same as **beta error, producer's risk** and **false negative**. It refers to the potential error that can be made in deciding a treatment does not have a **statistically significant** effect when, in fact, it is superior to **control**. It occurs when mistakenly accepting (not rejecting) the **null hypothesis** when it is false. The probability of making a type II error is called beta (β). Power = $1 - \beta$. For trials the probability of a β error is usually set at 0.20 or 20% probability. A 20% chance of missing a true difference.

type I mortality
A mortality schedule in which all hosts are assumed to live for a fixed number of years equal to the **life expectancy**.

type II mortality
A mortality schedule in which all hosts are assumed to die at a constant rate. This constant rate is equal to the inverse of the life expectancy.

type I variation
A minor variation, to the **marketing authorization**, defined in Article 2 of **Regulation (EC) No. 542/95**.

type II variation
A major variation, to the **marketing authorization**, as defined in Article 2 of **Regulation (EC) No. 542/95**, which cannot be deemed to be a **type I variation**.

type A reaction
An augmented pharmacologically predictable (in the majority of cases) reaction which is dose-dependent. It is generally associated with a high **morbidity** and a low **mortality**. These account for approximately 80% of all **adverse drug reactions**.
> See also **adverse drug reaction, adverse event**.

type B reaction
A bizarre reaction which cannot be explained on the basis of known **pharmacology** of the drug (is unpredictable pharmacologically), and is independent of dose and occurrence of **toxicity**. It is generally associated with a low **morbidity** and a high **mortality**. They are also termed **idiosyncratic adverse drug reactions**; it is important to note that this is a functional term which does not imply any specific mechanism.
> See also **adverse drug reaction, adverse event**.

UB-92
A universal claim form used for hospital billing of inpatient and outpatient services to both public payers and private payers.

UCC
Universal Copyright Convention.

UKCCR
UK Coordinating Committee on Cancer Research.

UK Clearing House on Health Outcomes (UKCHHO) (UK)
An organization, based within the Nuffield Institute for Health at the University of Leeds, that aims to develop approaches to outcomes assessment within routine health care practice and to promote the role of health outcomes within decision making in health care commissioning and provision. They have two databases available on the Internet; the other being an Outcomes Activities Database containing a wide range of outcomes related projects. This forms the basis for networking people working in similar areas or using similar measures.

Website: http://www.leeds.ac.uk/nuffield/infoservices/UKCH/home.html

UKDIPG see UK Drug Information Pharmacists' Group.

UK Drug Information Pharmacists' Group (UKDIPG)
A service provided on a national basis by specialist pharmacists, the majority of whom are based within hospital Trusts located across the UK. Their work is supported by regional drug information centres that provide additional resources and support to local centres. The principal pharmacists from the regional centres meet regularly within UKDIPG. Through cooperation and shared activity, UKDIPG coordinates the production of shared national information products, formulates strategy, and develops educational materials and training programmes.

An important function of the UKDIPG service is to provide a rapid and efficient enquiry answering service on all aspects of drug use. In general, enquiries relate to the selection, availability, identity, dose and administration of drugs for a wide spectrum of patient ages and disease states. In addition, many enquiries relate to such issues as **adverse drug reactions**, drug interactions, and within hospitals, policy documents for drug administration and the compatibilities of different drugs in intravenous solutions.

UK Drug Utilisation Research Group (UK DURG)
An organization whose aim is to promote drug utilization research and development in the British Isles, with particular concern for patient care, by encouraging cooperation and communication between those with an interest in this area including administrators, and providing a forum for the presentation of their work. It:
- is completely independent of industry and government
- offers twice-yearly scientific meetings to present the results and ideas at national level
- is affiliated to the **WHO** European Drug Utilization Research Group (EURODURG), with joint membership for all UK DURG members
- has the lowest membership fee and conference fees of any comparable national scientific society.

UKHFAN (UK)
UK Health For All Network.

UK HIV ADR Reporting Scheme see HIV ADR Reporting Scheme.

UK Medical Research Council (MRC) Collaborative Centre (UK)
A non-profit technology-transfer organization (a UK Registered Charity) affiliated to the UK Medical Research Council that acts as an interface between the MRC's research base and the pharmaceutical and biotechnology industries. The Centre delivers the technologies, scientific expertise and management that, through dedicated project teams, explore and develop original research ideas and discoveries for the benefit of medicine.

ULN see **upper limit of normal**.

UM see **utilization management**.

unbiased outcome (Clinical Trials)
An outcome not occurring by chance.

uncontrolled clinical trial
A trial with no active or **placebo** control and not designed as a **no-treatment concurrent** or **historical control study**.

unequal randomization (Clinical Trials)
A technique used to allocate subjects into groups at a differential rate; for example, three subjects may be assigned to a treatment group for every one assigned to the control group.

UNESCO
United Nations Educational and Scientific Organization.

UNICEF see **United Nations International Children's Emergency Fund**.

Unified Budget (UK)
A composite budget held by the **primary care group** combining the former General Medical Services and prescribing budgets.

United Nations International Children's Emergency Fund (UNICEF)
Founded in 1946, UNICEF advocates and works for the protection of children's rights, to help the young meet their basic needs and to expand their opportunities to reach their full potential.

United States Adopted Name (USAN) (US)
US approved names for drugs. These are assigned by the United States Adopted Name Council. Compare **British Approved Name**.

United States Patent and Trademark Office (PTO) (US)
A non-commercial entity which is a division of the US Department of Commerce. The role of the PTO is to promote the progress of science and the useful arts by securing, for limited times to authors and inventors, the exclusive right to their respective writings and discoveries. It does this through the issuance of patents and trademarks.
Website: http://www.uspto.gov.

United States Pharmacopoeia (USP)
1. Established in 1820, USP is a private, voluntary, not-for-profit organization. More than 1500 volunteer health care professionals, scientists, academics and government officials compose USP's 'family,' which is organized into three bodies:
   - Committee of Revision and Advisory Panellists
   - Officers and Trustees
   - Membership

The USP promotes the public health by establishing and disseminating officially recognized standards of quality and authoritative information for the use of medicines and other health care technologies by health professionals, patients and consumers.

2. The USP is a reference volume, published every 5 years by the US Pharmacopoeial Convention, which describes and defines approved therapeutic agents, and sets standards for purity, assay, etc. Agents are included on the basis of their therapeutic value. The USP is recognized by the **Food and Drug Administration** as the official standard for the therapeutic agents.

unlabelled adverse drug reaction see **unlisted adverse drug reaction**.

unlisted adverse drug reaction
An **adverse drug reaction** (ADR) that is not specifically listed as a suspected **adverse event** or ADR in the **company core safety information** (CCSI). This includes an ADR whose nature, severity, specificity or outcome is not consistent with the information in the CCSI. It also includes class-related reactions which are mentioned in the CCSI but are not specifically described as occurring with this product. Note the US equivalent term is 'unlabelled ADR'.
See also **adverse drug reaction, listed adverse drug reaction**.

upper limit of normal (ULN)
The top of the normal range for a particular laboratory: helps assure between-lab comparability.

upper margin of tolerance
The area in the agreement where companies can retain additional profit where this is strictly based on innovation, efficiency and competitiveness.

Uppsala Monitoring Centre (UMC) see **WHO Collaborative Centre for International Drug Monitoring**.

USAN see **United States Adopted Name**.

USC (US)
United States Code (Book of Laws).

USDA (US)
US Department of Agriculture.

user fee (US)
A fee paid by a drug or a biological **manufacturer** to the **Food and Drug Administration** (FDA) to cover the costs of processing a **submission** or in maintenance of an active licence. FDA uses these fees to hire more application reviewers and to accelerate reviews through the use of computer technology.

USGPO
United States Government Printing Office.

USP see **United States Pharmacopoeia**.

USTR (US)
US Trade Representative.

uterotonic agent
An agent that restores tone to the uterine muscles.

utility

1. In health outcomes analysis, utility is a number between 0 and 1 assigned to a health state or **outcome** as a way of giving a value to it. By convention, perfect health is assigned a utility of 1 and death a value of 0. Frequently, utilities are obtained using the standard gamble approach.
2. Patient preferences that are measured with techniques consistent with modern utility theory. It is based on specific axioms that describe how a rational decision maker ought to make a decision when the outcomes of that decision are uncertain. Commonly used measures of utility include the standard gamble or time-trade-off techniques.

utilization management (UM)

Any set of procedures that permit a payer to review the clinical appropriateness and cost-effectiveness of treatment prospectively, concurrently or retrospectively.

utilization review (UR)

1. The review of services delivered by a health care **provider** or supplier to determine whether those services were medically necessary; may be performed on a concurrent or retrospective basis.
2. The review of services delivered by a health care provider to evaluate the appropriateness, necessity, and quality of the prescribed services. The review can be performed on a prospective, concurrent, or retrospective basis.

V_D see **volume of distribution**.

VAERS (US)
Vaccine Adverse Event Reporting System.

VAI (US)
Voluntary Action Indicated (**Food and Drug Administration** Post-audit Inspection).

validation
The process by which a measurement is determined to be an appropriate way of quantifying a healthy state or outcome. Part of the validation process includes assessing **reliability** and **reproducibility**.

Good manufacturing practice (GMP) guides from the **European Commission**, the **World Health Organization** and the **Pharmaceutical Inspection Convention** define validation as the 'action of proving, in accordance with the principles of GMP, that any procedure, process, equipment, material, activity, or system actually leads to the expected results.' The Cooperation on International Traceability in Analytical Chemistry (CITAC) Guide to Quality in Analytical Chemistry and the Eurachem and Western European Laboratory Accreditation Cooperation (WELAC) Guidance on Interpretation of the EN 45 000 Series of Standards and ISO/IEC Guide 25 define validation of data and equipment in appendix C1.11 as 'the checking of data for correctness, or compliance with applicable standards, rules, and conventions (of data processing). In the context of equipment rather than data, validation involves checking for correct performance, etc.' The Organization for Economic Cooperation and Development (OECD) consensus document number 10 defines validation of a computerized system as 'the demonstration that a computerized system is suitable for its intended purpose'. The USP defines validation of analytical methods as 'the process by which it is established, by laboratory studies, that the performance characteristics of the method meet the requirements for the intended applications.'

The 1987 **Center for Drugs Evaluation and Review** guideline *General Principles of Validation* offers commonly accepted definitions of validation. It defines validation as 'establishing documented evidence which provides a high degree of assurance that a specific process will consistently produce a product meeting its predetermined specifications and quality attributes.' That definition is well thought out, and each word has special significance.

validation of data (Clinical Trials)
Procedure carried out to ensure that the data contained in the final clinical trial report match original observations and are free of errors.

validity
1. The extent to which a variable or intervention measures what it is supposed to measure or accomplishes what it is supposed to accomplish. The internal validity of a study refers to the integrity of the experimental design. The external validity of a study refers to the appropriateness by which its results can be applied to non-study patients or populations.
2. The accuracy of the relationship between two or more variables.

VAMP (UK)
A general practitioner computer information system supplier user group.

variability (variation) (Statistics)
'Noise' due to **random** (chance) and non-random (systematic) factors that obscure the actual factor of interest.

Biological variability

Natural variability either within an individual over time due to diurnal cycles and other rhythms, biological repair mechanisms, intermittent and varying food consumption, ageing, and so on or between individuals due to dietary differences, genetic differences, immune status differences, and so on. The natural variability of a physiologic parameter in a normal individual tested over time often equals that in a population of normal individuals tested at one time. The presence of biological variability in a group generally means that studies of that group must be large, particularly if the variability is large compared to the size of the difference in the biological parameter being measured. Because biological repair mechanisms tend to reduce a disease in an individual over time, this source of biological variability must be taken into account in study designs, particularly when individuals are compared with themselves over time. Otherwise, doing anything innocuous may appear to be associated with improvement, just as doing nothing would have been.

Laboratory variability

Variability in the laboratory setting due to changing environmental conditions, ageing and batch differences of testing components, personnel differences, and so on. Laboratory variability is minimized by testing samples collected over time from an individual at one time and by replicating the tests on a single sample with the personnel blind to the replications.

Observer variability

Variability due to differences in interpretation of measures that require any degree of subjective judgment (e.g. auscultation and palpation findings, radiographs, histology sections) either within the same observer over time or between observers. Observer variability is minimized by blinding observers to hypotheses, group assignment in trials, and other findings, by increasing objectivity of measures as much as possible, by providing standards and guidelines, and by training of observers. Observer variability can be random but is usually systematic (bias) and is usually due to human nature and the subtle effects of prior beliefs on perception rather than being due to deliberate deception.

variable

Any element, trait, characteristic, test, measurement, or factor that the research is designed to study, either as an experimental intervention or a possible outcome (or factor affecting the outcome) of that intervention.

variable, continuous

Variables that can assume all possible values along a continuum within a specified range, e.g. height, weight, blood pressure, CD4.

variable, dependent

A variable that has a value that is dependent upon the effect of one or more other independent variables. For example, diastolic blood pressure (dependent variable) can be dependent upon the effect of obesity (independent variable).

variable, discrete

Variable that has values that fall into a limited number of separate categories, e.g. gender (male/female), survival status (alive/dead), exposure status (exposed/non-exposed), blood type (A/B/AB/O).

variable, independent

A variable that influences the value of the dependent variable. For example, obesity (independent variable) can influence the level of diastolic blood pressure (dependent variable).

variable, quantile
A measure of variability which divides the distribution into equal, ordered subgroups. For example, terciles are thirds, quartiles are quarters, and quintiles are fifths.

variance (Statistics)
Square of the **standard deviation**. A measure of the amount by which a value differs from the mean. The degree to which a set of quantities vary: a measure of the spread of scores in a distribution of scores, that is, a measure of dispersion. The larger the variance, the further the individual cases are from the mean. The smaller the variance, the closer the individual scores are to the mean. Specifically, the population variance is the mean of the sum of the squared deviations from the mean score.

variation
1. As applied to **European Union** regulatory affairs, it is the term used to describe the process of making changes/amendments to an existing **marketing authorization** (MA) and consequently in the **SPC** of the product. It can be by application of the MA holder or at the instigation of the licensing authority. Two **Regulations** have been introduced for variations: **(EEC) No. 541/95** and **542/95**. To take account of the different needs for changes to an MA, variations are classified into two types: Type I (involving amendments to the contents such as they existed at the moment the decision was taken on the MA) and Type II (involving any change to the documentation, which is not Type I and does not require a new application procedure).
2. (Statistics) see **variability**.

VAS
Visual analogue scale.

vasoconstrictor agent
An agent that causes constriction of blood vessels.

vasodilator agent
An agent that causes dilation of blood vessels.

vasomotor
Causing constriction or dilation of the blood vessels.
See also **vasoconstrictor agent**, **vasodilator agent**.

vehicle
The carrier of the drug in a **drug product**. A substance that acts as a medium in which a drug is administered.

vehicle substances
Additives necessary in formulating a dosage form of a drug. They should be chemically inert and should not have any pharmacological effects in the dose used. They are used to produce a dosage form of the desired strength, volume form or consistency suitable for administration.

verification/validation of data (Clinical Trials)
The procedures carried out to ensure that the data contained in the final clinical trial report (**Final Report**) match original observations. These procedures may apply to raw data, hard copy or electronic **case record forms**, computer print-outs and statistical analyses and tables.
See also **audit**, **inspection**, **quality control**.

vermifuge
An agent that expels parasitic worms from the intestines.

vesicant see **epispastic**.

Veterinary Mutual Recognition Facilitation Group (VMRFG)
Established by the **Member States** (MSs) as a result of the need for a group that could coordinate and facilitate the operation of the decentralized **mutual recognition procedure**. The Group meets monthly before the **Committee for Veterinary Medicinal Products** meeting and comprises senior representatives from each MS. All features of this group are identical to the **MRFG**.

vial
A small glass vessel or bottle for holding medicines.

VICH
International Cooperation on Harmonization of Technical Requirements for Registration of Veterinary Products.

virucide see **antiviral**.

virulence
1. The relative ability of an organism to cause disease.
2. The case **mortality** rate of an infection.
3. The extent to which a pathogen harms its host.

These are different usages: what they have in common is that they refer to the effect on an already infected host, not to the degree of transmissibility to a subsequent susceptible.

VMD (UK)
Veterinary Medicines Directorate.

VMRFG see **Veterinary Mutual Recognition Facilitation Group**.

VNZ (Netherlands)
Association of the Sick funds.

volume of distribution (V_d)
The volume into which the drug distributes. It is the volume that would accommodate all drug in the body if its concentration throughout the body was the same as that in the plasma. Mathematically, it is calculated by dividing the 'Amount of drug in body' by 'plasma concentration'. This, however, assumes that the body behaves as a single, homogenous 'compartment'. In reality, drugs are rarely distributed into volumes which have these precise physiological values. Indeed, some drugs have V_d far in access of total body water. This is because distribution is not dilution throughout the body fluids but also of a sequestration or binding by various body tissues, e.g. muscle and fat. V_d can, therefore, vary from relatively small (e.g. 0.14 l/kg body weight for aspirin) to large (e.g. 10 l/kg body weight for digoxin). In general, V_d is small with:
- Low lipid solubility
- High plasma-protein binding
- Low tissue binding.

The converse is true.

volunteer(s) see **normal volunteers**.

volunteer bias
Volunteers may exhibit exposures or outcomes that may differ from non-volunteers (e.g. volunteers tend to be healthier).

VPC (UK)
Veterinary Products Committee.

VPRS (UK)
Voluntary Price Regulation Scheme that was introduced in the 1950s. Its name was later changed to **Prescription Pricing Regulation Scheme** in the mid 1970s.

vulnerable subjects
Individuals whose willingness to volunteer in a **clinical trial** may be unduly influenced by the expectation, whether justified or not, of benefits associated with participation, or of a retaliatory response from senior members of a hierarchy in case of refusal to participate. Examples are members of a group with a hierarchical structure, such as medical, **pharmacy**, dental and nursing students, subordinate hospital and laboratory personnel, employees of the pharmaceutical industry, members of the armed forces and persons kept in detention. Other vulnerable subjects include patients with incurable diseases, persons in nursing homes, unemployed or impoverished persons, patients in emergency situations, ethnic minority groups, homeless persons, nomads, refugees, minors and those incapable of giving consent.

warning (Clinical Trials)
Written advice given to the **investigator** to avoid the occurrence of **serious adverse events**, while allowing them to administer the investigational drug to a **subject**/patient who may benefit from it.

washout (Clinical Trials)
A treatment-free period at the outset of a **clinical trial** between two treatments of a cross-over trial. The purpose is to remove the effects of the previous treatment or avoid drug interactions. A baseline assessment is carried out at the end of the washout period to determine the patient's condition before the second active treatment is initiated.

weighted capitation (UK)
The current formula used to allocate the **National Health Service** resources to health authorities (HAs) and by some HAs to **GP fundholders**.

WELAC
Western European Laboratory Accreditation Cooperation.

well-being (of trial subjects) (Clinical Trials)
The physical and mental integrity of the subjects participating in a **clinical trial**.

WFPMM
World Federation of Proprietary Medicine Manufacturers.

WHO see **World Health Organization.**

WHO-ARD
WHO Adverse Reaction Dictionary.

WHO-ART
WHO Adverse Reaction Terminology.

WHO-ARTL
WHO Adverse Reaction Terminology List.

WHO Collaborative Centre for International Drug Monitoring (Uppsala Monitoring Centre (UMC))
A scheme whose main purpose and activity is the collection of data about **adverse drug reactions** from the worldwide community, especially from countries who are members of the **WHO** International Drug Monitoring Programme, and the generation of signals of drugs which might possibly have problematic **side-effects**. The objectives of the scheme are:
- To maintain and develop leading-edge excellence in the collection, processing and dissemination of information, with a priority commitment to data about the benefits and risks of **medicinal products**, and to research in the field.
- To stimulate and facilitate the definition and promotion of coherent, harmonized good-practice guidelines and methodology for **pharmacovigilance** and communications, and to observe and promote high level quality assurance procedures.
- To ensure the development and maintenance of the most efficient and effective systems for generating early warnings of **medicinal product** safety hazards.
- To facilitate a continuing programme of innovation in concepts and approaches, and in products, service and tools on the basis of the Centre's information and expertise and on the needs of the external world.
- To demonstrate through all the Centre's activities the highest standards of service and communications practice in all its relationships.

Activities:
- Receipt, analysis and recording of worldwide **adverse event** data.
- Maintenance and screening of international database (currently over 1.9 million records).
- Publication of previously unknown **adverse events** in SIGNAL.
- Quarterly publication of drug safety issues from National Centres in the WHO Adverse Reaction Newsletter.
- Editing, updating and publishing the Drug Dictionary.
- Developing and supplying DD Access software for searching the Drug Dictionary.
- Maintaining and publishing the Adverse Reaction Terminology (**WHO-ART**).
- Carrying out special searches of the database by request and providing on-line access to the database.
- Publishing a range of special reports.
- Assistance to potential members of the programme in developing their **pharmacovigilance** systems.
- Running annual training course for staff from National Centres.
- Organizing annual meeting for member and associate member countries.
- Publishing scientific articles.
- Contributing to international conferences.
- Product and Publication News.

WHO-DD
WHO Drug Dictionary.

WHO-DRL
WHO Drug Reference List.

WHO-EDL see **WHO Essential Drug List**.

WHO-EDM see **Essential Drugs and Medicines Policy (EDM)**.

WHO Essential Drug List
A list, published by the **World Health Organization**, of drugs which the Organization believes to provide safe, effective treatment for the majority of communicable and non-communicable diseases. WHO published the first Model List of Essential Drugs in 1977, in which it identified 208 individual drugs.

The 10th Model List of Essential Drugs, prepared by a WHO expert committee in 1997, contains 306 individual drugs. This number reflects the addition of 166 new drugs over the last twenty years and the deletion of 68 drugs no longer deemed appropriate. Today, the list contains safe, effective treatments for the infectious and chronic diseases that affect the vast majority of the world's population.

wholesale dealer's licence (WL)
A licence required to be obtained by wholesalers to authorize them to sell **medicinal products** to a person who buys the product for the purpose of sale or supply to someone else; it also covers sale to a practitioner for administration to his patients. WL is concerned primarily with the identification of the distributor, the suitability of the premises used for storage of products and adequacy of turnover of stock.

withdrawal
A substance-specific organic brain syndrome that follows the cessation of use or reduction in intake of a psychoactive substance that had been regularly used to induce a state of intoxication.

withdrawal bias (Clinical Trials)
Patients who withdraw from studies may differ systematically from those who remain.

within-patient differences see **inter-subject variation**.

WONCA
World Organization of National Colleges, Academies and Academic Associations of General Practitioners.

World Health Organization (WHO)
An agency of the United Nations whose mission is to promote global public health and well-being of all peoples throughout the world. It establishes and promotes medical standards and supports international health education and assistance programmes. WHO is defined by its Constitution as the directing and coordinating authority on international health work, its aim 'the attainment by all peoples of the highest possible level of health'.

WL
1. (US) Warning Letter (Most Serious **Food and Drug Administration** Post-audit Letter).
2. see **wholesale dealer's licence**.

WTO
World Trade Organization.

χ^2 (Statistics)
: Chi-squared test statistic.

xenobiotics
: Chemical substances that are foreign (*xenos* [Greek] = foreign) to an organism/the body, i.e. introduced into the body as in drugs.

X-ray see **radiography**

X-ray crystallography
: The use of X-ray diffraction to determine the three-dimensional (3D) molecular structure of a protein or chemical substance.

years of life lost (YLL)
The average annual years of life lost per 10 000 resident population under the age of 75.

Yellow Card Scheme (YCS) (UK)
This scheme, for **spontaneous reporting** of suspected **adverse drug reactions** (ADRs), was introduced in 1964, during the chairmanship of Sir Derek Dunlop of the **Committee on Safety of Medicines** (CSM), after the **thalidomide** tragedy highlighted the urgent need for routine post-marketing surveillance of medicines. Since then several hundred thousands of reports of suspected ADRs have been submitted to the (CSM)/**Medicines Control Agency** on a voluntary basis by doctors, dentists, pharmacists and coroners and by pharmaceutical companies under statutory obligations. The scheme has been (and continues to be) of the utmost importance for monitoring drug safety.

Under the scheme, doctors, dentists, hospital pharmacists and Her Majesty's Coroners are asked to provide details of suspected – NOT NECESSARILY PROVEN – ADRs they encounter during their regular work. They should report all reactions on new drugs. New drugs are labelled with a ▼ symbol (see **black triangle**) on product information and advertisements but these professionals should report only serious reactions on established drugs.

Reports received by the scheme are treated in strict confidence. Data are held securely and information revealing a reporter's identity is never released. The patient's full name need not be included in the report, however, the CSM encourages reporters to include the patient's initials, date of birth or age, sex and the hospital or clinic number. This facilitates identification of potential duplicate reports and allows for follow-up information to be requested, if necessary.

Reporting forms are distributed regularly with **Current Problems in Pharmacovigilance, British National Formulary**, The **ABPI Compendium of Data Sheets and SPCs, MIMS** (some issues) and at the back of prescription forms' pad.

A recent extension of the YCS is the **HIV Adverse Drug Reactions Reporting Scheme** (launched end of October 1997) which involves reporting suspected adverse drug reactions occurring in individuals infected with HIV which are then analysed and data are regularly fed back to reporters. The Scheme is a collaboration between the **MCA**, the Medical Research Council (MRC) HIV Clinical Trials Centre and the CSM.

See also **spontaneous reporting**.

YLL see **years of life lost**.

ZBB see **zero-based budgeting.**

zero-order kinetics
Kinetics for some drugs (e.g. ethanol) in which the drug saturates its **elimination** process and its rate of elimination is constant. For drugs that obey zero-kinetics, the half-life increases with increasing plasma concentration and the plasma concentration–time plot is linear.
Compare **first-order kinetics, half-life**.

zero time bias
The **bias** that occurs in a prospective study when individuals are found and enrolled in such a fashion that unintended systematic differences occur between groups at the beginning of the study (stage of disease, confounder distribution). **Cohort** studies are susceptible to zero time bias if the cohort is not assembled properly.